19TH EDITION

The Comprehensive NCLEX-RN® Review

Contributors

Lawrette Axley, PhD, RN, CNE

Adrienne Blanks, RN, BSN, MSN

Bridgette Bryan, DNP, MS, RN

Nicole Hancock, EdD, MSN, RN

Deborah Cardi, MSN, RN

Alison DeLong, MS, RN

Jo Ellen Greischar–Billiard, MS, RN

Dianne B. Harris, EdD, MSN, RN, CNE

Teresa LaFave, NP, MS, RN

Japonica Morris, EdD, MSN, RN

Rhonda Payne, PhD, RN, CNE

Shari Payne, MSN, RN

Kathleen Pollard, MSN, RN

Sheri Shields, RN, MSN

Faye Sigman, PhD, MSN, RN

Joy Weller, MS, RN

Intellectual Property Notice

REPRINTED AUGUST 2021

Director of development: Derek Prater
Project management: Siobhan Ryan
Coordination of content review: Lawrette Axley
Copy editing: Kelly Von Lunen, Melissa Treolo
Layout: Bethany Phillips
Cover design: Jason Buck

Important Notice to the Reader

User's Guide and Organization

Congratulations, graduate! You have successfully completed your program of nursing studies and are now eligible to take the licensing exam created by the National Council of State Boards of Nursing (NCSBN®).

Understanding the organizational format of this review book will help guide you through a focused review in preparation for NCLEX®. The book is intended to accompany a live review presentation and then be used as an outline for continued review prior to taking NCLEX. Each unit focuses on a specific area of nursing care. Unit 1 offers practical information about the exam, including how to prepare and test-taking strategies. The next eight units review essential content for the exam:

- Nursing Leadership and Management
- Community Health Nursing
- Pharmacology in Nursing
- Fundamentals for Nursing
- Adult Medical Surgical Nursing
- Mental Health Nursing
- Maternal and Newborn Nursing
- Nursing Care of Children

Tables and graphics are provided throughout to simplify more challenging content.

The content provided in this book is organized by specific areas of nursing and focuses on descriptions, contributing factors, manifestations, and collaborative care, which includes nursing interventions, diagnostics, medications, therapeutic measures, client education, and referral. The information is presented in a manner that promotes analysis and application of knowledge and reinforces priority of care when managing client care.

In the Practice Questions section, additional NCLEX-style questions are provided. Remember to apply clinical reasoning and use your test-taking strategies to select the correct answers.

It is important for new graduates to stay connected to content and practice questions until the NCLEX is taken. Implementing a focused review will create success on the NCLEX.

Feedback is always welcome. Therefore, please send suggestions for improvement, any noted errors, and personal testimonials of effectiveness to: *LRAdmin@atitesting.com*.

Table of Contents

UNIT ONE

Review of Test-Taking Strategies for the NCLEX® Exam

Information About NCLEX

A. **General Information**

1. The purpose of the NCLEX-RN is to determine whether a candidate is prepared to safely and effectively practice entry-level nursing.

2. The exam is designed to test essential nursing knowledge and a candidate's ability to apply that knowledge to clinical situations.

3. The exam is pass/fail, and no other score is given.

B. **Computerized Adaptive Testing (CAT)**

1. CAT is a system that selects test items for you based on answers selected up to that point in the exam.

2. When a question is answered, CAT selects items to administer that match the candidate's ability.

3. Passing or failing is determined when you reach a point in the test when minimal competency has been demonstrated.

C. **Exam Schedule**

1. The exam is given all year long.

D. **Number of Questions and Time Allowed**

1. There is no minimum amount of time for the exam, and the maximum time allowed is 6 hr. The average time for a candidate is 2.5 hr.

2. Candidates who have applied for licensure/registration with a participating BON/RB will be permitted to take the NCLEX eight times a year, but no more than once in any 45-day period.

3. The computer will automatically stop as soon as one of the following occurs.

   a. The candidate's measure of competency is determined to be above or below the passing standard.

   b. The candidate has answered all 265 test questions.

   c. The maximum amount of time has expired.

4. It is not possible to skip questions or return to previous questions.

5. The NCLEX-RN has a range of 75 to 265 questions. The exam includes 15 questions that are not scored.

6. The exam has a time limit of 6 hr. regardless of the number of items administrated. Two optional breaks are provided and count as part of the total testing time. Remember, a fresh mind is more alert!

7. About 2% of NCLEX candidates run out of time on their exams. So be aware of the time, but be sure to give every question your best effort. Do not randomly answer questions to finish quickly, as this can hinder your chance of passing.

The NCLEX-RN Test Plan

A. **The NCLEX-RN test plan is revised every 3 years.** The current test plan, available at www.ncsbn.org, identifies the major categories and nursing activities that guide the exam's content and questions.

B. **NCLEX questions are distributed and weighted according to client need categories in the current test plan.**

C. **The NCLEX-RN Registration Process**

1. Apply for licensure with one board of nursing (BON).

2. Register and pay fees with Pearson VUE via the internet (www.pearsonvue.com) or telephone.

3. Receive acknowledgment of receipt of registration from Pearson VUE.

4. The BON determines eligibility in the Pearson VUE system.

5. Receive Authorization to Test (ATT) email from Pearson VUE. (NOTE: Must test during the validity dates on the ATT.)

6. Schedule your exam appointment via the internet (by accessing your online account) or by telephone.

   a. Arrive 30 minutes before the exam appointment and present acceptable identification. Your signature, photograph, and palm vein scan will be obtained.

   b. Examples of acceptable forms of identification for domestic test centers are:

      1) Passport books and cards

      2) Driver's license

      3) Provincial/Territorial or state identification card

      4) Permanent residence card

      5) Military identification card

   c. The only identifications acceptable for international test centers are:

      1) Passport books and cards

7. If you are not successful on NCLEX, contact ATI for continued assistance and support.

It is recommended that you visit the Pearson VUE website to take the online NCLEX tutorial at www.pearsonvue.com.

You can learn more about the NCLEX at www.ncsbn.org.

NCLEX-RN Item Types

A. **Items include multiple choice, multiple response, fill-in-the-blank calculation, ordered response, and/or hot spots.** All item types may include multimedia (e.g., charts, tables, graphics, sound and video).

B. **Multiple Choice**

  1. Has four options, only one of which is correct.

  2. The correct answer is the **best** answer.

  3. The other three options are distractors.

  4. Distractors are options made to look like correct answers. They are intended to distract you from selecting the correct answer.

C. **Fill-in-the-Blank**

  1. Fill-in-the-blank items are calculation problems. The question may ask for an answer in a specific unit amount or a rounded decimal. If required, perform rounding at the end of the calculation.

  2. To answer these questions, a number should be typed into the answer box on the screen. You will not type in the unit of measurement.

  3. When answering the question, solve for the correct unit value.

  4. Write out the calculations on material provided.

  5. Click on the calculator button and verify your calculation.

D. **Drag and Drop/Ordered Response**

  1. Drag and drop/ordered response items list steps that must be placed in a correct order (e.g., numerical, alphabetical, chronological).

  2. Drag options in the left-hand column into the order of performance in the right-hand column.

  3. There is only one correct sequence.

E. **Multiple Response:** Select All That Apply

  1. Multiple response questions may have a single correct response, have more than one correct response, or require all responses to be correct.

  2. To answer these questions, click on all the answers that apply.

  3. Credit will only be given for completely correct answers. No partial credit is given.

  4. Consider each response as a true-false question.

F. **Hot Spot**

  1. Hot spot items use a "point-and-click" method that presents the candidate with a problem and a figure. The test taker selects the correct location on the figure.

  2. An "x" will appear on the area selected. Click on the area that constitutes the landmark to correctly answer the item.

  3. Read the question carefully, then analyze the image.

  4. The exam will allow the test taker to reclick on the image as many times as necessary.

  5. It is very important to remember that the screen is not a mirror image. If the question asks for an answer on the right or left side of the body, make sure to click on the appropriate side.

G. **Multimedia. All item types may include multimedia.**

  1. Charts or Tables

     a. First, read the question carefully. Use the mouse to click on each tab to open the document. When the tab is clicked, a separate window will open to display the data. Analyze the data provided in the charts or tables to correctly answer the question.

  2. Graphic Option

     a. The item and/or answer options are presented as graphics instead of text.

     b. The answers to these items are preceded by circles. Be sure to click on the circle to select the answer.

  3. Sound and Video

     a. When an audio item is presented on NCLEX, the candidate is prompted to apply headphones. The volume of the audio may be adjusted and replayed as often as needed.

Assess and Remediate

A. **New nursing graduates should review content and questions daily until they take the exam.** Adequate review depends on scores obtained on practice assessments, and NCLEX preparation after a live review may take from 2 to 8 weeks.

B. **For content review, use this NCLEX-RN review book that outlines content.** Use other nursing reference materials for more detailed information.

C. **Your practice assessment score reports will identify and help direct review of content.**

D. **Begin with areas that are most difficult or least familiar.**

E. **When studying body systems and the associated diseases:**

  1. Define the disease in terms of the pathophysiological process that is occurring.

  2. Identify a client's early and late manifestations.

  3. Identify the most important or life-threatening complications.

  4. Review the prescribed medical plan, including prescribed diagnostic and laboratory tests, expected lab value alterations, medications, and prescribed treatments.

  5. Identify and prioritize the nursing interventions associated with early and late manifestations.

  6. Identify client teaching that the nurse should provide to the client/family to prevent or adapt to the disease process and/or clinical condition.

Test-Taking Strategies

NOTE: Although the majority of NCLEX-RN items are written at the application and analysis level, there are some knowledge and comprehension items on the test. Make certain that you have a broad knowledge in all client need categories so that you can demonstrate a minimal level of competency when asked to apply your knowledge to the care of the clients in the scenario presented on the exam.

A nurse prepares to administer medications to a client who has asthma. Which of the following effects should the nurse recognize as an adverse response to bronchodilator therapy?

1. Limited routes of administration
2. Hyperkalemia
3. Increased myocardial oxygen use
4. Hypoglycemia

NOTE: Knowledge-based questions test recall and recognition.

An older adult client reports recurring calf pain after walking one to two blocks that disappears with rest. The client has weak pedal pulses, and the skin on the lower legs is shiny and cool to touch. Which of the following nursing interventions is appropriate at this time?

1. Position the legs dependently.
2. Elevate the left leg above the heart.
3. Immobilize the left leg to prevent further injury.
4. Assess dorsiflexion and extension of the left foot.

NOTE: Application and analysis questions require use of nursing knowledge to solve client problems.

A. **The amount of information in the stem and distractors can be overwhelming.** A useful approach is to break the analysis of the question into a series of steps. Remember to focus on the fact that there is always something you know in the question and answer options. This helps you stay in control of the exam.

B. **Use the STOP approach.**

1. **Story:** Identify the issue and client in the question.

   a. The issue in a question is the problem that is presented. Examples of the issue:

      1) Medication: digoxin
      2) Nursing problem: a client who is at risk for infection or in pain
      3) Behavior: restlessness, agitation
      4) Disorder: diabetes mellitus, ulcerative colitis
      5) Procedure: glucose tolerance test, cardiac catheterization
      6) The client in the question usually has a health problem.
      7) The client may be a relative, significant other, or another member of the health care team with whom the nurse is interacting.
      8) The correct answer to the question must relate to the client in the question.

2. **Think:** About the type of stem and key words.

   a. Identify the type of stem in the question.

      1) True-response stem requires an answer that is a true statement.

         a) Example: A nurse is preparing to administer a bolus feeding to a client through a nasogastric (NG) tube and observes that the exit mark on the tube has moved since the last feeding. Which of the following actions should the nurse take?

      2) False-response stem requires an answer that is a false statement.

         a) Example: A newly licensed nurse is preparing to remove a client's abdominal wound sutures. The manager recognizes a need for further education when the nurse does which of the following?

      3) Answering questions that focus on priorities.

         a) The majority of NCLEX questions will be priority-setting questions, which ask the test taker to identify what comes first, is most important, or gets the highest priority.

         b) The NCLEX will use stems that ask, "What will the nurse do **first**?"

            (1) For example:

               (a) What is the nurse's initial response?
               (b) A nurse should give immediate consideration to which of the following?
               (c) Which of the following nursing actions should receive the highest priority?
               (d) Which of the following actions should the nurse take first?

            (2) Example: A nurse is preparing an automated external defibrillator (AED) for a client receiving CPR after a cardiac arrest. Which of the following actions should the nurse perform first?

   b. Key words focus attention on important details.

      1) During the **early** period, which of the following nursing **procedures** is **best**?
      2) The nurse should **expect** to find which of the following characteristics in an **adult** who has **diabetes mellitus**?
      3) Which of the following nursing **actions** is **essential**?
      4) Which of the following nursing **actions** should the nurse take **first**?

3. **Options:** Consider potential responses/answers.

   a. Develop answers in your mind before looking at the options provided.

   b. Review each answer option one at a time.

4. **Pick:** The correct answer.

  a. Identify the option that best matches your answer or that best answers the question.

  b. Make your selection and do not change it.

5. Apply the STOP strategy to the following question.

  a. A client who has recently undergone surgery for a tracheostomy is now at home. The nurse recognizes a need for immediate intervention when the caregiver does which of the following?

    1) Places an air humidifier at the bedside.

    2) Suctions intermittently for 15 seconds.

    3) Cuts a 4x4 gauze pad to put around the tracheostomy tube.

    4) Removes the ties before cleaning the tracheostomy.

C. **Use priority-setting guidelines to answer questions.**

  1. **Maslow's Hierarchy of Needs** indicates that physiological needs come first, followed by safety and security; love and belonging; self-esteem; and self-actualization.

  2. **"ABCs"**—airway, breathing, circulation needs will frequently take priority. Never perform ABC checks blindly without considering whether ABC issues are acute vs. chronic or stable vs. unstable. For example, a client who is quadriplegic and receiving ventilation has chronic airway/breathing problems. However, if there is not an acute consideration such as pneumonia, the client should be considered chronic and stable. This client would not be the nurse's first priority.

  3. **Sources of safety and risk reduction** issues need to be identified.

  4. **The nursing process** indicates that assessment is a priority.

  5. Consider options that are **least restrictive or least invasive**.

  6. Determine the survival potential of the client. Is the issue emergent, urgent, nonurgent, or expectant? It is not unusual to want to care for the client who, in your mind, is the sickest. However, this may be an inappropriate choice in a triage situation. Clients who are so sick that they cannot be saved should not be treated first.

  7. **Acute** client problems take priority over **chronic** problems.

  8. Determine if the client is **stable** or **unstable**.

D. **Default test-taking strategies help you make decisions.**

  1. Use time to your advantage.

    a. **Early vs. late signs and symptoms**: Early clinical manifestations are generalized and nonspecific, whereas late signs are specific and serious. Eliminate incorrect answer choices using this strategy.

      1) Example: An adolescent was admitted 12 hr ago following a motor vehicle crash. Multiple skeletal fractures were sustained. The client is in balanced-suspension traction. Which of the following assessment findings requires immediate intervention by the nurse?

        1. Disorientation

        2. Shallow respirations

        3. Chest pain with positioning

        4. Bloody drainage at the pin site

    b. **Pre, post, intra**: You may be asked about complications associated with certain procedures. What should you do if you know little or nothing about the procedure? Pay attention to whether the question is asking about "preprocedural" or "postprocedural" concerns. Eliminate the options that do not correspond to what is being asked.

      1) Example: A nurse is caring for a client who is scheduled for electroconvulsive therapy (ECT). Which of the following medications should the nurse withhold prior to therapy?

        1. Atropine sulfate

        2. Phenytoin

        3. Methohexital

        4. Succinylcholine

    c. **Time elapsed**: The priority nursing action will change based on the time interval stipulated. The closer the client is to the origination of risk, the higher the risk for complications. The time issue may be stated in terms of hours or days. In other instances, the physical location of the client will tell you how long it has been since the origination of risk. Pay attention. Is the client in the PACU, postsurgical unit, or somewhere else? The time issue buried in those words should help you eliminate incorrect answers that don't match what is being asked.

      1) Example: A home health nurse is performing an admission assessment on a client who had a knee arthroplasty 1 week ago. Which of the following client statements should concern the nurse most?

        1. "I am so glad to be off those blood thinners."

        2. "I will keep a pillow under my knee when I am in bed."

        3. "I am planning to use a wheelchair to help me get around."

        4. "I plan to take ibuprofen instead of the prescribed hydrocodone for pain control."

d. Remember: the **most complete answer** = least room for error.

1) You'll encounter questions on NCLEX that will ask you to choose the instruction or documentation that is most accurate. What should you do if you don't remember much about the subject matter? Choosing an answer that is most complete will typically result in the least room for error and subsequent delivery of safe and effective care.

2) To help you determine which answer is the most complete, evaluate answer options based on how much objectivity (fact) vs. subjectivity (opinion) there is in the answer choices. A specific value, like a blood pressure, is factual, whereas a client's report of past incidences of "high" blood pressure is subjective. Responses that are subjective are generally not correct.

   a) Example: A client has not voided 8 hr following the removal of an indwelling bladder catheter. Which of the following should be the nurse's initial action?

      1. Increase fluids.
      2. Perform bladder scan.
      3. Place indwelling catheter.
      4. Provide assistance to bathroom.

e. Read the question and options closely for words asking about **direction** or **magnitude**. For instance, stop and concentrate on the terms intra vs. inter; hyper vs. hypo; increase vs. decrease; lesser vs. greater; and gain vs. lose. It is common to misread these terms by simply skimming over them too quickly.

   1) Example: A nurse irrigates a postoperative client's NG tube twice with 30 mL normal saline solution. At the end of the shift, the NG collection device contains 475 mL. Record the amount of NG drainage.

f. When in doubt, always choose a nursing action that could **prevent harm to the client**. Even if you don't know whether it is related to the stem, it is still a life-saving maneuver that, in all likelihood, is correct.

   1) Example: A nurse is caring for a client who has a chest tube. The nurse notes that the chest tube has become disconnected from the chest drainage system. Which of the following actions should the nurse take?

      1. Reposition the client to a high-Fowler's position.
      2. Increase the suction to the chest drainage system.
      3. Place the client on low flow oxygen via nasal cannula.
      4. Immerse the end of the chest tube in a bottle of sterile water.

g. Seldom will a correct answer have the nurse physically leave the client. Choose an answer that **keeps the nurse with the client**.

   1) Example: When an older adult client dies from complications of a cerebrovascular accident (CVA), the client's partner is present at the bedside. Which of the following actions should the nurse take?

      1. Escort the partner to the hallway outside the room.
      2. Ask the chaplain to come be with the partner.
      3. Stay with the partner at the bedside.
      4. Give the partner time alone.

h. In some instances, rule out an option if you know it is associated with something else. For example, you may not know about the laboratory values for warfarin therapy, but you do know the laboratory values for heparin and aspirin. Those values can be eliminated because you are **using what you know.**

   1) Example: A client who has just been diagnosed with rheumatoid arthritis is required to receive 3 months of methotrexate therapy. The nurse recognizes that which of the following are associated with the therapy? (Select all that apply.)

      1. WBC count 1,200/mm³
      2. Weight gain 2.27 kg (5 lb)
      3. Oral temperature of 37.2° C (99° F)
      4. Urine specific gravity 1.003
      5. Platelets 5,000/mm³

i. **Safe and effective delegation** of tasks and client care assignments are extremely important when setting priorities for client care.

   1) RNs perform all initial client teaching. The licensed practical nurse (LPN) may reinforce teaching performed by the RN.

   2) RNs should perform all admission assessments and vital signs so that an accurate baseline is established.

   3) Client care assignments are made by the RN, not by support staff.

      a) Example: A nurse is organizing care for a group of clients. Which of the following should the nurse assign to the assistive personnel (AP)?

         1. Record a client's vital signs during the transfusion of blood.
         2. Assist a client who is requesting a bedpan 1 day post hysterectomy.
         3. Offer a pamphlet regarding advanced directives to a newly admitted client.
         4. Ask a client if pain was relieved after administration of acetaminophen.

j. You may want to answer questions based on the way you saw procedures done while you were in a clinical setting at school, during summer employment, or working as an intern. NCLEX items must be answered to be consistent with nationwide practice standards, not necessarily with what may have been done within your particular institution or geographic area.

The Day of the Exam

A. **Plan for everything.**

B. **Assemble everything needed for the exam the night before.**

C. **Identification:** When candidates arrive at the test center, they are required to present one form of acceptable identification. The first and last names on the ID must exactly match the first and last names on the application sent to the board of nursing. Visit the NCSBN website (www.ncsbn.org) for acceptable forms of ID.

D. **Candidates are required to arrive at least 30 minutes before the scheduled testing time.**

E. **Verify the route to the exam site, and take a test drive several days prior.**

F. **Pay close attention to your physiological needs.**

   1. Dress in layers to accommodate your comfort in the testing center. No hats, scarves, gloves, or coats are allowed in the testing room.

   2. Get a good night's sleep the night before the exam.

   3. Eat a nourishing meal that includes protein and long-acting carbohydrates.

   4. Avoid stimulants and depressants.

   5. Meet elimination needs prior to beginning the exam.

G. **During the exam:**

   1. Listen to and carefully read the instructions.

   2. Avoid distraction. Focus on answering one question at a time.

   3. Think positively.

H. **Manage anxiety.**

   1. Mild levels of anxiety increase effectiveness.

   2. Avoid cramming the night before the exam.

   3. Do something enjoyable and relaxing the night before the exam.

   4. Learn and practice measures to manage your anxiety level during the exam, as needed.

      a. Take a few deep breaths.

      b. Tense and relax muscles.

      c. Visualize a peaceful scene.

      d. Visualize your success.

UNIT TWO

Nursing Leadership and Management

Leadership and Management

A. **Leadership:** A way of behaving that influences others to respond, not because they have to, but because they want to. Leaders help others to identify and focus on the achievement of goals. Leadership is an interaction that focuses on the personal development of the members of the group.

1. Essential Components of Leadership
   a. Effective communication
   b. Conflict manager
   c. Knowledge/competence
   d. Role model
   e. Delegation
   f. Identifies goals/objectives
   g. Motivation
   h. Proactive
   i. Flexible

2. **Leadership Styles**
   a. Authoritative
   b. Democratic
   c. Laissez-faire

3. All nurses need leadership skills to initiate and maintain effective working relationships, coordinate care, delegate, and resolve conflict. Transactional leaders focus on immediate problems using rewards as motivation. Transactional leaders empower and motivate followers toward a common vision.

B. **Management:** A problem-oriented process with a focus on the activities needed to achieve a goal; supplying the structure, resources, and direction for the activities of the group. Management involves personal interaction, but the focus is on the group's process. The most effective managers are also effective leaders. The organization grants power and authority to the manager.

1. Functions of Management
   a. Planning
   b. Organizing
   c. Staffing
   d. Directing
   e. Controlling

2. Characteristics of Managers
   a. Hold formal position of authority and power
   b. Coach subordinates
   c. Work toward shared goals of quality, efficiency, and excellence
   d. Promote innovation

DETERMINE THE LEADERSHIP STYLE
(AUTHORITATIVE, DEMOCRATIC, OR LAISSEZ-FAIRE) USED IN EACH SCENARIO

Scenario 1: A nurse manager does not participate, but delegates the staff scheduling to the nurses on the unit.	☐ AUTHORITATIVE ☐ LAISSEZ-FAIRE ☐ DEMOCRATIC
Scenario 2: A nurse manager allows the staff nurses to participate in trial use of new IV pumps and contribute input when choosing a new product.	☐ AUTHORITATIVE ☐ LAISSEZ-FAIRE ☐ DEMOCRATIC
Scenario 3: A nurse manager makes a decision for the staff to wear blue scrubs without consulting the staff nurses.	☐ AUTHORITATIVE ☐ LAISSEZ-FAIRE ☐ DEMOCRATIC
Scenario 4: A nurse manager allows the staff to choose which holiday they would prefer to take off before completing the work schedule.	☐ AUTHORITATIVE ☐ LAISSEZ-FAIRE ☐ DEMOCRATIC
Scenario 5: A nurse manager instructs the staff nurses to "work out the problem between yourselves" when a conflict arises between two nurses.	☐ AUTHORITATIVE ☐ LAISSEZ-FAIRE ☐ DEMOCRATIC
Scenario 6: A nurse manager changes the policy regarding sterile dressing changes and directs the staff to follow the new procedure.	☐ AUTHORITATIVE ☐ LAISSEZ-FAIRE ☐ DEMOCRATIC

Answer key: 1. Laissez-faire; 2. Democratic; 3. Authoritative; 4. Democratic; 5. Laissez-faire; 6. Authoritative

3. **Nursing interventions**: Nurses should learn management skills and identify their own personal leadership styles. Nurses should know the differences between being an authoritative and democratic leader. The most effective management style in a health care environment is the democratic leader who uses an interdisciplinary approach to encourage open communication and collaboration, which will promote individual autonomy and accountability.

C. **Professional communication:** Involves sending, receiving, and interpreting written, face-to-face, and nonverbal information between at least two people.

1. Influence outcomes with good communication.
   a. Reduce errors.
   b. Improve continuity of care.
   c. Build teamwork/collaboration.

2. Coordination of Care
   a. Leadership and management
   b. Setting priorities
   c. Delegation
   d. Conflict resolution
   e. Problem-solving
   f. Documentation
   g. Consultation
   h. Transfers
   i. Discharge

3. **Therapeutic communication:** The purposeful use of communication to build and maintain helping relationships with clients, families, and significant others. Therapeutic communication is client-centered, purposeful, planned, and goal-directed.

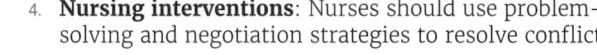

4. **Nursing interventions**: Effective communication requires commitment, effort, focus, and cooperation, especially when dealing with complex clinical issues and people who have diverse backgrounds and perspectives. It is essential to understand and use effective communication skills to successfully manage others.

D. **Conflict:** Arises when there are two or more opposing views, feelings, expectations, or other divergent issues.

1. Types of Conflict
   a. Intrapersonal: individual
   b. Interpersonal: between two or more people
   c. Intergroup: department, organization
2. Causes of Conflict
   a. Ineffective communication
   b. Unmet/unclear expectations
   c. Change
   d. Differences in values/beliefs
3. Conflict Management Strategies
   a. Avoiding/withdrawing
   b. Cooperating/accommodating
   c. Compromising/negotiating
   d. Competing/coercing
   e. Collaborating
   f. Smoothing
4. **Nursing interventions**: Nurses should use problem-solving and negotiation strategies to resolve conflict.

Teamwork and Collaboration

A. Foster a culture that values collaboration and cooperation.
B. Communicate that teamwork is expected.
C. Publicly celebrate team success.
D. Offer assistance during crises.
E. Assist team members with client care.
F. Participate in team conferences.

Quality

A. **Quality improvement:** A philosophy that promotes implementation of a plan to continually improve health care services and client outcomes.

B. **Performance improvement (Quality Improvement, Quality Control):** The process used to identify and resolve performance deficiencies, focusing on assessment of outcomes to improve delivery of quality care.

1. Steps in the performance improvement process:
   a. A standard is developed and approved by facility committee.
   b. Standards are made available to employees by way of policies and procedures.
   c. Quality issues are identified by staff, management, or risk management department.
   d. An interprofessional team is developed to review the issue.
   e. The current state of structure and process related to the issue is analyzed.
   f. Data collection methods are determined.
   g. Data are collected, analyzed, and compared with the established benchmark.
   h. If the benchmark is not met, possible influencing factors are determined. A root cause analysis may be done.
      1) Investigates the consequence and possible causes
      2) Analyzes the possible causes and relationships that may exist
      3) Determines additional influences at each level of relationship
      4) Determines the root cause or causes
   i. Potential solutions or corrective actions are analyzed, and one is selected for implementation.
   j. Educational or corrective action is implemented.
   k. The issue is re-evaluated at a pre-established time to determine the efficacy of the solution or corrective action.

III Variance/Incident/Irregular Occurrence

A variance, or incident, is an event that occurs outside the usual expected normal events or activities of the client's stay, unit functioning, or organizational processes.

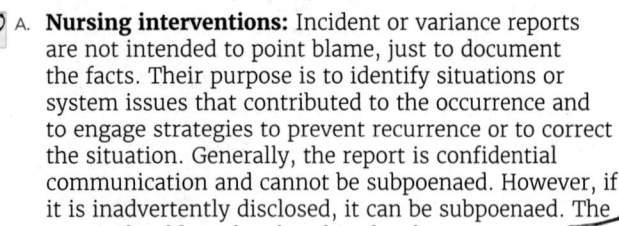

A. **Nursing interventions:** Incident or variance reports are not intended to point blame, just to document the facts. Their purpose is to identify situations or system issues that contributed to the occurrence and to engage strategies to prevent recurrence or to correct the situation. Generally, the report is confidential communication and cannot be subpoenaed. However, if it is inadvertently disclosed, it can be subpoenaed. The report should not be placed in the chart.

B. **Reportable incidents**

1. Medication errors
2. Procedure/treatment errors
3. Equipment-related injuries/errors
4. Needlestick injuries
5. Client falls/injuries
6. Visitor/volunteer injuries
7. Threat made to client or staff
8. Loss of property (e.g., dentures, jewelry, personal wheelchair)

IV Resource Management

Budgeting and resource allocation are determined based on human, financial, and material resources.

A. **Considerations**

   a. Budgeting: personnel, operational, capital
   b. Resource allocation: distribution of goods and services
   c. Cost-effective care: efficiency without compromise to standards and/or quality

1. The Budget Process
   a. **Planning:** Assess what the needs are.
   b. **Setting goals:** Determine what should be accomplished.
   c. **Preparation:** Develop a plan (time frame).
   d. **Monitoring and approval:** Implement the plan (ongoing monitoring and analysis).
   e. **Modification:** Evaluate the outcome (revise and modify as needed).

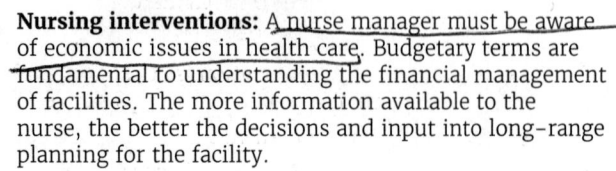

B. **Nursing interventions:** A nurse manager must be aware of economic issues in health care. Budgetary terms are fundamental to understanding the financial management of facilities. The more information available to the nurse, the better the decisions and input into long-range planning for the facility.

V Case Management

Case management provides client care coordination with the interprofessional team.

A. The principles of case management include a collaborative process to provide quality and continuity of care by minimizing fragmentation and high cost. Furthermore, the case manager is an advocate for the client and family.

VI Continuity of Care

Focuses on the experience of the client as the client moves through the health care system; guiding the client through this experience requires coordination, integration, collaboration, and facilitation of all the events along the continuum.

A. **Nursing's Role in Continuity of Care**

1. Coordinate care with the interprofessional team.
2. Act as a liaison and be a client advocate.
3. Complete admission, transfer, discharge, and postdischarge prescriptions.
4. Initiate, revise, and evaluate the plan of care.
5. Report the client's status.
6. Coordinate discharge planning.
7. Facilitate referrals and use of community resources.

VII Consultation and Referral

A. **Consultation:** A professional provides expert advice in a particular area and determines what treatment or services the client requires.

1. Examples of consultation: an orthopedic surgeon for a client with a hip fracture; a psychiatrist for a client whose risk for suicide must be assessed
2. **Nursing interventions:** Notify the primary care provider of the client's needs, provide the consultant with pertinent information, include consultant's information in the plan of care, and facilitate coordination with other health care providers in order to protect the client from conflicting and potentially dangerous prescriptions.

B. **Referral:** A formal request for a special service by another care provider so that the client can access the care identified by the primary care provider or consultant. The intervention becomes that specialist's responsibility, but the nurse continues to be responsible for monitoring the client's response and progress.

1. Examples of referrals: inpatient—physical therapy, wound care nurse; outside of the facility—hospice

C. **Nursing interventions:** The processes of consultation and referral are integral for effective use of services along the continuum, and they establish collaboration with the interdisciplinary team. The nurse should support the client/family with appropriate consultation and referral to contacts in the community.

Delegation and Prioritization

I Delegation/Assignment/Supervision/Accountability

A. **Delegating:** Transferring the authority to perform a selected nursing task in a selected situation to another team member while maintaining accountability.

B. **Assigning:** Transferring the authority, accountability, and responsibility to another member of the health care team (such as when an RN directs another RN to assess a client, the second RN is already authorized to assess clients in the RN scope of practice).

C. **Supervising:** Monitoring the progress toward completion of delegated tasks; the amount of supervision required depends on the direction of the delegation, the abilities of the person being delegated to, and the location of the ultimate responsibility for outcomes.

D. **Accountability:** Moral responsibility for consequences of actions

E. **Five Rights of Delegation**
   1. Right person
   2. Right task
   3. Right circumstances
   4. Right direction and communication
   5. Right supervision and evaluation

F. **Nursing interventions:** It is essential for a nurse to understand legal responsibilities when managing and delegating nursing care to a wide variety of health care workers. The nurse must delegate activities thoughtfully, taking into account individual job descriptions, knowledge base, and skills demonstrated. Remember, the professional nurse is accountable for determining the extent and complexity of client needs and for assigning work that is consistent with the individual's position, description, and duties.

G. **The RN Cannot Delegate**
   1. Nursing process — ADPIE
   2. Client education
   3. Tasks that require nursing judgment (including care of unstable clients)

II Roles and Responsibilities for Levels of Staff

A. **Assistive Personnel (AP)/Unlicensed Assistive Personnel (UAP)**
   1. Training is often on the job.
   2. An AP may complete a certification program—certified nursing assistant.
   3. An AP functions under the direction of the licensed practical nurse (LPN) or RN.
   4. Skills
      a. Performs basic hygiene care and grooming.
      b. Reports to the LPN or RN.
      c. Provides assistance with ADLs such as nutrition, elimination, and mobility.

DELEGATION WORKSHEET

Which tasks are most appropriately delegated to a licensed practical nurse (LPN) or unlicensed assistive personnel (UAP)?

Task	LPN	UAP
1. Activities of daily living	☐ LPN	☒ UAP
2. Ambulating	☐ LPN	☒ UAP
3. Tracheostomy care	☒ LPN	☐ UAP
4. Suctioning	☒ LPN	☐ UAP
5. Feeding	☐ LPN	☒ UAP
6. Positioning	☐ LPN	☒ UAP
7. Inserting urinary catheter	☒ LPN	☐ UAP
8. Checking nasogastric tube patency	☒ LPN	☐ UAP
9. Medication administration	☒ LPN	☐ UAP
10. Sterile specimen collection	☒ LPN	☐ UAP
11. Vital signs (on stable clients)	☐ LPN	☒ UAP
12. Intake and output	☐ LPN	☒ UAP
13. Reinforcing client teaching	☒ LPN	☐ UAP

Answer Key: 1. UAP; 2. UAP; 3. LPN; 4. LPN; 5. UAP; 6. UAP; 7. LPN; 8. LPN; 9. LPN; 10. LPN; 11. UAP; 12. UAP; 13. LPN

   d. Performs basic skills such as taking vital signs, including pulse oximetry, and calculating I&O.
   e. Emphasis is on maintaining a safe environment and recognizing situations to report to immediate superior.
   f. Performs skills that are noninvasive and do not require sterile technique.

B. **Licensed Practical Nurse (LPN)/Licensed Vocational Nurse (LVN)**
   1. Education is approximately 12 to 18 months in an accredited program.
   2. LPNs must complete and pass the NCLEX-PN® exam for licensure.
   3. Supervised by the RN or provider
   4. Scope of practice is determined by nurse practice acts, which vary by state (requirements to maintain an active license are determined by each state).
      a. Meets the health needs of clients
      b. Cares for clients whose condition is considered to be stable and/or chronic with an expected outcome
      c. Performs reinforcement teaching
      d. Contributes to care plan through discussing client problems/findings with RN
      e. Calculates and monitors IV flow rate
      f. Administers IVPB medications
      g. Monitors IV fluids

C. **Registered Nurse (RN)**
  1. May be diploma, associate degree, baccalaureate degree, or higher.
  2. Education ranges from 2 or more years.
  3. RNs must complete and pass the NCLEX-RN® exam for licensure.
  4. Functions under the direction of the health care provider.
  5. Advanced clinical skills in caring for the acute client with complex care needs; outcome uncertain.
  6. Scope of practice is determined by nurse practice acts, which vary by state (requirements to maintain an active license are determined by each state).

D. **Advanced Practice Nurse**
  1. May be non-degree, master's degree, or higher.
  2. Education ranges from 18 months to more than 4 years (in addition to basic RN program).
  3. Must complete and pass a certification exam (in addition to the NCLEX-RN exam) applicable to the specialty and practice (adult nurse practitioner, diabetic educator).
  4. Functions vary according to the state practice act, which may be either autonomous or under the direct or indirect supervision of a provider.
  5. Skills vary according to the state practice act and may include the ability to prescribe, diagnose, and treat.

E. **Health Care Provider**
  1. May be a provider, provider's assistant, or nurse practitioner.
  2. In general, only an attending provider has admitting privileges to a facility, although another care provider in the practice may direct the care given to the client.

III Prioritization Principles

A. **Nurses must continually set and reset priorities in order to safely care for multiple clients.**
  1. Assessments are completed.
  2. Interventions are provided.
  3. Steps in a client procedure are completed.
  4. Components of client care are completed.

B. **Establishing priorities in nursing practice requires that these decisions be made based on evidence obtained:**
  1. During shift reports and other communications with members of the health care team.
  2. Through careful review of documents.
  3. By continually and accurately collecting client data.

PRIORITIZATION PRINCIPLES IN CLIENT CARE

PRINCIPLE	EXAMPLES
Prioritize systemic before local ("life before limb").	Prioritizing interventions for a client in shock over interventions for a client with a localized limb injury
Prioritize acute (less opportunity for physical adaptation) before chronic (greater opportunity for physical adaptation).	Prioritizing the care of a client with a new injury/illness (e.g., mental confusion, chest pain) or an acute exacerbation of a previous illness over the care of client with a long-term chronic illness
Prioritize actual problems before potential future problems.	Prioritizing administration of medication to a client experiencing acute pain over ambulation of a client at risk for thrombophlebitis
Prioritize according to Maslow's Hierarchy of Needs.	Prioritizing the care of the client needs according to Maslow's Hierarchy (e.g., physiological needs, such as nutrition, are a higher priority than self-esteem)
Recognize and respond to trends vs. transient findings.	Recognizing a gradual deterioration in a client's level of consciousness and/or Glasgow Coma Scale score
Recognize signs of emergencies and complications vs. "expected client findings."	Recognizing signs of increasing intracranial pressure in a client newly diagnosed with a stroke vs. the clinical findings expected following a stroke
Apply clinical knowledge to procedural standards to determine the priority action.	Recognizing that the timing of administration of antidiabetic and antimicrobial medications is more important than administration of some other medications

Nursing Process
- Assessment
  Diagnosis
  Outcome Identification
  Planning
  Implementation
  Evaluation

Self Actualization
esteem
love + belonging
Safety
physiological needs

Glasgow Coma Scale

eye opening
Spontaneous 74
to sound 73
to pressure 72
none 71

verbal response
oriented 75
confused 74
words 73
sounds 72
none 71

Motor response
obey commands 76
localising 75
normal flexion 74
abnormal flexion 73
extension 72
none 71

PRIORITIZATION WORKSHEET

Select the client from each group that the nurse should assess first after morning report and select a principle of prioritization that applies to that client.

Group A

☒ 1. A client receiving morphine sulfate via a PCA pump with respirations of 8/min

☐ 2. A client 2 days postoperative right knee replacement who has not had a bowel movement

☐ 3. A client with a left below-the-knee amputation who is having difficulty with body image

☐ 4. A client who has a heart rate of 110 beats per minute after an albuterol respiratory treatment

Group B

☐ 1. A client who has diabetes mellitus and whose capillary blood glucose is 150 mg/dL before breakfast

☒ 2. A client 2 days postoperative colon resection with an oral temperature of 39.8° C (103.6° F) *above 101*

☐ 3. A client in Buck's traction who refuses to take the daily prescribed stool softener

☐ 4. A client with cervical fusion needing to ambulate the length of the hallway

Group C

☐ 1. A client who has chronic kidney disease and a creatinine level of 2.3   *0.7–1.3 creatinine*   *capillary refills*

☐ 2. A client who is 2 hr post cardiac catheterization with capillary refill less than 3 seconds   *2 sec or less*

☐ 3. A client with a swollen, reddened, and painful intravenous site after receiving antibiotics

☒ 4. A client with expiratory wheezes after receiving intravenous contrast for a CT scan

Answer Key

Group A: The client receiving morphine should be seen first. Respiratory depression is an adverse effect of morphine. Several principles can be used in the scenario: ABCs, which include airway and breathing; unexpected problem before an expected problem; actual problem before potential problem; and physiological needs from Maslow's Hierarchy of Needs. Place this client as the highest priority. The postoperative client who has not had a bowel movement has a potential problem, but not an actual problem at this point, placing the client at a lower priority. A client who has impaired body image falls under self-esteem or socialization in Maslow's Hierarchy of Needs, placing this client at a lower priority. The client who has a heart rate of 110/min after an albuterol treatment is experiencing an expected reaction to this medication, which places this client at a lower priority.

Group B: The client 2 days postoperative colon resection with a temperature of 39.8° C (103.6° F) should be seen first. An elevated temperature in the first few days postoperative may indicate an infection and should be addressed immediately. This is a safety issue according to Maslow's Hierarchy of Needs, and it is an unexpected event. It also could be systemic and cause sepsis. Capillary blood sugar glucose 150 mg/dL is elevated but expected for most clients who have diabetes mellitus. The client in Buck's traction who refuses to take his stool softener may have a potential problem, but does not have an actual problem at this time. A client who has cervical fusion and needs to ambulate also has a potential problem of thrombosis, but does not have an actual problem. Actual problems are higher priority than potential problems.

Group C: The client who has expiratory wheezes should be seen first, as the finding may indicate allergic reaction to the contrast. The client has an actual airway problem (ABCs and Maslow's physiological needs), which is an unexpected finding indicating a systemic complication and places this client at highest priority. The client who has chronic kidney disease and a creatinine level of 2.3 mg/dL has an expected elevation for the condition. The client with a capillary refill of less than 3 seconds has an expected outcome. A client with a swollen, reddened, and painful IV site has an actual safety problem (Maslow's Hierarchy of Needs), but the condition is local, not systemic, placing the client at lower priority.

---

mild | moderate | severe
13-15 | 9-12 | 3-8

Best score - 15
Comatosed < 8
Unresponsive - 3

THE COMPREHENSIVE NCLEX-RN® REVIEW

Ethical Issues

I Ethical Practice

A. **Ethical Principles**

1. **Autonomy**: The right to make one's own decisions

2. **Beneficence**: The obligation to do good for others

3. **Confidentiality**: The obligation to observe the privacy of another and maintain strict confidence

4. **Fidelity**: The obligation to be faithful to agreements and responsibilities, to keep promises

5. **Justice**: The obligation to be fair to all people (when allocating limited resources)

6. **Nonmaleficence**: The obligation not to harm others (Hippocrates states, "First, do no harm.")

7. **Paternalism**: Assuming the right to make decisions for another

8. **Veracity**: The obligation to tell the truth

B. **Ethical dilemmas:** Ethical dilemmas are problems for which more than one choice can be made, and the choice is influenced by the values and beliefs of the decision-makers. Ethical dilemmas are very common in health care, and nurses must be prepared to apply ethical theory and decision-making.

C. **The American Nurses Association's (ANA)** *Code of Ethics for Nurses:* Sets guidelines to use when providing client care, outlines the nurse's responsibility to the client and the profession of nursing, and assists the nurse in making ethical decisions.

D. **Ethical decision-making:** A process in which the nurse, client, client's family, and health care team make decisions, taking into consideration personal and philosophical viewpoints, the *ANA Code of Ethics for Nurses*, and ethical principles. Frequently, this requires that a balance be struck between science and morality.

E. **Advocacy:** A process by which the nurse assists the client to grow and develop toward self-actualization. Advocacy is a critical leadership role and emphasizes the values of caring, autonomy, respect, and empowerment.

II Organ Donation

A. **Organ and tissue donation is regulated by state and federal laws.** Facilities will have specific policies and procedures to follow during the process.

B. Federal law requires health care facilities to provide access to trained specialists who make the request to clients and/or family members and provide information regarding consent, organ and tissues that can be donated, and how burial or cremation will be affected by donation.

C. Provide emotional support and answer questions.

III Advance Directives

A document in which a client who is competent is able to express wishes regarding future acceptable health care (including the desire for extraordinary lifesaving measures: resuscitation, intubation, and artificial hydration and nutrition) and/or designate another person to make decisions when the client becomes physically or mentally unable to do so. The Patient Self-Determination Act requires all clients admitted to a health care facility be asked if they have advance directives.

A. **Planning guides for seriously ill clients**

1. **Living will**: Legal document that instructs health care providers and family members about what, if any, life-sustaining treatment an individual wants if at some time the individual is unable to make decisions.

2. **Durable power of attorney for health care**: Legal document that designates another person to make health care decisions for the client when the client becomes unable to make decisions independently.

3. **Nursing interventions**: Ensure communication to the health care team when clients have provided advance directives (available in the medical record). Clients who do not have advance directives must be given written information outlining rights related to health care decisions.

Legal Issues

I Informed Consent

Obtained after a client receives complete disclosure of all pertinent information provided by the provider regarding the surgery or procedure to be performed. Obtained only if the client understands the potential benefits and risks associated with the surgery or procedure.

A. **Elements of Informed Consent**

1. Individual giving consent must fully understand the procedure that will be performed, the risks involved, expected/desired outcomes, expected complications/side effects, and alternate treatments or therapies available.

2. Consent is given by a competent adult, legal guardian or designated power of attorney (DPOA), emancipated or married minor, parent of a minor, or a court order.

3. A trained medical interpreter must be provided when the person giving consent is unable to communicate due to a language barrier.

B. **Nurse's role:** Witness the client's signature and ensure the provider gave the necessary information and that the client understood and is competent to sign; notify the provider if clarification is needed.

C. **Documentation:** Thorough documentation includes reinforcement of information given by the provider, any irregular occurrences, and use of an interpreter.

II Client Rights

A. **Patient bill of rights:** Right to humane care and treatment

B. **Americans with Disabilities Act (ADA):** Eliminates discrimination against Americans who have physical or mental disabilities

C. **Confidentiality:** The right to privacy with respect to one's personal medical information

  1. **Legislation:** Health Insurance Portability and Accountability Act (HIPAA) of 1996

     a. A uniform, federal act providing privacy protection for health consumers.

     b. State laws that may provide additional protections to consumers are not affected by HIPAA.

     c. Guarantees that clients are able to access their medical records.

     d. Provides clients with control over how their personal health information is used and disclosed.

     e. Outlines limited circumstances in which personal health information can be disclosed without first obtaining consent of the client or the client's family:

        1) Suspicion of child or elder abuse

        2) When otherwise required by law (such as suspicion of criminal activity)

        3) Incidences of state agency or health department requirements; reportable communicable disease

III Legal Responsibilities

A. **Sources of law:** The Constitution, statutes, administrative agencies, and court decisions

B. **Types of Laws and Courts**

  1. Criminal law

     a. Felony—serious crime

     b. Misdemeanor—less serious crime

  2. Civil laws

     a. Tort law

        1) **Unintentional torts:** negligence, malpractice

        2) **Quasi-intentional torts:** breach of confidentiality, defamation of character

        3) **Intentional torts:** assault, battery, false imprisonment

  3. State laws: Nursing practice is regulated by state law. Each state's board of nursing has rules, regulations, and standards that vary based on statutes defining practice.

C. **Nurse Practice Act**

  1. Varies from state to state

D. **Good Samaritan Law**

  1. Health care providers are protected from potential liability if volunteering away from their place of employment, as long as the nurses' actions are not grossly negligent.

E. **Mandatory Reporting**

  1. Abuse

     a. Nurses are mandated to report abuse of vulnerable populations (children, older adults). Any suspicion of abuse must be reported based on facility policy.

  2. Communicable Disease

     a. A complete list is available from the CDC. Report to public health department to ensure appropriate medical treatment, and plan for prevention and control, including public education.

F. **Impaired Coworker**

  1. A nurse who suspects a coworker of using drugs or alcohol while working has the duty to report to the appropriate supervisory personnel according to institutional policy.

G. **Malpractice (Professional Negligence)**

  1. The failure of a person with professional training to act in a reasonable and prudent manner within the identified scope of practice and/or within the guidelines identified by the state regulating agency.

H. **Negligence**

  1. The omission to do something that a reasonable person would do, or doing something that a reasonable person would not do

  2. Negligence can be mitigated by: following practice standards, communicating effectively with the health care team, and accurate/timely documentation.

I. **Nursing interventions:** Nurses who are able to recognize the rights and responsibilities in legal matters are better able to protect themselves against liability or loss of licensure.

! Point to Remember

One of the most vital and basic functions of a professional nurse is the duty to intervene when the safety or well-being of a client or another person is obviously at risk.

Information Technology

I Informatics

The use of information technology as a communication and information-gathering tool that supports clinical decision-making and scientifically based nursing practice.

A. Allows candidates to test for nursing licensure (NCLEX®) with rapid results

B. Permits verification of licensure online for nurses and other health care professionals

C. Informatics: Technology resources are used to gather data in a systematic way to support clinical decision-making and scientifically based nursing practice.

D. Client care: Electronic documentation, medication dispensing, and client education resources.

E. Professional education (medications, diseases, procedures, treatments)

F. Client portals: Allows integration of e-health and collaboration between client and health care providers.

II Data Security

A. Passwords are necessary to prevent improper access to computers and medication systems.

B. Only individuals who have a professional relationship with a client may access the client's personal health information, per HIPAA regulations.

C. Computer terminals must be logged off and locked when not in immediate use.

D. Monitor screens must be shielded or situated so that unauthorized individuals cannot see the information.

III Use of Technology in Health Care

A. Documentation

B. Databases for teaching and learning

C. Electronic Health Record

D. Mobile applications

E. Telehealth/telemedicine

! Point to Remember

A nurse should not share computer passwords with another person, including coworkers and family members.

! Point to Remember

Nurses should instruct clients to review valid and credible websites. The author, institution, and credentials should be reviewed.

UNIT THREE

Community Health Nursing

The Nurse's Role in Community Nursing

I Community Assessment: Individuals, Families, and Aggregates

A comprehensive assessment clarifying the client problem by evaluating:

A. Biological factors
B. Social factors
C. Cultural factors
D. Physical factors
E. Environmental factors
F. Social systems
G. Financial constraints (The client's eligibility for service and situational constraints must also be considered.)

II Community Nurse Referrals

Assist in linking the community resource with the client to provide holistic care; must have thorough knowledge of resource individuals and organizations.

A. Use computerized records, databases, and telecommunication technologies for physical, audio, and visual data.
B. Responsible for coordination, providing continuity of care, and evaluating the outcome.
C. Examples of community nursing referrals
   1. Psychological services
   2. Support groups
   3. Medical equipment providers
   4. Meal delivery services
   5. Transportation services
   6. Life care planner
D. Examples of community health nurse practice settings
   1. Home health nurse
   2. Hospice nurse
   3. Occupational health nurse
   4. Parish nurse
   5. School nurse
   6. Case managers

III Community Health Nursing

Goal is to preserve, protect, promote, and maintain health of individuals, families, and groups in the community.

A. **Vulnerable groups**
   1. Migrant workers and immigrants
   2. Poor and homeless persons
   3. Victims of violence or abuse
   4. Substance abusers
   5. Severely mentally ill individuals
   6. Older adults
   7. Pregnant adolescents
   8. Individuals with communicable diseases

Disaster Planning

I Disaster

A serious disruption of the functioning of a community that causes widespread human, material, economic, or environmental losses that exceed the ability of the affected community or society to cope with using its own resources. Prevention, preparedness, response, and recovery are the four stages of disaster management.

A. **Internal disasters** are events in the health care facility that threaten to disrupt the care environment.
   1. Structural (e.g., fire, loss of power)
   2. Personnel-related (e.g., strike, high absenteeism)
B. **External disasters** are events outside the health care facility and may be human-made or natural.
   1. Human-made disasters
      a. Transportation-related incidents (e.g., car, train, plane, and subway crashes)
      b. Terrorist attacks, including bombs (e.g., suicide bombs and dirty bombs) and bioterrorism
      c. Industrial accidents
      d. Chemical spills or toxic gas leaks
      e. Structural fires
   2. Natural disasters
      a. Extreme weather conditions, including blizzards, ice storms, hurricanes, tornadoes, and floods
      b. Ecological disasters, including earthquakes, landslides, tsunamis, volcanoes, and forest fires
      c. Microbial disasters such as epidemics and pandemics
      d. A combined internal/external disaster situation can arise when an external disaster, such as a severe weather condition, causes mass casualties and prevents health care providers from getting to the facility, perhaps due to traffic or road conditions.

II Disaster Prevention

A. **Reducing risk from natural and human-made hazards**
1. Protecting buildings and infrastructure
2. Improving security and public health awareness

III Disaster Preparedness

A. **Occurs at the national, state, and local levels**
B. **Interagency cooperation within the community is essential in a disaster and requires:**
1. Communitywide planning for emergencies and/or hazards that may affect the local area.
2. Coordination between community emergency system and health care facilities.
3. Developing a local emergency communications plan and/or network.
4. Identification of potential emergency public shelters.

C. **Role of the nurse**
1. In the health care facility
    a. The Joint Commission mandates specific standards for hospital preparedness, including an Emergency Operation Plan (EOP).
    b. An EOP includes training for personnel, criteria for activation, and specific actions for various emergency/disaster scenarios.
    c. Disaster drills should be conducted at least twice annually; one involving communitywide resources and actual or simulated clients.
2. In the community
    a. Education provided to families about disaster planning
        1) A family disaster plan should include:
            a) What to do in an evacuation
            b) Plans for family pets
            c) Where to meet in case of an emergency
        2) A family disaster kit should include:
            a) A flashlight with extra batteries
            b) A battery-powered radio
            c) Nonperishable food that requires no cooking (along with a nonelectric can opener)
            d) One gallon of water per person
            e) Basic first-aid supplies
            f) Matches in a waterproof container
            g) Household liquid bleach for disinfection
            h) Emergency blanket and/or sleeping bag and pillow
            i) Rain gear
            j) Clothing and sturdy footwear
            k) Prescription and OTC medications
            l) Toiletries
            m) Important documents and money

3. **Nursing interventions**
    a. Assess community for risks.

IV Disaster Response

A. **Emergency management system**
1. Provides public access to immediate health care (911)
2. Dispatch communication center
3. Trained first responders: emergency medical technicians
4. Transportation to medical resources: ground (ambulance) and/or air (helicopter)

B. **Declaration of a disaster**
1. **Disaster area**: Local officials request that the governor of the state take appropriate action under state law and the state's emergency plan and declare a disaster area.
2. **Federal disaster area**: The governor of the affected state requests declaration of a disaster area by the president to qualify the affected area for federal disaster relief.
3. **Internal disaster**: The nursing or administrative supervisor may declare an internal disaster in case of a facility-related issue.

C. **Disaster relief organizations**
1. Federal Emergency Management Agency (FEMA)
    a. FEMA is part of the U.S. Department of Homeland Security.
        1) Manages federal response and recovery efforts
2. American Red Cross
    a. Not a government agency, but authorized by the government to provide disaster relief
    b. The American Red Cross provides:
        1) Shelter and food to address basic human needs
        2) Health and mental services
        3) Food to emergency and relief workers
        4) Blood and blood products to disaster victims
    c. The American Red Cross also handles inquiries from concerned family members outside the disaster area.
3. Hazardous material response team (Hazmat)
    a. Hazardous materials may be radioactive, flammable, explosive, toxic, corrosive, or biohazardous, or may have other characteristics that make them hazardous in specific circumstances.
    b. Hazmat team members are specially trained to respond to these situations and wear protective equipment.
    c. In a toxic exposure disaster, Hazmat will coordinate the decontamination effort.
4. Other agencies include: U.S. Department of Homeland Security (DHS), Center for Disease Control (CDC), and Office of Emergency Management (OEM).

v Role of the Nurse

A. **Triage**: Process of prioritizing which clients should receive care first

   1. **Non-mass casualty situation**: The nurse prioritizes client care so that clients who have conditions of the highest acuity are evaluated and treated first. Emergency services are presented with a large number of casualties. However, they are still functional and able to provide care to victims on all three levels.

      a. **Emergent:** immediate threat to life; critically injured

      b. **Urgent:** major injuries that require immediate treatment

      c. **Nonurgent:** minor injuries that do not require immediate treatment; slightly injured

   2. **Mass casualty disaster triage**: The field and/or emergency services are presented with a number of casualties and/or ground conditions and are unable to treat everyone. The staff must provide the greatest good for the greatest number. Consists of four levels:

      a. **Emergent or Class I (red tag)**: immediate threat to life; do not delay treatment

      b. **Urgent or Class II (yellow tag)**: major injuries that require treatment; can delay treatment 30 min to 2 hr

      c. **Nonurgent or Class III (green tag)**: minor injuries that do not require immediate treatment, can delay treatment 2 to 4 hr

      d. **Expectant or Class IV (black tag)**: expected and allowed to die; prepare for morgue

---

MASS CASUALTY DISASTER TRIAGE

Select the appropriate triage category after a mass casualty disaster triage (red, yellow, green, black).

	RED	YELLOW	GREEN	BLACK
1. Airway obstruction	☒ RED	☐ YELLOW	☐ GREEN	☐ BLACK
2. "Walking wounded"	☐ RED	☐ YELLOW	☒ GREEN	☐ BLACK
3. Requires immediate attention	☒ RED	☐ YELLOW	☐ GREEN	☐ BLACK
4. Closed fracture	☒ RED	☐ YELLOW	☒ GREEN	☐ BLACK
5. Shock	☒ RED	☐ YELLOW	☐ GREEN	☐ BLACK
6. Expected and allowed to die	☐ RED	☐ YELLOW	☐ GREEN	☒ BLACK
7. Contusions	☐ RED	☐ YELLOW	☒ GREEN	☐ BLACK
8. Massive head trauma	☐ RED	☐ YELLOW	☐ GREEN	☒ BLACK
9. Need treatment within 30 min to 2 hr	☐ RED	☒ YELLOW	☐ GREEN	☐ BLACK
10. Cardiac arrest	☐ RED	☐ YELLOW	☐ GREEN	☒ BLACK
11. Open fracture with a distal pulse	☐ RED	☒ YELLOW	☐ GREEN	☐ BLACK
12. Treatment can be delayed more than 2 hr	☐ RED	☐ YELLOW	☒ GREEN	☐ BLACK

Answer Key: 1. Red; 2. Green; 3. Red; 4. Green; 5. Red; 6. Black; 7. Green; 8. Black; 9. Yellow; 10. Black; 11. Yellow; 12. Green

---

B. **Health care facility disaster plan**

   1. A nursing or administrative supervisor may implement the disaster plan due to extreme weather conditions or an anticipation of mass casualties.

   2. Plans to implement

      a. Establishment of an incident command center

      b. Premature discharge of clients who are stable from the facility

      c. Transfer of clients who are stable from the intensive care unit

      d. Postponement of scheduled admissions and elective operations

      e. Mobilization of personnel (call in off-duty individuals)

      f. Protection of personnel and visitors

      g. Evacuation plan

   3. Role of the charge nurse during a disaster

      a. Preparation of a discharge list that features clients who can safely and quickly be discharged, such as the most stable, non-bedridden clients (e.g., clients admitted for observation, scheduled for diagnostic tests, or those who can be cared for at home or at a rehab facility)

      b. Personnel sent to the command center, if required

      c. Off-duty personnel called in, if requested

      d. Disaster victims prepared for admittance

vi Disaster Recovery

Begins when danger no longer exists and the "stand down" order has been given.

A. **Crisis intervention**

   1. Mental health response team employs advanced crisis intervention techniques to help victims, survivors, and their families better handle the powerful emotional reactions associated with crises and disasters.

   2. Goals

      a. Reduce the intensity of an individual's emotional reaction.

      b. Assist individuals in recovering from the crisis.

      c. Help to prevent serious long-term problems from developing.

B. **Posttraumatic stress disorder (PTSD)**: A mental health condition that can develop following any traumatic or catastrophic life experience.

   1. PTSD symptoms can develop in survivors of a disaster weeks, months, or even years following the catastrophic event.

c. **Critical incident stress debriefing and administrative review**

1. Health care providers who respond to a highly stressful event that is extremely traumatic or overwhelming may experience significant stress reactions.

2. The critical incident stress debriefing process is designed to prevent the development of posttraumatic stress among first responders and health care professionals.

   a. Defusing: discussion of feelings shortly after the disaster/critical incident (such as at the end of a shift)

   b. Formal debriefing: discussion some hours or days after the disaster/critical incident, in a large group setting, with mental health teams of peer support personnel serving as the leaders

3. Administrative review to identify areas of the agency response plan that were effective and areas that need improvement

VII Agents of Bioterrorism

A. **Three categories (A, B, C) of priority based on ease of transmission and morbidity and mortality rates.**

1. **Category A:** highest priority and threat to national security because agents are easily transmitted and have high mortality rates. Include: smallpox, botulism, anthrax, tularemia, hemorrhagic viral fevers (e.g., Ebola), and plague.

2. **Category B:** second-highest priority, agents are moderately easy to disseminate and have moderate morbidity rates and low mortality rates. Include: typhus fever, ricin toxin, diarrheagenic *E. coli*, and West Nile virus.

3. **Category C:** third-highest priority, emerging pathogens that could be engineered for mass dissemination. Agents are easy to produce and have a potential for high morbidity and mortality rates. Include: hantavirus, influenza virus, tuberculosis, and rabies virus.

Culturally Competent Care

I Cultural Care

A. **Culture:** Knowledge, beliefs, values, and traditions that are shared by a group of people about life and the world, which passes to the next generation.

B. **Cultural competence:** The ability to provide care that respects and integrates aspects of culture to meet client needs.

C. **Cultural humility:** Continuing self-reflection and awareness of cultural biases, assumptions, and values; better knowing of one's self that results in better care.

II Cultural Competence

There are twelve standards to serve as a guide for providing culturally competent care.

A. Social justice

B. Critical reflection

C. Knowledge of cultures

D. Culturally competent practice

E. Cultural competence in health care systems and organizations

F. Client advocacy and empowerment

G. Multicultural workforce

H. Education and training in culturally competent care

I. Cross-cultural communication

J. Cross-cultural leadership

K. Policy development

L. Evidence-based practice and research

III Cultural Assessment

Assessment to identify values, beliefs, meaning, and behavior of clients

A. What is the client's ethnic affiliation, and what is its importance in the client's daily life?

B. Does the client speak, write, read, and understand English?

C. What dietary preferences or prohibitions does the client follow?

D. Are there rituals or customs that the client wishes to keep related to transitions such as birth and death?

E. Does the client want or need to have family involved in care?

F. Is the client using herbal or other traditional remedies?

G. What behaviors or views are important to the spirituality of the client?

IV Cultural Factors Affecting Health

A. **Time Orientation**

1. Past: Cultures that focus on past orientation look to the past to provide direction for current situations. Review weekly progress to assist clients with health promotion and disease prevention.

2. Present: Place greater value on quality of life and view present time as being more important than future time. Focus on immediate benefits versus long-term outcomes as an effective approach when discussing disease prevention.

3. Future: Delays immediate gratification until future goals are met. Focus on long-term goals.

B. **Language and Communication:** Verbal and Nonverbal

1. Speak in a low, moderate voice.

2. Discuss one topic at a time.

3. Eye contact and the use of touch varies among cultural groups.

4. Language and communication barriers may impact a client's utilization of health care.

5. Recognize nonverbal cures of poor understanding.

   a. Blank expression

   b. Inappropriate laughter

   c. Absence of questions

C. **Space:** Preferred Distance Between Individuals

1. Take cues from the client and be aware of spatial distance preferences.

2. Clients may move closer or farther away from the nurse depending on personal space preference.

D. **Beliefs and practices:** An individual's beliefs regarding health affects actions taken to treat and prevent disease.

1. Biomedical beliefs: Focus is on identifying a cause for every effect on the body. This is the basis for the current United States health system.

2. Naturalistic beliefs: Relates the individual as a part of nature or creation. An imbalance in nature is believed to cause disease, such as in Eastern medicine.

3. Magico-religious beliefs: Illness and health are linked to supernatural forces. Some Christian religions share this belief as faith healing.

4. Folk healer beliefs: Clients may seek help from a spiritual healer, folk doctor, or shaman.

V Nursing Interventions

A. Address the client by their last name, unless the client gives permission to use another name.

B. Recognize individual uniqueness and the diversity within cultures.

C. Respect the client's values, beliefs, and practices.

D. Remain sensitive to the client's spiritual beliefs.

1. Spirituality is a subjective concept that implies connectedness.

2. Spirituality may or may not include religion.

3. Addressing clients' spiritual needs is required for all health care facilities by the Joint Commission.

E. Provide a diet that is consistent with client's customs and preferences.

F. Allow family to be involved in care, if desired.

G. Review the client's herbal and/or alternative methods to provide client education and prevent interactions with currently prescribed medications or treatments.

H. Consider cultural factors that affect health when providing care, such as time orientation, language and communication, space, and beliefs and practices.

I. Provide a qualified interpreter if necessary.

VI National CLAS Standards

The U.S. Department of Health and Human Services has identified culturally and linguistically appropriate services standards (CLAS) to promote equitable care and improve quality of health services. CLAS standards include:

A. Offering language and communication assistance to those with limited proficiency in English at no charge to the individual and ensuring that they are informed regarding availability of services

B. Ensuring that only qualified people provide language assistance

C. Providing written materials in the languages of commonly-served populations

D. Ensuring continuous quality improvement and accountability in the implementation of CLAS standards

E. Partner with the local community to establish and implement services that ensure cultural and linguistic appropriateness

VII Using an Interpreter

The nurse should use a qualified interpreter when it is difficult for a nurse or client to understand the other's language.

A. Observe the client for nonverbal messages.

B. Address the client, as well as the interpreter.

C. Interpreters should have knowledge of health-related terminology.

D. Have the interpreter translate written materials into the client's primary language.

E. Consider client preferences when selecting the age and gender of an interpreter.

F. Federal government mandates require agencies to have a plan that will improve access to federal health care programs for individuals who have limited English proficiency.

G. Review the material with the client to ensure that nothing has been missed or misunderstood.

H. The use of family members as interpreters should be avoided because clients may need privacy in discussing sensitive matters. Family members can have difficulty understanding medical terminology.

RELIGIOUS/SPIRITUAL INFLUENCES ON HEALTH

	BIRTH PRACTICES	DEATH PRACTICES	DIETARY RESTRICTIONS	HEALTH PRACTICES
Buddhism	Believe in reincarnation. Contraception to prevent conception is acceptable.	Ensure a calm, peaceful environment. Chanting is common. Monk delivers last rites. Organ donation is encouraged. Cremation is common.	Vegetarian diet practiced by many. Avoidance of alcohol.	A quiet, peaceful environment allows client to rest and practice meditation and prayer. May refuse care on holy days.
Catholicism	Contraception, abortion, and sterilization are prohibited. Baptism is required.	Priest administers last rites. Organ donation is acceptable. Suicide may prevent burial in Catholic cemetery.	Some may abstain from eating meat on Ash Wednesday and on Fridays during Lent.	Most want to see a priest when hospitalized. May request communion or confession to aid in healing. May wear cross or medal or display religious statues.
Christian Science	Abortion is prohibited. A client may choose to give birth at home.	Unlikely to seek medical help to prolong life. Organ donation is discouraged.	Must abstain from alcohol.	Medications and blood products are avoided. Healing ministers practice spiritual healing and do not use medical or psychological techniques.
Hinduism	Contraception is acceptable. Abortion may be prohibited. Males are not circumcised. Child is not named until the tenth day of life.	Believe in reincarnation. Allowing a natural death is traditional. Client may want to lie on floor while dying. A thread is placed around the neck/wrist. Organ donation is acceptable. Prefer cremation.	Vegetarian diet is encouraged. Most abstain from beef and pork. Right hand is used for eating and left hand for toileting and hygiene. Several days a year are set aside for fasting.	Personal hygiene is very important. Future lives are influenced by how one faces illness, disability, and death.
Islam (Muslim)	Contraception is acceptable. Abortion is permitted in certain circumstances. A prayer is said into the infant's ear at birth. Circumcision is customary.	Client may want to confess sins prior to death. A dying client may wish to be placed facing Mecca (usually east). Organ donation and autopsy is acceptable by some. Devout Muslims may refuse both, fearing desecration of the dead. Rituals include traditional bathing with burial within 24 hr. Cremation is prohibited.	Food must be halal (lawful). Pork, alcohol, and some shellfish are prohibited. Ramadan is a period of fasting during the ninth lunar month. Halal (permitted) meats are from animals that have been slaughtered during a payer ritual. Haram (prohibited) foods include pork, gelatin, alcohol, and animals with fangs.	A client may wish to pray five times a day, facing Mecca, and may have a prayer rug. Privacy during prayer is important. Women are very modest and wear clothes that cover their entire body. Women may refuse/avoid male health care workers.

	BIRTH PRACTICES	DEATH PRACTICES	DIETARY RESTRICTIONS	HEALTH PRACTICES
Judaism	Abortion is permitted. Ritual circumcision of males is called a bris, performed on the eighth day of life. Orthodox Jewish males are not allowed in the delivery room.	An autopsy is discouraged. Organ donation is permitted. Someone stays with the body at all times. Ritual bathing and burial within 24 hr. Cremation is prohibited.	Food is required to be kosher. Milk and meat cannot be served at the same meal or prepared on the same dishes. Pork and shellfish prohibited. Fasting required on Yom Kippur. Lactose intolerance is common among Jews of European origin.	Saving a life overrides nearly all religious obligations. Prayers of well-being of the sick may be said. Anything that can be done to ease the client's suffering is encouraged. During the Sabbath, Orthodox Jews refrain from using electrical appliances.
The Church of Jesus Christ of Latter-day Saints (Mormon)	Contraception is at the discretion of the man and woman. Abortion is opposed except in certain maternal circumstances. Infants are not baptized.	Organ donation is permitted. An autopsy is permitted. Life continues beyond death.	Alcohol, coffee, and tea are prohibited. Fasting is required once a month.	May want to use herbal remedies in addition to medical care. When blessing the sick, a person is anointed with oil by two elders.
Seventh-Day Adventist	Abortion is acceptable in some circumstances. Opposed to infant baptism.	An autopsy is acceptable. Organ donation is acceptable.	Vegetarian diet is encouraged. Alcohol, coffee, and tea are prohibited.	Healing accomplished through medical intervention and divine healing. Prayer and anointing with oil may be performed.

UNIT FOUR

Pharmacology in Nursing

Calculations and Conversions

Basic medication dose conversion and calculation skills are essential to providing safe nursing care. Standard conversions are used to solve dosage calculation problems. Nurses are responsible for the administration of the correct amount of medication based on the type of medication being administered.

A. **Standard Conversion Factors**

1. 1 mg = 1,000 mcg
2. 1 g = 1,000 mg
3. 1 kg = 1,000 g
4. 1 kg = 2.2 lb
5. 60 mg = 1 gr
6. 30 mL = 1 oz
7. 1 L = 1,000 mL
8. 5 mL = 1 tsp
9. 15 mL = 1 tbsp
10. 1 tbsp = 3 tsp

B. **Temperature Conversions**

1. $37.0°\ C = 98.6°\ F$
2. $°C = (°F - 32) \times (5/9)$
3. $°F = (°C \times 9/5) + 32$

C. **Calculations for IV Administration**

1. Number of hours = total volume/mL/hr
2. gtt per min = total volume × gtt/mL in administration set/total number of minutes

D. **Calculations for Dosage**

1. Dosage on hand (H)/mL = Dosage desired (D)/mL

PRACTICE TEST QUESTIONS

1. A client has the following food for lunch: 8 oz ice chips, 1 cup tea, 1 cup coffee, and 240 mL milk. The client eats the ice chips, and drinks all of the tea, coffee, and half of the milk. The total intake for lunch is ____.

2. A client has a prescription for 0.25 mg digoxin. The dose on hand is 0.5 mg tablets of digoxin. How many tablets will the client receive?

3. A client's IV infusion rate is 75 mL/hr. How many hours will it take for a 500 mL bag of IV fluid to infuse?

4. The IV rate is 100 mL/hr and the administration set is 15 drops/mL. How many drops per minute will deliver the required fluids?

5. A client has a prescription for heparin sodium 7,000 units IV. The vial contains 10,000 units/mL. How many milliliters of heparin will the nurse administer?

6. A nurse is preparing 300,000 units of procaine penicillin. The vial contains 1,500,000 units/2 mL. How many milliliters will the nurse administer?

7. A client weighs 180 lb and has a prescription for 0.5 mL of medication per kilogram of body weight. How many milliliters of medication will the client receive?

8. A client is receiving dextrose 5% in water at 50 mL/hr in one IV and D$_5$W 75 mL/hr in another IV. The client also receives IV piggyback medication every 8 hr prepared in 100 mL of fluid. What is the total amount of IV fluid the client will receive in 8 hr?

9. The IV administration set delivers 10 drops/mL. The rate of flow in drops/min for 1,000 mL dextrose 5% in water to infuse in 8 hr is ____.

10. When measuring a client's output, the nurse records 300 mL of urine at 0800, 450 mL of liquid stool at 1130, 225 mL of urine at 1300, and 35 mL of emesis at 1430. What is the client's total output for this shift?

11. A client receiving an IV infusion has a prescription for 1,000 mL in 12 hr. Using a microdrip system that delivers 60 microdrops/mL, the nurse should regulate the infusion for how many drops per minute?

    A. 45

    B. 68

    C. 83

    D. 96

12. A client's temperature is 100° F. What is this temperature in degrees centigrade?

13. A nurse has available meperidine 50 mg/mL. The prescription is to administer meperidine 35 mg. How many milliliters will the nurse safely administer?

14. A nurse is preparing an IV antibiotic in 100 mL dextrose 5% in water to infuse over 20 min. The infusion set is calibrated for 10 drops/mL. What drip rate should the nurse use?

Answer Key: 1. 720; 2. 0.5; 3. 6.7; 4. 25; 5. 0.7; 6. 0.4; 7. 41; 8. 1,100; 9. 21; 10. 1,010; 11. C (83); 12. 37.8; 13. 0.7; 14. 50

Medication Therapies

I Medication Actions, Interactions, and Reactions

A. **Medication properties (pharmacokinetics):** The absorption, distribution, metabolism, and excretion of a medication; describes the onset of action, peak level, duration of action, and bioavailability

B. **Medication interaction:** When a medication is given with another medication and alters the effect of either or both medications

C. **Adverse reactions:** Negative effects experienced by a client as the result of a specific medication; may be hazardous, tolerated, or subside with continued use

II Pharmacotherapy Across the Life Span

A. **Medications and pregnancy:** A majority of medications cross the placental barrier, thereby increasing the risk of teratogenicity. All medications should be given with extreme caution to ensure safety to the developing fetus.

B. **Medications and breastfeeding:** Most medications taken by a mother who is breastfeeding appear in breast milk. Medication levels tend to be the highest in the newborn immediately after the medication is administered to the mother. Mothers who are breastfeeding are advised to breastfeed before taking the medication. For additional guidelines, review Unit 8.

C. **Medication in children:** Pharmacokinetics are influenced by a child's age, size, and maturity of the targeted organ. To reduce the risk of toxicity, these factors must be considered: safe calculation of the child's dosage (mg/kg/day), medication that is age-appropriate, monitoring of IV medications to prevent fluid overload (smaller solution containers should be used to avoid infusing too much fluid), and the administration of inhalants using a metered-space device. For additional guidelines, review Unit 9.

D. **Medication in older adults:** Age-related changes affect therapeutic effects of medications in older adult clients. Older adult clients experience more adverse effects than younger adults due to aging body systems. Confusion, lethargy, falls, and weakness may be mistaken for senility, rather than adverse reactions. If the adverse reaction is not identified, unnecessary medication may be prescribed to treat complications caused by the medication. As the client continues to receive medications, the risk for toxicity increases, especially in cases of polypharmacy. Toxicity in older adults is a greater risk when taking diuretics, antihypertensives, digoxin, steroids, anticoagulants, hypnotics, and over-the-counter medications.

III Safe Medication Administration

A. **The RN is prepared to administer medications using the enteral, parenteral, and transcutaneous routes.**

B. **The RN must assess the client's:**
   1. Allergies and adverse effects
   2. Current medication regimen for potential interactions
   3. Physiologic status compared to baseline assessment data

C. **The RN follows the six rights of medication administration** (i.e., right client, right drug, right dose, right route, right time, right documentation) to protect the safety of the client and follow the scope of practice to maintain professional licensure.

IV Laboratory Profiles in Pharmacology

Laboratory testing may be indicated for specific medications. The nurse is accountable for collaborating with the health care provider in ensuring client safety when laboratory testing is prescribed.

A. **Therapeutic Drug Monitoring**
   1. Measures blood drug levels to determine effective medication dosages and prevent medication toxicity. The test may also be used to identify noncompliance with medication regimens.
   2. Blood testing is preferred because it provides information about current therapeutic levels, whereas urine levels reflect the presence of a drug over several days.

B. **Peak levels reflect the highest concentration.**

AVERAGE TIMES FOR DRAWING PEAK LEVELS

ROUTE OF ADMINISTRATION	TIME SPECIMEN IS DRAWN AFTER ADMINISTRATION
Oral intake	1 to 2 hr
Intramuscular	1 hr
Intravenous	30 min

C. **Trough levels** reflect the lowest concentration or residual level and are usually obtained within 15 min prior to administration of the next scheduled dose. The scheduled dose of medication should not be administered until the trough level is confirmed.

> **NOTE:** The timing for drawing a peak and trough level varies based on the half-life (time required for the body to decrease the medication blood level by 50%) for the medication.

D. **Culture and Sensitivity:** Cultures are obtained to detect the presence of pathogens within the specimen collected. If a culture produces organisms, testing is performed in the laboratory to identify the appropriate antibiotic therapy (sensitivity). Begin antibiotic therapy after obtaining lab sample.

> **NOTE:** When prescribed, cultures should be obtained prior to initiating antibiotic therapy (definitive therapy). When cultures cannot be drawn prior, the provider will prescribe a broad-spectrum antibiotic (empirical therapy). Monitoring culture results is imperative to ensure proper antimicrobial treatment.

v Intravenous Therapy

Administration of fluids via an intravenous catheter (peripheral or central vein access) for the purpose of providing medication, fluid, electrolyte, or nutrient replacement

A. **Guidelines for Safe IV Administration**
   1. Review medication guidelines for precautions related to IV administration for compatibility, rate of administration, necessity of infusion pump, and serious adverse reactions.
   2. Never administer medications through tubing being used for blood administration.
   3. Implement standard precautions and follow policies related to IV site changes.
   4. Fluids should be infused within 24 hr (discard unused portion) to prevent infection.
   5. Maintain patency of IV access.

B. **Types of IV Access**
   1. Peripheral vein
   2. Central venous catheters
      a. PICC (peripherally inserted central catheter)
      b. Nontunneled percutaneous central venous catheter
      c. Tunneled central venous catheter (Hickman, Groshong)
      d. Implanted port

C. **Prevent complications associated with IV infusion.**

COMPLICATIONS ASSOCIATED WITH IV INFUSION

COMPLICATION	NURSING INTERVENTIONS
Infiltration	**Prevention:** Use smallest catheter for prescribed therapy, stabilize port-access, assess blood return. **Treatment:** Stop infusion, remove peripheral catheters, apply cold compress, elevate extremity, insert new catheter in opposite extremity.
Extravasation	**Prevention:** Know vesicant potential before giving medication. **Treatment:** Stop infusion, discontinue administration set, aspirate drug if possible, apply cold compress, document condition of site (may photograph).
Phlebitis/ thrombophlebitis	**Prevention:** Rotate sites every 72 to 96 hr, secure catheter, use aseptic technique; for PICCs, avoid excessive activity with the extremity. **Treatment:** Stop infusion, remove peripheral IV catheters, apply heat compress, insert new catheter in opposite extremity.
Hematoma	**Prevention:** Avoid veins not easily seen or palpated; obtain hemostasis after insertion. **Treatment:** Remove IV device and apply light pressure if bleeding; monitor for signs of phlebitis and treat.
Catheter embolus	**Prevention:** Do not reinsert stylet needle into catheter. **Treatment:** Immediately apply tourniquet high on extremity to limit venous flow. Prepare for removal under x-ray.

D. **Complications Associated with Central Venous Catheters**

COMPLICATIONS OF CENTRAL VENOUS CATHETERS

COMPLICATION	NURSING INTERVENTIONS
Pneumothorax (during insertion)	**Prevention:** Use ultrasound to locate veins, avoid subclavian insertion when possible. **Treatment:** Administer oxygen, assist provider with chest tube insertion.
Air embolism	**Prevention:** Have client lie flat when changing administration set or needleless connectors, ask client to perform Valsalva maneuver if possible. **Treatment:** Place client in left lateral Trendelenburg, administer oxygen.
Lumen occlusion	**Prevention:** Flush promptly with NS between, before, and after each medication. **Treatment:** Use 10 mL syringe with a pulsing motion.
Bloodstream infection	**Prevention:** Maintain sterile technique. **Treatment:** Change entire infusion system, notify provider, obtain cultures, and administer antibiotics.

E. **Complications Associated with PICC Line**

COMPLICATIONS ASSOCIATED WITH PICC LINE

COMPLICATION	NURSING INTERVENTIONS
Catheter occlusions	Prevent kinks, reposition arm, confirm blood return, flush catheter between medications, administer approved antithrombolytic.
Catheter dislodges	Assess blood return, discomfort in jaw, chest, or ear, contact provider.
Phlebitis	Apply low degree heat, discontinue if not resolved.
Catheter embolism	Secure catheter, avoid pulling, follow safe practices for catheter removal.
Infection	Use aseptic technique, keep dressing clean and dry, intervene immediately for any sign of infection.

vi Total Parenteral Nutrition (TPN)

Hypertonic solution containing dextrose, proteins, electrolytes, minerals, trace elements, and insulin prescribed according to the client's needs and administered via central venous device (PICC line, subclavian, or internal jugular vein)

A. **Care and Maintenance of TPN**
   1. Before administering, verify prescription and solution with another nurse.
   2. Administer via infusion pump.
   3. Monitor weight daily.
   4. Monitor and record I&O, noting fluid balance.
   5. Monitor serum glucose levels every 4 to 6 hr.
   6. Monitor for signs of infection.
   7. Change dressing every 48 to 72 hr per facility protocol.
   8. Change IV tubing and fluid every 24 hr.
   9. If TPN solution is temporarily unavailable, administer dextrose 10% in water to prevent hypoglycemia.

VII Antidote/Reversal Agents

A. **Acetaminophen:** acetylcysteine
B. **Benzodiazepine:** flumazenil
C. **Curare:** edrophonium
D. **Cyanide poisoning:** methylene blue
E. **Digitalis:** digoxin immune FAB
F. **Ethylene poisoning:** fomepizole
G. **Heparin and enoxaparin:** protamine sulfate
H. **Iron:** deferoxamine
I. **Lead:** succimer
J. **Magnesium sulfate:** calcium gluconate 10%
K. **Narcotics:** naloxone
L. **Warfarin:** phytonadione (vitamin K)

VIII Therapeutic Drug Levels

A. **Aminophylline:** 10 to 20 mcg/mL
B. **Carbamazepine:** 5 to 12 mcg/mL
C. **Digoxin:** 0.8 to 2.0 ng/mL   *Saunders 0.5-2.0*
D. **Gentamicin:** 5 to 10 mcg/mL
E. **Lidocaine:** 1.5 to 5.0 mcg/mL
F. **Lithium:** 0.4 to 1.4 mEq/L
G. **Magnesium sulfate:** 4 to 8 mg/dL
H. **Phenobarbital:** 10 to 40 mcg/mL
I. **Phenytoin:** 10 to 20 mcg/mL
J. **Salicylate:** 100 to 250 mcg/mL
K. **Theophylline:** 10 to 20 mcg/mL
L. **Tobramycin:** 5 to 10 mcg/mL
M. **Trough Drug Levels**
   1. Gentamicin: 1 to 2 mcg/mL
   2. Tobramycin: 1 to 2 mcg/mL
   3. Vancomycin: 15–20 mcg/mL

IX Toxic Drug Levels

A. **Acetaminophen:** greater than 250 mcg/mL
B. **Aminophylline:** greater than 20 mcg/mL
C. **Amitriptyline:** greater than 500 ng/mL
D. **Digoxin:** greater than 2.4 ng/mL   *(2.0)*
E. **Lidocaine:** greater than 5 mcg/mL
F. **Lithium:** greater than 2.0 mEq/L
G. **Magnesium sulfate:** greater than 9 mg/dL
H. **Methotrexate:** greater than 10 mcmol over 24 hr
I. **Phenobarbital:** greater than 40 mcg/mL
J. **Phenytoin:** greater than 30 mcg/mL
K. **Salicylate:** greater than 300 mcg/mL
L. **Theophylline:** greater than 20 mcg/mL

X Common Drug Class Suffixes

COMMON DRUG CLASS SUFFIXES

SUFFIX	MEDICATION CATEGORY
-dipine	Ca+ channel blocker
-afil	Erectile dysfunction
-caine	Anesthetics
-pril	ACE inhibitor
-pam, -lam	Benzodiazepine
-statin	Antilipidemic
-asone, -solone	Corticosteroid
-olol	Beta blocker
-cillin	Penicillin
-ide	Oral hypoglycemic
-prazole	Proton pump inhibitor
-vir	Antiviral
-ase	Thrombolytic
-azine	Antiemetic
-phylline	Bronchodilator
-arin	Anticoagulant
-dine	Antiulcer
-zine	Antihistamine
-cycline	Antibiotic
-mycin	Aminoglycoside
-floxacin	Antibiotic
-tyline	Tricyclic antidepressants
-pram, -ine	SSRIs

SIDE EFFECTS AND ADVERSE REACTIONS

This worksheet will build upon your knowledge of medication side effects and adverse reactions. NCLEX will expect you to be able to manage clients experiencing side effects and adverse reactions to medications. Match the side effect or adverse reaction with the medication or classification. Each should only be used once.

A 1. ACE inhibitors
I 2. Benzodiazepines
B 3. Beta blockers
E 4. Ciprofloxacin
C 5. Digoxin
F 6. Doxycycline
D 7. Furosemide
J 8. Lithium
G 9. Tobramycin
H 10. Valacyclovir

A. Angioedema
B. Bronchospasm
C. Yellow tinge to vision
D. Hypokalemia
E. Tendon rupture
F. Tooth discoloration
G. Ototoxicity
H. Thrombotic thrombocytopenic purpura
I. Anterograde amnesia
J. Tremors

Answer Key: 1. A; 2. I; 3, B; 4. E; 5. C; 6. F; 7. D; 8. J; 9. G; 10. H

THE MEDICATION CATEGORIES

This worksheet will build on your overall knowledge of medications. Learning medications by categories will help you group medications and reduce the number you have to memorize. This list is not all-inclusive, but is a great place to start. NCLEX® will expect you to know entry-level pharmacology. Column one lists generic medication categories or classifications. In column two, write the commonly used "ending" for the medication classification. In column three, write an example of a medication that would be included in the classification.

MEDICATION CATEGORY	"ENDING"	MEDICATION
1. ACE inhibitors		
2. Antivirals		
3. Antifungals		
4. Antilipidemics		
5. Angiotensin II receptor blockers (ARBs)		
6. Beta blockers		
7. Calcium-channel blockers		
8. Erectile dysfunction medications		
9. Histamine$_2$ receptor antagonists		
10. Proton pump inhibitors		

Answer Key for Endings: 1. –pril; 2. –vir; 3. –azole; 4. –statin; 5. –sartan; 6. –olol; 7. –dipine; 8. –afil; 9. –dine; 10. –prazole
Medications: Answers for medications may vary.

SECTION 3

Medications for the Cardiovascular System

Antihypertensives

Treatment for clients with hypertension includes lifestyle modification and medications.

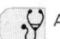

A. **Nursing interventions for clients taking antihypertensive medications include:**

1. Assess weight, vital signs, and hydration status.
2. Assess blood pressure in supine, sitting, and standing positions.
3. Assess laboratory profiles: renal function, coagulation.
4. Teach clients to take medication at same time each day.
5. Clients should avoid hot tubs and saunas.
6. Do not discontinue medication abruptly.
7. Prevent orthostatic hypotension.

B. **Angiotensin-Converting Enzyme (ACE) Inhibitors and Angiotensin II Receptor Blockers (ARBs)**

1. **Action**
   a. ACE inhibitors: block the conversion of angiotensin I to angiotensin II.
   b. ARBs: selectively block the binding of angiotensin II to AT1 receptors found in tissues.

ACE INHIBITORS	ARBS
Captopril	Losartan
Enalapril	Valsartan
Enalaprilat (intravenous route)	Irbesartan
Fosinopril	
Lisinopril	

2. **Therapeutic use**: hypertension, heart failure, MI, diabetic nephropathy

3. **Precautions/Interactions**
   a. Use with caution if diuretic therapy is in place.
   b. Monitor potassium levels.

4. **Side/Adverse Effects**
   a. Persistent nonproductive cough with ACE inhibitors
   b. Angioedema; hypotension
   c. Should not be used in second and third trimester of pregnancy

5. **Nursing Interventions and Client Education**
   a. Captopril should be taken 1 hr before meals.
   b. Monitor blood pressure.
   c. Monitor for angioedema and promptly administer epinephrine 0.5 mL of 1:1,000 solution subcutaneously.

C. **Calcium-Channel Blockers**

1. **Action:** Slows movement of calcium into smooth-muscle cells, resulting in arterial dilation and decreased blood pressure

2. **Medications**
   a. Nifedipine
   b. Verapamil
   c. Diltiazem
   d. Amlodipine

3. **Therapeutic Use**
   a. Angina, hypertension
   b. Verapamil and diltiazem may be used for atrial fibrillation, atrial flutter, or SVT.

4. **Precautions/Interactions**
   a. Use cautiously in clients taking digoxin and beta blockers.
   b. Contraindicated for clients who have heart failure, heart block, or bradycardia.
   c. Do not consume grapefruit juice (toxic effects).

5. **Side/Adverse Effects**
   a. Constipation
   b. Reflex tachycardia
   c. Peripheral edema
   d. Toxicity

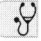

6. **Nursing Interventions and Client Education**
   a. Do not crush or chew sustained-release tablets.
   b. Administer IV injection over 2 to 3 min.
   c. Slowly taper dose if discontinuing.
   d. Monitor heart rate and blood pressure.

D. **Alpha Adrenergic Blockers (Sympatholytics)**
   1. **Action:** Selectively inhibit alpha1 adrenergic receptors, resulting in peripheral arterial and venous dilation that lowers blood pressure
   2. **Medications**
      a. Prazosin
      b. Doxazosin mesylate
   3. **Therapeutic Use**
      a. Primary hypertension
      b. Doxazosin mesylate may be used in treatment of BPH.
   4. **Precautions/Interactions**
      a. Increased risk of hypotension and syncope if given with other antihypertensives, beta blockers, or diuretics.
      b. NSAIDs may decrease the effect of prazosin.
   5. **Side/Adverse Effects**
      a. Dizziness
      b. Fainting
   6. **Nursing Interventions and Client Education**
      a. Monitor heart rate and blood pressure.
      b. Take medication at bedtime to minimize effects of hypotension.
      c. Advise to notify prescriber immediately about adverse reactions.
      d. Consult prescriber before taking any OTC medications.

E. **Centrally Acting Alpha$_2$ Agonists**
   1. **Action:** Stimulate alpha adrenergic receptors (alpha$_2$) in the brain to reduce peripheral vascular resistance, heart rate, and systolic and diastolic blood pressure
   2. **Medications**
      a. Clonidine
      b. Guanfacine HCl
      c. Methyldopa
   3. **Therapeutic Use**
      a. Primary hypertension—may be used in combination with diuretics or other antihypertensives
      b. Hypertensive crisis
      c. Severe cancer pain (parenteral administration via epidural)
   4. **Precautions/Interactions**
      a. Contraindicated with anticoagulant therapy, hepatic failure.
      b. Do not administer to clients taking MAOIs.
      c. Do not administer methyldopa through IV line with barbiturates or sulfonamides.
      d. Use cautiously in CVA, MI, diabetes mellitus, major depression, or chronic renal failure.
      e. Do not use during lactation.

5. **Side/Adverse Effects**
   a. Dry mouth
   b. Drowsiness and sedation (resolves over time)
   c. Rebound hypertension
   d. Black or sore tongue
   e. Leukopenia

6. **Nursing Interventions and Client Education**
   a. Monitor for adverse CNS effects.
   b. Monitor CBC, heart rate, and blood pressure.
   c. Assess for weight gain or edema.
   d. Monitor closely for rebound hypertension when medication is discontinued (48 hr).
   e. Instruct to never skip a dose.
   f. Take at bedtime to minimize effects of hypotension.
   g. Notify prescriber of any involuntary jerky movements, prolonged dizziness, rash, yellowing of skin.

F. **Beta Adrenergic Blockers (Sympatholytics)**
   1. **Action:** Inhibit stimulation of receptor sites, resulting in decreased cardiac excitability, cardiac output, myocardial oxygen demand; lower blood pressure by decreasing release of renin in the kidney

   NOTE: Beta$_1$ receptors are primarily in the cardiac and renal tissues. Beta$_2$ receptors are found primarily in the lungs, gastrointestinal tract, liver, uterus, vascular smooth muscle, and skeletal muscle.

   2. **Medications:** May be selective or nonselective
      a. Cardioselective Beta$_1$ Medications
         1) Metoprolol
         2) Atenolol
         3) Metoprolol succinate
      b. Nonselective (Beta$_1$ and Beta$_2$) Medications
         1) Propranolol
         2) Nadolol
         3) Labetalol
   3. **Therapeutic Use**
      a. Primary hypertension
      b. Angina
      c. Tachydysrhythmias, heart failure, and MI
   4. **Precautions/Interactions**
      a. Contraindicated in clients who have AV block and sinus bradycardia.
      b. Do not administer nonselective beta blockers to clients who have asthma, bronchospasm, or heart failure.
      c. Propranolol may mask effects of hypoglycemia in clients who have diabetes mellitus.
      d. Do not administer labetalol in same IV line with furosemide.

5. **Side/Adverse Effects**
   a. Bradycardia
   b. Nasal stuffiness
   c. AV block
   d. Rebound myocardium excitation if stopped abruptly
   e. Bronchospasm

6. **Nursing Interventions and Client Education**
   a. Administer 1 to 2 times daily as prescribed.
   b. Do not discontinue without consulting provider.
   c. Do not crush (or chew) extended-release tablets.
   d. Hold medication and notify provider if systolic blood pressure is less than 100 mm Hg or pulse is less than 60/min.
   e. Monitor clients who have diabetes mellitus for indications of hypoglycemia.

G. **Vasodilators**

1. **Action:** Direct vasodilation of arteries and veins resulting in rapid reduction of blood pressure (decreased preload and afterload)

2. **Medications**
   a. Nitroglycerin
   b. Enalaprilat
   c. Nitroprusside
   d. Hydralazine

3. **Therapeutic Use**
   a. Hypertensive emergencies

4. **Precautions/Interactions**
   a. Clients who have hepatic or renal disease
   b. Older adults
   c. Electrolyte imbalances

5. **Side/Adverse Effects**
   a. Dizziness
   b. Headache
   c. Profound hypotension
   d. Cyanide toxicity
   e. Thiocyanate poisoning

6. **Nursing Interventions and Client Education**
   a. Nitroprusside may not be mixed with any medication.
   b. Apply protective cover to container.
   c. Discard unused fluid after 24 hr.
   d. Provide continuous ECG and blood pressure monitoring.

II Cardiac Glycosides

Used in the treatment of clients who have cardiac failure or ineffective pumping mechanism of the heart muscle.

A. **Action**

1. Increase the force and velocity of myocardial contractions to improve stroke volume and cardiac output.
2. Slow the conduction rate, allowing for increased ventricular filling.

B. **Medication**

1. Digoxin

C. **Therapeutic Uses**

1. Heart failure
2. Atrial fibrillation

D. **Precautions/Interactions**

1. Thiazide or loop diuretics increase risk of hypokalemia and precipitate digoxin toxicity.
2. ACE and ARBs increase risk of hyperkalemia.
3. Verapamil increases risk of toxicity.

E. **Side/Adverse Effects**

1. Digoxin toxicity: GI effects (anorexia, nausea, vomiting, abdominal pain); CNS effects (fatigue, weakness, diplopia, blurred vision, yellow-green or white halos around objects)

F. **Nursing Interventions and Client Education**

1. Assess apical pulse for 1 min prior to administration.
2. Notify provider if HR is less than 60 (adult), less than 70 (child), or less than 90 (infant).
3. Monitor for signs of digoxin toxicity, hypokalemia, and hypomagnesemia.
4. Notify provider of any sudden increase in pulse rate that previously had been normal or low.
5. Maintain therapeutic digoxin level.

G. **Management of Digoxin Toxicity**

1. Discontinue digoxin and potassium-wasting medications.
2. Treat dysrhythmias with phenytoin (or lidocaine).
3. Treat bradycardia with atropine.
4. For excess overdose, administer digoxin immune FAB to prevent absorption.

III Antianginal Medications

The use of organic nitrates, beta adrenergic blocking agents, and calcium channel blockers to treat pain related to imbalances between myocardial oxygen supply and demand

A. **Organic Nitrates**
   1. **Action**
      a. Relax peripheral vascular smooth muscles, resulting in dilation of arteries and veins, thus reducing venous blood return (reduced preload) to the heart, which leads to decreased oxygen demands on the heart
      b. Increase myocardial oxygen supply by dilating large coronary arteries and redistributing blood flow
   2. **Medications**
      a. Sublingual tablet
      b. Sustained-release tablet
      c. Transdermal ointment
      d. Transderm unit (patch)
B. **Therapeutic Use**
   1. Acute angina attack
   2. Prophylaxis of chronic stable or variant angina
C. **Precautions/Interactions**
   1. Contraindicated in clients with head injury
   2. Hypotensive risk with antihypertensive medications
   3. Contraindicated if taking erectile dysfunction medications—life-threatening hypotension
D. **Side/Adverse Effects**
   1. Headache
   2. Orthostatic hypotension
   3. Reflex tachycardia
   4. Tolerance
E. **Nursing Interventions and Client Education**
   1. Nitrostat/Nitrolingual
      a. Administer sublingual.
      b. Rest for 5 min. If pain not relieved by first tablet, call 911, then take a second tablet. May use up to three tablets taken 5 min apart. Keep Nitrostat in original dark container.
      c. Nitrolingual may be used prophylactically 5 to 10 min before exercise.
      d. Do not shake Nitrolingual canister (forms bubbles).
      e. Replace NTG tablets every 6 months.
      f. Wear medical alert identification.
   2. Nitro-Bid (topical ointment)
      a. Wear gloves for administration.
      b. Do not massage or rub area.
      c. Apply to area without hair (chest, flank, or upper arm preferable).
      d. Cover the area where the patch is placed with a clear plastic wrap and tape in place.
      e. Gradually reduce the dose and frequency of application over 4 to 6 weeks.
   3. Nitro-Dur (transderm patch)
      a. Skin irritation may alter medication absorption.
      b. Optimal locations for patch are upper chest or side; pelvis; and inner, upper arm.
      c. Rotate skin sites, usually worn for 12 to 14 hr then removed.

IV Antidysrhythmic Agents

A. **Action:** Antidysrhythmic agents are complex agents with multiple mechanisms of action. They are classified according to their effects on the electrical conduction system of the heart (Class I, II, III, IV).
B. **Medications**
   1. Adenosine: slows conduction time through the AV node, interrupts AV node pathways to restore NSR.
   2. Amiodarone: prolongs repolarization, relaxes smooth muscles, decreases vascular resistance.
   3. Atropine: increases the heart rate by counteracting the muscarine-like actions of acetylcholine and other choline esters.
C. **Precautions/Interactions**
   1. Toxicity is a major concern due to additive effects.
   2. Caution is needed when used with an AV block.
   3. Caution is needed when using anticholinergic medications.

ANTIDYSRHYTHMIC MEDICATIONS

Adenosine

THERAPEUTIC USE	Convert SVT to sinus rhythm
SIDE/ADVERSE EFFECTS	Flushing, nausea Bronchospasm, prolonged asystole
NURSING INTERVENTIONS	Rapid IV (1 to 2 seconds) push Flush immediately with normal saline

Amiodarone

THERAPEUTIC USE	Ventricular fibrillation, unstable ventricular tachycardia
SIDE/ADVERSE EFFECTS	Bradycardia Cardiogenic shock Pulmonary disorders
NURSING INTERVENTIONS	Incompatible with heparin May be given in PO maintenance dose Monitor for respiratory complications

Atropine

THERAPEUTIC USE	Bradycardia, known exposure to chemical nerve agent, reduce secretions
SIDE/ADVERSE EFFECTS	When used for life-threatening emergency, has no contraindications
NURSING INTERVENTIONS	Monitor for dry mouth, blurred vision, photophobia, urinary retention, and constipation

V Antilipemic Medications

A. **Action:** Aid in lowering low-density lipoprotein (LDL) levels and increase high-density lipoprotein (HDL) levels. Therapy includes diet, exercise, and weight control.

B. **Therapeutic Uses**

1. Primary hypercholesterolemia
2. Prevention of coronary events
3. Protection against MI and stroke in clients who have diabetes mellitus

C. **Precautions/Interactions**

1. Should be discontinued during pregnancy.
2. Use with caution in renal dysfunction.

D. **Side/Adverse Effects**

1. Muscle aches
2. Hepatotoxicity
3. Rhabdomyolysis
4. Peripheral neuropathy

 E. **Nursing Interventions and Client Education**

1. Take medication in the evening (cholesterol synthesis increases).
2. Monitor liver and renal function laboratory profiles.
3. Low-fat/high-fiber diet.
4. Note dietary precautions with specific classes.

F. **Statin Medications**

1. **Action:** Interfere with hepatic enzyme HMG-CoA to reduce formation of cholesterol precursors

2. **Medications**

   a. Atorvastatin
   b. Simvastatin
   c. Lovastatin
   d. Pravastatin sodium
   e. Rosuvastatin
   f. Fluvastatin

3. **Precautions/Interactions**

   a. Prolonged bleeding in clients taking warfarin
   b. Multiple drug interactions: digoxin, warfarin, thyroid hormones, thiazide diuretics, phenobarbital, NSAIDs, tetracycline, beta-blocking agents, gemfibrozil, glipizide, glyburide, oral contraceptives, and phenytoin

 4. **Nursing Interventions and Client Education**

   a. Do not administer with grapefruit juice.

G. **Cholesterol Absorption Inhibitor**

1. **Action:** Inhibits the absorption of cholesterol secreted in the bile and from food. Often used in combination with other antilipemic medications.

2. **Medications**

   a. Ezetimibe

 3. **Nursing Interventions and Client Education**

   a. Take 2 hr before or 4 hr after other antilipemics.
   b. Risk of liver damage increased when combined with statins.

Medications for the Respiratory System

Medications used to treat chronic inflammatory conditions caused by asthma, bronchitis, and emphysema

A. **Treatment for chronic respiratory disorders often includes multiple drug therapies.** When administered as inhalation therapies, the following guidelines should be implemented.

1. Advise to take the beta$_2$ agonist before the inhaled glucocorticoid to increase steroid absorption.

2. Instruct on procedures for inhalation:

   a. Remove the mouthpiece cap.
   b. If appropriate for medication, shake container.
   c. Stand up or sit upright; exhale deeply.
   d. Place the mouthpiece between teeth, and close lips tightly around the inhaler.
   e. While breathing in, press down on the inhaler to activate and release the medication; continue breathing in slowly for several more seconds (slow, long, steady inhalation is better than quick, short breaths).
   f. Hold breath for 5 to 10 seconds.
   g. Breathe in/out normally.

3. Examine mouth for irritation.

4. Perform frequent oral care.

I Beta$_2$ Adrenergic Agonists

A. **Action:** Promote bronchodilation by activating beta$_2$ receptors in bronchial smooth muscle

BETA$_2$ ADRENERGIC AGONISTS MEDICATIONS

Albuterol

ROUTE/ONSET	Inhaled (short-acting) 5 to 15 min
USE	Acute bronchospasm

Formoterol, salmeterol

ROUTE/ONSET	Inhaled (long-acting) Formoterol: onset: 1 to 3 min; duration: 10 hr Salmeterol: onset: 10 to 20 min; duration: 12 hr
USE	Long-term control of asthma

Terbutaline

ROUTE/ONSET	Oral (long-acting)
USE	Long-term control of asthma

B. **Precautions/Interactions**
1. Contraindicated for clients with tachydysrhythmias.
2. Caution: diabetes mellitus, hyperthyroidism, heart disease, hypertension, angina.
3. Beta blockers will reduce effects.
4. MAOIs will increase effects.

C. **Side/Adverse Effects**
1. Tachycardia, palpitations
2. Tremors

D. **Nursing Interventions and Client Education**
1. Caution against using salmeterol more frequently than every 12 hr.

II Methylxanthines

A. **Action:** Relaxation of bronchial smooth muscle, resulting in bronchodilation

B. **Medications**
1. Aminophylline
2. Theophylline

C. **Therapeutic Uses**
1. Relief of bronchospasm
2. Long-term control of asthma

D. **Precautions/Interactions**
1. Contraindicated with active peptic ulcer disease.
2. Caution: diabetes mellitus, hyperthyroidism, heart disease, hypertension, angina.
3. Do not mix parenteral form with other medications.
4. Phenobarbital and phenytoin decrease theophylline levels.
5. Caffeine, furosemide, cimetidine, fluoroquinolones, acetaminophen, and phenylbutazone falsely elevate therapeutic levels.

E. **Side/Adverse Effects**
1. Irritability and restlessness
2. Toxic effects: tachycardia, tachypnea, seizures

F. **Nursing Interventions and Client Education**
1. Monitor therapeutic levels for aminophylline and theophylline.
2. Avoid caffeine intake.
3. Monitor for signs of toxicity.
4. Smoking will decrease effects.
5. Alcohol abuse will increase effects.

G. **Treatment of Toxicity**
1. Stop parenteral infusion.
2. Activated charcoal to decrease absorption in oral overdose.
3. Lidocaine for dysrhythmias.
4. Diazepam to control seizures.

III Inhaled Anticholinergics

A. **Action:** muscarinic receptor blocker resulting in bronchodilation

B. **Medications**
1. Ipratropium
2. Tiotropium

C. **Therapeutic Uses**
1. Prevent bronchospasm
2. Manage allergen- or exercise-induced asthma
3. COPD

D. **Precautions/Interactions**
1. Contraindicated for clients with peanut allergy (contains soy lecithin).
2. Use extreme caution with narrow-angle glaucoma and BPH.
3. Do not use for treatment of acute bronchospasms.

E. **Side/Adverse Effects**
1. Dry mouth and eyes
2. Urinary retention

F. **Nursing Interventions and Client Education**
1. Instruct client that maximum effects may take up to 2 weeks.
2. Shake inhaler well before administration.
3. When using two different inhaled medications, wait 5 min between.
4. If administered via nebulizer, use within 1 hr of reconstitution.

IV Glucocorticoids

A. **Action:** Prevent inflammatory response by suppression of airway mucus production, immune responses, and adrenal function

GLUCOCORTICOID MEDICATIONS

Oral	Inhalation	Intravenous
Prednisone	Beclomethasone dipropionate	Hydrocortisone sodium succinate
Prednisolone		
Betamethasone	Budesonide	Methylprednisolone sodium succinate
	Fluticasone propionate	Betamethasone sodium phosphate
	Triamcinolone acetonide	

B. **Respiratory Therapeutic Uses**
1. Short term
   a. IV agents: status asthmaticus
   b. Oral: treatment of symptoms following an acute asthma attack
2. Long term
   a. Inhaled: prophylaxis of asthma
   b. Oral: treatment of chronic asthma

C. **Precautions/Interactions**

1. Clients who have diabetes mellitus may require higher doses.
2. Never stop medication abruptly.

D. **Side/Adverse Effects**

1. Euphoria, insomnia, psychotic behavior
2. Hyperglycemia
3. Peptic ulcer
4. Fluid retention
5. Withdrawal symptoms
6. Increased appetite

E. **Nursing Interventions and Client Education**

1. Assess client activity and behavior.
2. Administer medication with meals.
3. Teach symptoms to report.
4. Do not take with NSAIDs.
5. Teach client about gradual reduction of dose to prevent Addisonian crisis.

v Leukotriene Modifiers

A. **Action:** Prevent effects of leukotriene, resulting in decreased inflammation, bronchoconstriction, airway edema, and mucus production

B. **Medications**

1. Montelukast
2. Zileuton
3. Zafirlukast

C. **Therapeutic Uses**

1. Long-term management of asthma in adults and children
   a. Montelukast can be given to clients over age 1.
   b. Zileuton can be given to clients 12 years and older.
   c. Zafirlukast can be given to clients 5 years and older.
2. Prevention of exercise-induced bronchospasm

D. **Precautions/Interactions**

1. Do not use for acute asthma attack.
2. Zileuton or zafirlukast: high risk of liver disease, increased warfarin effects, and theophylline toxicity.
3. Phenobarbital will decrease circulating levels of montelukast.
4. Chewable tablets contain phenylalanine.

E. **Side/Adverse Effects**

1. Elevated liver enzymes (zileuton or zafirlukast)
2. Warfarin and theophylline toxicity (zileuton or zafirlukast)
3. May increase levels of beta blockers leading to hypotension and bradycardia (propranolol)

F. **Nursing Interventions and Client Education**

1. Never abruptly substitute for corticosteroid therapy.
2. Teach client to take daily in the evening.
3. Do not decrease or stop taking other prescribed asthma drugs until instructed.
4. If using oral granules, pour directly into mouth or mix with cold soft foods (never liquids).
5. Use open packets within 15 min of taking medication.

vi Antitussives, Expectorants, Mucolytics

DRUG ACTIONS AND THERAPEUTIC USE BY CLASS

Antitussives: hydrocodone, codeine

ACTION	Suppress cough through action in the CNS
THERAPEUTIC USE	Chronic nonproductive cough

Expectorants: guaifenesin

ACTION	Promote increased mucus secretion to increase cough production
THERAPEUTIC USE	Often combined with other agents to manage respiratory disorders

Mucolytics: acetylcysteine, hypertonic saline

ACTION	Enhance the flow of secretions in the respiratory tract
THERAPEUTIC USE	Acute and chronic pulmonary disorders with copious secretions Cystic fibrosis Antidote for acetaminophen poisoning

A. **Precautions/Interactions**

1. Only saline solutions should be used in children younger than 2 years.
2. Opioid antitussives have potential for abuse.
3. Caution with OTC medications—potentiate effects.

B. **Side/Adverse Effects**

1. Drowsiness
2. Dizziness
3. Aspiration and bronchospasm risk with mucolytics
4. Constipation

C. **Nursing Interventions and Client Education**

1. Monitor cough frequency, effort, and ability to expectorate.
2. Monitor character and tenacity of secretions.
3. Auscultate for adventitious lung sounds.
4. Teach client why multiple therapies are needed.
5. Promote fluid intake.

V Thyroid Hormone Antagonist

A. **Action:** Inhibits synthesis of thyroid hormone

B. **Medication**

1. Methimazole

C. **Therapeutic Uses**

1. Hyperthyroidism
2. Preoperative thyroidectomy
3. Thyrotoxic crisis
4. Thyroid storm

D. **Precautions/Interactions**

1. Administer with caution to clients who have bone marrow depression, hepatic disease, or bleeding disorders.
2. Discontinue prior to radioactive iodine uptake testing.
3. Contraindicated with breastfeeding.

E. **Side/Adverse Effects**

1. Skin rash, pruritus
2. Abnormal hair loss
3. GI upset
4. Paresthesias
5. Periorbital edema
6. Joint and muscle pain
7. Jaundice
8. Agranulocytosis
9. Thrombocytopenia

F. **Nursing Interventions and Client Education**

1. Administer with food at the same time each day.
2. Increase fluids to 3 L/day.
3. Instruct client to avoid OTC products containing iodine.
4. Instruct client to take medication as prescribed.
5. If discontinuing, dose must be tapered off.
6. Monitor client for therapeutic response: weight gain, decreased pulse, blood pressure, and T_4 levels.
7. Monitor client for signs of overdose and signs of hypothyroid: periorbital edema, cold intolerance, mental depression.

VI Anterior Pituitary/Growth Hormones

A. **Action:** Increase production of insulin–like growth factor throughout the body

B. **Medications**

1. Somatropin

C. **Therapeutic Use**

1. Treat growth hormone deficiencies
2. Turner's syndrome

D. **Precautions/Interactions**

1. Contraindicated in clients who are severely obese.
2. Therapy must be discontinued prior to epiphyseal closure.
3. Avoid concurrent use of glucocorticoids.

E. **Side/Adverse Effects**

1. Hyperglycemia
2. Hypothyroidism

F. **Nursing Interventions and Client Education**

1. Monitor growth patterns.
2. Reconstitute medication per manufacturer instructions.
3. Administer subcutaneous per protocol.
4. Dose is individualized.

VII Posterior Pituitary Hormones/ Antidiuretic Hormones

A. **Action:** Promote reabsorption of water with the kidneys; vasoconstriction of vascular smooth muscle

B. **Medications**

1. Desmopressin (DDAVP): oral, intranasal, subcutaneous, IV
2. Vasopressin: intranasal, subcutaneous, IV

C. **Therapeutic Uses**

1. Diabetes insipidus
2. Cardiac arrest
3. Nocturnal enuresis
4. Hemophilia (Desmopressin)

D. **Precautions/Interactions**

1. Contraindicated in clients with chronic nephritis or high risk for myocardial infarction

E. **Side/Adverse Effects**

1. Hyponatremia
2. Seizures
3. Coma

F. **Nursing Interventions and Client Education**

1. Monitor urine specific gravity.
2. Monitor blood pressure.
3. Monitor urinary output.
4. Prevent hyponatremia due to water intoxication.
5. Instruct for use of nasal spray.

VIII Adrenal Hormone Replacement

A. **Action:** Anti-inflammatory, suppresses immune response

B. **Medications**
1. Dexamethasone
2. Hydrocortisone sodium succinate
3. Fludrocortisone acetate
4. Prednisone

C. **Therapeutic Uses**
1. Acute and chronic replacement for adrenocortical insufficiency (Addison's disease)
2. Inflammation, allergic reactions, cancer

D. **Precautions/Interactions**
1. Contraindicated in clients who have systemic fungal infection.
2. Caution in clients who have hypertension, gastric ulcers, diabetes, osteoporosis.
3. Requires higher doses in acute illness or extreme stress.

E. **Side/Adverse Effects**
1. Adrenal suppression when administered for inflammation, allergic reactions
2. Infection
3. Hyperglycemia
4. Osteoporosis
5. GI bleeding
6. Fluid retention

F. **Nursing Interventions and Client Education**
1. Do not skip doses.
2. Monitor blood pressure.
3. Monitor fluid and electrolyte (F&E) balance, weight, and output.
4. Monitor for signs of bleeding and GI discomfort.
5. Teach client to take calcium supplements and maintain vitamin D levels.
6. Give with food.
7. Taper off dose regimen when discontinuing medication.
8. Provide immunoprotection.

Medications for the Hematologic System

I Blood and Blood Products

A. **Examples**
1. Whole blood
2. Packed red blood cells (RBCs)
3. Platelet concentrations

ADMINISTRATION OF BLOOD PRODUCTS

Whole blood

TIME COMPLETED	2 to 4 hr	
ACTION/ THERAPEUTIC USE	Replace volume › Hemorrhage › Surgery › Trauma	› Burns › Shock
MONITOR FOR REACTION	Acute hemolytic Febrile Anaphylactic	Mild allergic Hypervolemia Sepsis

Packed RBCs

TIME COMPLETED	2 to 4 hr	
ACTION/ THERAPEUTIC USE	Increase available RBC Severe anemia Hemoglobinopathies	Hemolytic anemia Erythroblastosis fetalis
MONITOR FOR REACTION	Acute hemolytic Febrile Anaphylactic	Mild allergic Sepsis

Platelets

TIME COMPLETED	15 to 30 min	
ACTION/ THERAPEUTIC USE	Increase platelet count Active bleeding Thrombocytopenia	Aplastic anemia Bone marrow suppression
MONITOR FOR REACTION	Febrile	Sepsis

FFP

TIME COMPLETED	30 to 60 min	
ACTION/ THERAPEUTIC USE	Replace clotting factors › Hemorrhage › Burns › Shock	› Thrombotic thrombocytopenic purpura (TTP) › Reverse effects of warfarin
MONITOR FOR REACTION	Acute hemolytic Febrile Anaphylactic	Mild allergic Hypervolemia Sepsis

ADMINISTRATION OF BLOOD PRODUCTS (CONTINUED)

Pheresed granulocytes

TIME COMPLETED	45 to 60 min	
ACTION/ THERAPEUTIC USE	Severe neutropenia Neonatal sepsis	Neutrophil dysfunction
MONITOR FOR REACTION	Acute hemolytic Febrile Anaphylactic	Mild allergic Hypervolemia Sepsis

Albumin

TIME COMPLETED	5% (1 to 10 mL/min)	25% (4 mL/min)
ACTION/ THERAPEUTIC USE	Expand volume via oncotic changes Hypovolemia Hypoalbuminemia	Burns Severe nephrosis Hemolytic disease of the newborn
MONITOR FOR REACTION	Risk for hypervolemia and pulmonary edema	

B. **Nursing Interventions and Client Education**

1. Client ID, name, and blood type must be verified by two nurses.

2. Prior to administration, assess baseline vital signs, including temperature.

3. Establish IV access, 18- to 20-gauge catheter.

4. Must have 0.9% sodium chloride primed tubing.

5. For the first 15 min, stay with the client and infuse slowly, monitoring for any reaction. If a reaction occurs, perform the following interventions.

   a. Stop blood immediately and take vital signs.

   b. Infuse 0.9% sodium chloride.

   c. Notify the provider.

   d. Follow facility policy (send urine sample, CBC, and bag and tubing to laboratory for analysis).

6. Complete infusion of product within 4 hr.

II Hematopoietic Growth Factors

A. **Action:** Stimulate the bone marrow to synthesize the specific blood cells

MEDICATIONS FOR HEMATOPOIETIC GROWTH FACTORS

Epoetin alfa

THERAPEUTIC USES	Stimulate RBC production Anemia related to: Chronic kidney disease Retrovir therapy Chemotherapy
SIDE/ADVERSE EFFECTS	Hypertension
NURSING INTERVENTIONS	Subcutaneous or IV Do not agitate vial Monitor hematocrit and hemoglobin

Filgrastim, injection
Pegfilgrastim, IV over 2 to 4 hr

THERAPEUTIC USES	Stimulate WBC production Neutropenia related to cancer
SIDE/ADVERSE EFFECTS	Bone pain Leukocytosis
NURSING INTERVENTIONS	Subcutaneous or IV Do not agitate vial Monitor CBC

Oprelvekin

THERAPEUTIC USES	Stimulate platelet production Thrombocytopenia related to cancer
SIDE/ADVERSE EFFECTS	Fluid retention Blurred vision Cardiac dysrhythmia
NURSING INTERVENTIONS	Administer within 6 to 24 hr after chemotherapy Subcutaneous

III Iron Preparations

A. **Action:** Treat iron deficiency

B. **Medications**

1. Oral

   a. Ferrous sulfate

   b. Ferrous gluconate

   c. Ferrous fumarate

   d. Dilute liquid preparations with juice or water and administer with a plastic straw or medication dosing syringe (avoid contact with teeth).

   e. Encourage orange juice fortified with vitamin C (vitamin C facilitates absorption).

   f. Avoid antacids, coffee, tea, dairy products, or whole grain breads concurrently and for 1 hr after administration due to decreased absorption.

   g. Monitor the client for constipation and gastrointestinal upset.

2. Parenteral

   a. Iron dextran

   b. Used for client unable to take oral medication

   c. Intramuscular

      1) Use a large-bore needle (19- to 20-gauge, 3-inch).

      2) Change needle after drawing up from vial.

      3) Z-track (ventrogluteal preferable), never in deltoid muscle.

      4) Do not massage injection site.

   d. IV (preferred over IM)

      1) Administer a small test dose (25 mg over 5 min). Observe patient for 15 min, then slowly administer additional preparation.

      2) Use manufacturer's recommendation for specific product.

IV Anticoagulant

A. **Action:** Modify coagulation by altering the clotting cascade or dissolving an existing clot

1. Parenteral

   a. Modify or inhibit clotting or cellular properties to prevent clot formation (heparin)

   b. Prevents conversion of prothrombin to thrombin by inactivating coagulation enzymes (low molecular weight heparin: enoxaparin)

2. Oral

   a. Prevent synthesis of coagulation factors VII, IX, X, and prothrombin (warfarin)

   b. Inhibiting thrombin formation (dabigatran)

   c. Inhibit factor Xa (rivaroxaban)

B. **Medications and Therapeutic Uses**

1. Parenteral

   a. Stroke

   b. Pulmonary embolism

   c. Deep-vein thrombosis

   d. Cardiac catheterization

   e. MI

   f. DIC

2. Oral (warfarin)

   a. Venous thrombosis

   b. Prevent thrombus formation for clients who have atrial fibrillation or prosthetic heart valves

   c. Prevent recurrent MI

   d. Prevent transient ischemic attacks (TIAs)

3. Oral (dabigatran etexilate)

   a. Reduce risk of stroke/embolism for clients with nonvalvular atrial fibrillation

4. Oral (rivaroxaban)

   a. Reduce risk of stroke/embolism for clients with nonvalvular atrial fibrillation

   b. Prevention of DVT and PE in clients undergoing total hip or knee arthroplasty.

C. **Precautions/Interactions**

1. Parenteral

   a. Administer subcutaneous or IV.

   b. Incompatible with many medications (any bicarbonate base).

   c. Avoid NSAIDs, aspirin, or medications containing salicylates.

2. Oral (warfarin)

   a. Not safe for use during pregnancy (category X).

   b. Contraindications: thrombocytopenia, vitamin K deficiency, liver disease, alcohol use disorder.

   c. Decreased effects with phenobarbital, carbamazepine phenytoin, and oral contraceptives.

   d. Food sources high in vitamin K may decrease effects.

3. Oral (dabigatran)
   a. Caution if changing anticoagulation medication.
   b. Discontinue 1 to 2 days prior to surgical procedures.
4. Oral (rivaroxaban)
   a. No antidote for severe bleeding (prepare to administer activated charcoal to prevent further absorption).
   b. Wait 6 hr before restarting after removal of epidural catheters.

D. **Side Effects/Interactions**
   1. Parenteral
      a. Hemorrhage
      b. Heparin-induced thrombocytopenia
      c. Toxicity/overdose
   2. Oral (warfarin)
      a. Hemorrhage
      b. Toxicity/overdose
   3. Oral (dabigatran, rivaroxaban)
      a. Bleeding
      b. GI discomfort (dabigatran)
      c. Bleeding, bruising, headache, or eye pain (rivaroxaban)

E. **Nursing Interventions/Client Education**
   1. Parenteral
      a. Heparin: Monitor aPTT every 4 to 6 hr for IV administration.
      b. Monitor for signs of bleeding.
      c. Safety precautions to prevent bleeding.
      d. Administer subcutaneous heparin to abdomen, 2 inches from umbilicus (do not aspirate or massage).
      e. Rotate injection sites and observe for bleeding or hematoma.
      f. Administer protamine sulfate for heparin toxicity (1 mg neutralizes 100 units of heparin).
   2. Oral (warfarin)
      a. Administer once daily.
      b. Monitor INR or PT.
      c. Teach client that bleeding risk remains up to 5 days after discontinued therapy.
      d. Teach client to avoid NSAIDs and medications with aspirin.
      e. Teach client to wear medical alert bracelet.
      f. Client may self-monitor for PT/INR using a coagulation monitor.
      g. Teach measures to prevent injury and bleeding.
      h. Administer vitamin K for warfarin toxicity.
      i. Garlic, ginger, ginkgo (may increase bleeding), and ginseng (may decrease effectiveness).
      j. Avoid alcohol.

3. Oral (dabigatran, rivaroxaban)
   a. Teach client to take medication daily and avoid skipping doses.
   b. If a dose is missed, it should not be taken within 6 hr of the next scheduled dose.
   c. Tablets should not be crushed, broken, or chewed.
   d. Teach client to avoid NSAIDs and medications with aspirin.
   e. Teach client to monitor for signs of bleeding and report to provider.
   f. Teach client to monitor for signs of GI bleeding.

V Antiplatelet Medications

A. **Action:** Prevent platelets from aggregating (clumping together) by inhibiting enzymes and factors that normally promote clotting

B. **Medications**
   1. Aspirin
   2. Abciximab
   3. Clopidogrel
   4. Ticlopidine
   5. Pentoxifylline
   6. Dipyridamole

C. **Therapeutic Uses**
   1. Prevention of acute myocardial infarction or acute coronary syndromes
   2. Prevention of stroke
   3. Intermittent claudication

D. **Precautions/Interactions**
   1. Contraindicated in thrombocytopenia
   2. Caution with peptic ulcer disease

E. **Side/Adverse Effects**
   1. Prolonged bleeding
   2. Gastric bleeding
   3. Thrombocytopenia

F. **Nursing Interventions and Client Education**
   1. Monitor for signs of prolonged bleeding.
   2. Teach client to report tarry stool, ecchymosis.

VI Thrombolytic Medications

A. **Action:** Dissolve clots that have already formed by converting plasminogen to plasmin, which destroys fibrinogen and other clotting factors

B. **Medications**
   1. Alteplase
   2. Tenecteplase
   3. Reteplase

C. **Therapeutic Uses**
   1. Acute myocardial infarction
   2. Deep-vein thrombosis (DVT)
   3. Massive pulmonary emboli (PE)
   4. Ischemic stroke (alteplase)

D. **Precautions/Interactions**

1. Contraindicated for intracranial hemorrhage, active internal bleeding, aortic dissection, and brain tumors.

2. Use caution when using in clients who have severe hypertension.

3. Concurrent use of anticoagulants or antiplatelet medications increases risk for bleeding.

E. **Side/Adverse Effects**

1. Serious bleeding risks from recent wounds, puncture sites, weakened vessels

2. Hypotension

3. Possible anaphylactic reaction

F. **Nursing Interventions and Client Education**

1. Administration must take place within 4 to 6 hr of symptom onset.

2. Continuous monitoring is required.

3. Clients will begin anticoagulant therapy to prevent repeated thrombotic event.

SECTION 7

Medications for the Gastrointestinal System

I Antacids

A. **Action:** Neutralize gastric acid and inactivate pepsin

MEDICATIONS FOR THE GASTROINTESTINAL SYSTEM

	SIDE/ADVERSE EFFECTS
Aluminum hydroxide	Constipation
	Hypophosphatemia
Magnesium hydroxide (Milk of Magnesia)	Diarrhea
	Renal impairment
	Hypermagnesemia
Sodium bicarbonate	Constipation

B. **Therapeutic Uses**

1. Peptic ulcer disease

2. GERD

C. **Precautions/Interactions**

1. Prolonged use can result in hypophosphatemia.

2. Can decrease absorption of certain medications.

D. **Nursing Interventions and Client Education**

1. Clients who have renal impairment should only use aluminum-based preparations.

2. Other medications should be taken 1 hr before or after antacids.

3. Older adults with poor nutritional status are at high risk of hypophosphatemia.

4. Do not self-prescribe antacid use for longer than 2 weeks

II Antisecretory/Blocking Agents

A. **Action:** Prevent or block selected receptors within the stomach

B. **Medications**

1. **Proton Pump Inhibitors (PPI)**

   a. Omeprazole

   b. Lansoprazole

   c. Rabeprazole sodium

   d. Esomeprazole

2. Histamine$_2$ Receptor Antagonists (H$_2$ Blocker)

   a. Ranitidine hydrochloride

   b. Cimetidine

   c. Nizatidine

   d. Famotidine

C. **Therapeutic Uses**

1. Gastric and duodenal ulcers

2. GERD

3. Zollinger-Ellison syndrome

D. **Precautions/Interactions**

1. Contraindicated during lactation.

2. Must be used with caution if client has COPD.

E. **Side Effects/Adverse Effects**

1. Can increase the risk for osteoporosis with long-term use, pneumonia in COPD clients, and acid rebound (PPI)

2. Decreased libido/impotence (H$_2$ Blocker)

3. Lethargy, depression, confusion (H$_2$ Blocker)

F. **Nursing Interventions and Client Education**

1. Teach client to seek appropriate care (many take OTC preparations).

2. Review medication regimen and teach client about precautions related to time of administration as required.

3. Do not crush, chew, or break tablets.

4. Notify prescriber of any sign of GI bleeding.

5. Modify diet as prescribed.

III Mucosal Protectants

A. **Sucralfate**

1. **Action:** Adheres to injured gastric ulcers upon contact with gastric acids; protective action for up to 6 hr; has no systemic effects

B. **Therapeutic Use**

1. Gastric and duodenal ulcers

2. GERD

C. **Precautions/Interactions**

1. Chronic renal failure

D. **Nursing Interventions and Client Education**

1. Administer on an empty stomach at least 1 hr before meals.

2. Do not administer within 30 min of antacids.

iv Antiemetics

A. **Action:** Multiple classifications of medications that affect the GI tract or the "vomiting center" of the brain to reduce nausea/vomiting

B. **Therapeutic Uses**
   1. Postoperative
   2. Chemotherapy
   3. Nausea/vomiting associated with disease process

ANTIEMETIC MEDICATIONS

Promethazine

SIDE/ADVERSE EFFECTS	Drowsiness	EPS
	Anticholinergic effects	Potentiates effects when given with narcotics
	Severe respiratory depression in children less than 2	
PRECAUTIONS/ INTERACTIONS	Cardiovascular and hepatic disease	
NURSING INTERVENTIONS	Monitor vital signs	IM—large muscle
	Safety precautions	

Metoclopramide

SIDE/ADVERSE EFFECTS	Drowsiness	EPS
	Diarrhea	Tardive dyskinesia
	Restlessness	
PRECAUTIONS/ INTERACTIONS	Seizures, cardiovascular disease, pheochromocytoma	
NURSING INTERVENTIONS	Instruct client about rapid GI emptying	
	Discontinue with signs of EPS	

Ondansetron

SIDE/ADVERSE EFFECTS	Headache	EPS
NURSING INTERVENTIONS	Administer tablets 30 min prior to chemotherapy and 1 to 2 hr before radiation	
PRECAUTIONS/ INTERACTIONS	Risk for dysrhythmia	
	Do not administer to clients with prolonged QT interval	

Scopolamine

SIDE/ADVERSE EFFECTS	Blurred vision	Anticholinergic effects
	Sedation	
PRECAUTIONS/ INTERACTIONS	Increased mydriatic effect causes increased ocular pressure	
	Use with caution for client with glaucoma	
NURSING INTERVENTIONS	Apply transdermal patches behind ear	
	Use lubricating eye drops	

v Antidiarrheals

A. **Action:** Activate opioid receptors in the GI tract to decrease intestinal motility and to increase the absorption of fluid and sodium in the intestine

B. **Medications**
   1. Diphenoxylate plus atropine
   2. Loperamide
   3. Paregoric

C. **Therapeutic Uses**
   1. Management of diarrhea

D. **Precautions/Interactions**
   1. Increased risk of megacolon for clients who have IBS
   2. Contraindicated in clients with COPD (paregoric)

E. **Side/Adverse Effects**
   1. Constipation
   2. Drowsiness
   3. Dry mouth
   4. Blurred vision

F. **Nursing Interventions and Client Education**
   1. Monitor F&E.
   2. Avoid caffeine intake (increases GI motility).

vi Stool Softeners/Laxatives

A. **Action:** Facilitates peristalsis and bowel movements

STOOL SOFTENER/LAXATIVE MEDICATIONS

	THERAPEUTIC USES
Psyllium	Decrease diarrhea (bulk-forming)
Docusate sodium	Relieve constipation (surfactant)
Bisacodyl	Preprocedure colon evacuation (stimulant)
Magnesium hydroxide (Milk of Magnesia)	Prevent painful elimination (low-dose osmotic)
	Promote rapid evacuation (high-dose osmotic)

B. **Precautions/Interactions**
   1. Contraindicated in clients with fecal impaction, bowel obstruction
   2. Most laxatives are contraindicated in clients with ulcerative colitis and diverticulitis (psyllium may be used)

C. **Side/Adverse Effects**
   1. F&E imbalances
   2. GI irritation
   3. Can lead to toxic levels of magnesium
   4. Fluid retention (laxatives with sodium)

D. **Nursing Interventions and Client Education**
   1. Contraindicated with fecal impaction, bowel obstruction, and acute surgical abdomen.
   2. Encourage regular exercise and promote regular bowel elimination.
   3. Monitor for chronic laxative use/abuse.
   4. Provide adequate fluid and fiber intake to avoid obstruction.

Medications Affecting the Urinary System

I Diuretics

A. **Action:** Increase the amount of fluid excretion via the renal system

DIURETIC MEDICATIONS

Loop	Thiazide	Potassium Sparing
Furosemide	Hydrochlorothiazide	Spironolactone
Bumetanide	Chlorothiazide	Triamterene

B. **Therapeutic Use**

1. Pulmonary edema caused by heart failure
2. Edema unresponsive to other diuretics
3. Hypertension unresponsive to other diuretics

C. **Precautions/Interactions**

1. Use cautiously in clients who have diabetes mellitus.
2. Contraindicated in pregnancy.
3. NSAIDs reduce diuretic effect.

D. **Side/Adverse Effects**

1. Loop and thiazide diuretics
   a. Hypovolemia
   b. Ototoxicity (loop diuretics)
   c. Hypokalemia
   d. Hyponatremia
   e. Hyperglycemia
   f. Digoxin toxicity
   g. Lithium toxicity
2. Potassium-sparing diuretics
   a. Hyperkalemia
   b. Endocrine effects (impotence, menstrual irregularities)

E. **Nursing Interventions and Client Education**

1. Monitor I&O.
2. Monitor vital signs.
3. Monitor for F&E imbalances.
4. Administer early morning to prevent nocturia.
5. Instruct clients taking loop/thiazide diuretics to increase intake of foods high in potassium.
6. Instruct clients taking potassium-sparing diuretics to avoid foods high in potassium such as salt substitutes.

II Osmotic Diuretics

A. **Action:** Pull fluid back into the vascular and extravascular space by increasing serum osmolality to promote osmotic changes

B. **Medication**

1. Mannitol

C. **Therapeutic Uses**

1. Prevent renal failure related to hypovolemia
2. Decrease intracranial pressure related to cerebral edema
3. Decrease intraocular pressure

D. **Precautions/Interactions**

1. Use with caution in heart failure.

E. **Side/Adverse Effects**

1. Pulmonary edema
2. F&E imbalances
3. Thirst, dry mouth

F. **Nursing Interventions and Client Education**

1. Monitor daily weight, I&O, and electrolytes.
2. Monitor for signs of hypovolemia.
3. Monitor neurological status.

III Alpha Adrenergic Blockers for Urinary Hesitancy

A. **Tamsulosin**

1. **Action:** Inhibits smooth muscle contraction in the prostate, which improves the rate of urine flow for clients with BPH
2. **Precautions/Interactions**
   a. Must rule out bladder cancer prior to administering tamsulosin.
   b. Combined use with cimetidine may facilitate toxicity.
   c. Use cautiously with medications causing hypotension (such as sildenafil)

B. **Bethanechol**

1. **Action:** Increases detrusor muscle tone to allow strong start to voiding for clients with postoperative urinary hesitancy
2. **Precautions/Interactions**
   a. Contraindicated for clients who have urinary tract obstruction.
   b. Contraindicated for clients with hypotension or decreased cardiac output. May cause bradycardia.

ALPHA ADRENERGIC BLOCKERS

Tamsulosin

SIDE/ADVERSE EFFECTS	May cause decreased libido, headache, and dizziness
NURSING INTERVENTIONS AND CLIENT EDUCATION	Take 30 min after meal at same time each day
	If dose is missed for several days, restart at the lowest dose
	Can cause orthostatic hypotension

Bethanechol

SIDE/ADVERSE EFFECTS	Excessive salivation, abdominal cramps, diarrhea
NURSING INTERVENTIONS	Administer on empty stomach

IV Anticholinergic Medications for Overactive Bladder

A. **Action:** Antispasmodic actions to decrease detrusor muscle spasms and contractions

B. **Medications**
   1. Oxybutynin
   2. Tolterodine
   3. Darifenacin
   4. Solifenacin
   5. Trospium
   6. Fesoterodine

C. **Therapeutic Use**
   1. Urinary incontinence
   2. Urinary urgency and frequency

D. **Precautions/Interactions**
   1. Do not use for clients who have intestinal obstruction.
   2. Use with other anticholinergics can increase anticholinergic effects.
   3. Risk for cognitive impairment in older clients.

E. **Side/Adverse Effects**
   1. Anticholinergic symptoms
   2. Drowsiness
   3. Dyspepsia

 F. **Nursing Interventions and Client Education**
   1. Instruct client to manage anticholinergic side effects.
   2. Instruct client to report constipation lasting longer than 3 days.

V Sexual Dysfunction

A. **Action:** Enhances the effect of nitric oxide to promote relaxation of penile muscles, allowing increased blood flow to produce an erection

B. **Medications**
   1. Sildenafil
   2. Tadalafil
   3. Vardenafil

C. **Therapeutic Uses**
   1. Erectile dysfunction
   2. Less commonly used in the treatment of pulmonary arterial hypertension

D. **Precautions/Interactions**
   1. Contraindicated for clients taking nitrate drugs, alpha blockers for BPH, or antihypertensives.
   2. Contraindicated for clients who have history of stroke, hypo/hypertension, or heart failure.

E. **Side/Adverse Effects**
   1. Hypotension
   2. Priapism (erection lasting longer than 4 hr)
   3. Vision impairment
   4. Hearing loss
   5. Headache
   6. Flushing

F. **Nursing Interventions and Client Education**
   1. Administer 1 hr before sexual activity; do not use more than once daily.
   2. Instruct client to notify provider of all medications currently taken, including herbal preparations.
   3. Instruct client to avoid intake of any organic nitrates.
   4. Instruct client to stop taking medication and notify prescriber immediately for erection lasting longer than 4 hr or any loss of vision.

Medications for the Immune System

I Immunizations

A. **Action:** Stimulate production of antibodies to prevent illness

CHILDHOOD IMMUNIZATIONS*

TYPE	SIDE/ADVERSE EFFECTS**	CONTRAINDICATION
DTaP, Tdap	Fever Irritability Seizures	Occurrence of seizures within 3 days of vaccine
Hib	Low-grade fever	Age younger than 6 weeks
Rotavirus	Irritability, diarrhea, vomiting, and intussusception	History of intussusception Maximum age for the final dose is 8 months, 0 days
IPV	Anaphylactic reaction to neomycin, streptomycin, or polymyxin B	
MMR	Joint pain Anaphylaxis Thrombocytopenia	Allergy to eggs, gelatin, or neomycin Immunocompromised, pregnancy
Varicella	Vesicles on skin Pruritus	Pregnancy Allergy to gelatin and neomycin Immunocompromised
Seasonal influenza	Fever	Nasal spray contraindicated for children younger than 2, adults older than 50 years, and clients who are immunocompromised History of Guillain-Barré
Hepatitis A, B	Anaphylaxis	Hep A: pregnancy Hep B: allergy to yeast
Meningococcal vaccine		History of Guillain-Barré
HPV—up to age 26		Pregnancy Allergy to yeast

* Schedule is determined by the Centers for Disease Control and Prevention.
** Risk in addition to localized inflammation

ADULT IMMUNIZATIONS (AGES 18 YEARS AND OLDER)*

TYPE	SCHEDULE
Tetanus booster	Every 10 years
MMR	One or two doses at ages 19 to 49
Varicella	Two doses if no history of disease
Pneumococcal (PPSV)	Once after age 65 Recommended for immunocompromised, COPD, living in long-term care facility
Hepatitis A	Two doses for high-risk clients
Hepatitis B	Three doses for high-risk clients
Seasonal influenza	Annually
Meningococcal vaccine	Students entering college Adults older than 56 years Repeat every 5 years for high-risk clients
Herpes zoster	Over age 60

* Schedule is determined by the Centers for Disease Control and Prevention.

B. **Nursing Interventions and Client Education**
  1. Consult CDC guidelines for schedule of administration.
  2. Educate clients about the purpose of immunizations and keeping records.
  3. Instruct parents to avoid administration of aspirin for management of adverse effects in children.
  4. Instruct clients regarding side/adverse effects and management.

II Antimicrobials

A. **Action:** Inhibit growth, destroy, or otherwise control replication of microbes

MULTIGENERATION ANTIBIOTICS

Aminoglycosides

MEDICATIONS	Amikacin Gentamicin sulfate Streptomycin
THERAPEUTIC USE	Septicemia, meningitis, pneumonia
PRECAUTIONS	High risk for ototoxicity, nephrotoxicity Monitor creatinine and BUN Monitor trough levels

Cephalosporins

MEDICATIONS	Cephalexin Cefaclor Cefotaxime
THERAPEUTIC USE	Upper respiratory, skin, urinary infections Used as prophylaxis for clients at risk
PRECAUTIONS	Cross-sensitivity with penicillins Monitor for signs of Clostridium difficile

Fluoroquinolones

MEDICATIONS	Ciprofloxacin Levofloxacin
THERAPEUTIC USE	Bronchitis, chlamydia, gonorrhea, PID, UTI, pneumonia, prostatitis, sinusitis
PRECAUTIONS	Caution with hepatic, renal, or seizure disorders

Macrolides

MEDICATIONS	Azithromycin Clarithromycin Erythromycin
THERAPEUTIC USE	Upper respiratory infections, sinusitis, Legionnaires' disease, whooping cough, acute diphtheria, chlamydia
PRECAUTIONS	Used for clients who have penicillin allergy Administer with meals

Nitrofurantoin

THERAPEUTIC USE	UTI
PRECAUTIONS	Broad-spectrum Contraindicated in renal dysfunction Urine will have brown discoloration

Penicillins

MEDICATIONS	Amoxicillin Ampicillin
THERAPEUTIC USE	Pneumonia, upper respiratory infections, septicemia, endocarditis, rheumatic fever, GYN infections
PRECAUTIONS	Hypersensitivity with possible anaphylaxis

Sulfonamides

MEDICATIONS	Trimethoprim/sulfamethoxazole
THERAPEUTIC USE	UTI, bronchitis, otitis media
PRECAUTIONS	Consume at least 3 L/day of fluid Use backup contraceptives Avoid sun exposure

Tetracyclines

MEDICATIONS	Doxycycline calcium Tetracycline HCl
THERAPEUTIC USE	Fungal, bacterial, protozoal, rickettsial infections
PRECAUTIONS	Consume at least 3 L/day of fluid Use backup contraceptives Avoid sun exposure Permanent tooth discoloration if given to children younger than 8 years

Glycopeptide

MEDICATION	Vancomycin
THERAPEUTIC USE	MRSA, bacterial, C. difficile infections
PRECAUTIONS	Contraindication: Allergy to corn Caution: Ototoxicity, nephrotoxicity Administer over 1 hr IV to prevent red man syndrome Monitor trough levels

SPECIAL CLASSES OF ANTIMICROBIALS

Antifungal

MEDICATIONS	Fluconazole
THERAPEUTIC USE	Candidiasis infections
PRECAUTIONS	Monitor hepatic and renal function Refrigerate suspensions Increased risk of bleeding for clients taking anticoagulants

Antimalarials

MEDICATIONS	Hydroxychloroquine Quinine sulfate
THERAPEUTIC USE	Prevent malarial attacks, rheumatoid arthritis Systemic lupus
PRECAUTIONS	Increased risk of psoriasis Monitor for drug-induced retinopathy

Antiprotozoal

MEDICATIONS	Metronidazole
THERAPEUTIC USE	Trichomoniasis and giardiasis, *clostridium difficile*, amebic dysentery, PID, vaginosis
PRECAUTIONS	Take with food Do not consume alcohol during therapy or 48 hr after completion of regimen

Antituberculars

MEDICATIONS	Isoniazid (INH) Rifampin
THERAPEUTIC USE	Prevention and treatment of TB Latent TB INH: 6 to 9 months Active TB: multiple therapy up to 24 months
PRECAUTIONS	Risk of neuropathies and hepatotoxicity Consume foods high in vitamin B6 Avoid foods with tyramine (INH) Increased risk of phenytoin toxicity (INH) Avoid alcohol Discoloration of urine, saliva, sweat, and tears (rifampin)

Antiretrovirals

MEDICATIONS	Acyclovir Valacyclovir HCl Zidovudine
THERAPEUTIC USE	Genital herpes, shingles, HIV
PRECAUTIONS	Acyclovir and valacyclovir: administer with food Increase fluid intake Begin therapy with first onset of symptoms

C. **Nursing Interventions and Client Education**

1. Assess history of medication allergies and treatment.
2. Monitor for signs of medication reaction.
3. Monitor for signs of secondary infections.
4. Administer medications at appropriate time intervals to maintain therapeutic effects.
5. If C&S is prescribed, perform test before initiating therapy.
6. Instruct client to complete entire medication regimen.

SECTION 10

Medications for the Musculoskeletal System

I Bisphosphonates

A. **Action:** Decrease the number and action of osteoclasts, resulting in bone resorption

B. **Medications**

1. Alendronate: daily or weekly
2. Risedronate: daily, weekly, monthly
3. Ibandronate: monthly or every 3 months
4. Zoledronate: IV annually

C. **Therapeutic Use**

1. Prevention and treatment of osteoporosis
2. Paget's disease
3. Hypercalcemia related to malignancy

D. **Precautions/Interactions**

1. Contraindicated during lactation.
2. Clients who have esophageal stricture or difficulty swallowing may only use zoledronate.
3. Absorption is decreased when taken with calcium supplements, antacids, orange juice, and caffeine.

E. **Side/Adverse Effects**

1. Musculoskeletal pain
2. Esophagitis and GI discomfort
3. Jaw pain (zoledronate)
4. Atrial fibrillation (zoledronate)

F. **Nursing Interventions and Client Education**

1. Administer medication in the morning on an empty stomach.
2. Instruct client to consume at least 8 oz water (not carbonated).
3. Client must remain upright (sitting or standing) for 30 min after taking medication.
4. Consume adequate amounts of vitamin D.

II Antirheumatics

A. **Action:** Provide symptomatic relief and delay in disease progression by inhibiting or modulating inflammatory processes

ANTIRHEUMATIC DRUG CATEGORIES

Disease-modifying antirheumatic drugs (DMARDs)

MEDICATIONS	Methotrexate Hydroxychloroquine Etanercept Infliximab Adalimumab
ACTION	Interrupt complex immune responses, preventing disease progression

Glucocorticoids

MEDICATIONS	Prednisone Prednisolone
ACTION	Decrease inflammation by suppressing leukocytes and fibroblasts, and reversing capillary permeability

NSAIDs

MEDICATIONS	Ibuprofen Indomethacin Naproxen Celecoxib
ACTION	Inhibit prostaglandin synthesis, resulting in decreased inflammatory responses

III DMARDs

A. **Therapeutic Use**

   1. Slow joint degeneration and progression of rheumatoid arthritis

B. **Precautions/Interactions**

   1. Methotrexate: Contraindicated in pregnancy, kidney or liver failure, psoriasis, alcohol use disorder, or hematologic dyscrasias.

C. **Side/Adverse Effects**

   1. Methotrexate: Increased risk of infection, bone marrow suppression, GI ulceration

   2. Hydroxychloroquine: retinal damage (blindness)

D. **Nursing Interventions and Client Education**

   1. Instruct client about measures to prevent infection.

   2. Monitor liver function tests.

   3. Instruct client to use reliable contraception.

   4. Instruct client that initial effects may take 3 to 6 weeks, and full therapeutic effects may take several months.

   5. Administer with food.

   6. Instruct clients taking hydroxychloroquine about the critical importance of retinal examination every 6 months.

IV Glucocorticoids

A. **Therapeutic Use**

   1. Provide symptomatic relief of inflammation and pain.

B. **Precautions/Interactions**

   1. Contraindicated in systemic fungal infection.

   2. Do not administer live virus vaccines during therapy.

   3. Should only be used for a short duration.

C. **Side/Adverse Effects**

   1. Risk of infection

   2. Osteoporosis

   3. Adrenal suppression

   4. Fluid retention

   5. GI discomfort

   6. Hyperglycemia

   7. Hypokalemia

D. **Nursing Interventions and Client Education**

   1. Do not skip doses.

   2. Monitor blood pressure.

   3. Monitor F&E balance and weight.

   4. Monitor for signs of bleeding, GI discomfort.

   5. Teach client to take calcium supplements and maintain vitamin D levels.

   6. Give with food.

   7. Never stop abruptly.

   8. Provide immunoprotection.

V NSAIDs

A. **Therapeutic Use**

   1. Provide rapid, symptomatic relief of inflammation and pain.

B. **Precautions/Interactions**

   1. Hypersensitivity to aspirin or other NSAIDs.

   2. May increase the risk of MI and stroke (non-aspirin NSAIDS).

C. **Side/Adverse Effects**

   1. GI discomfort

   2. GI ulceration

   3. Renal impairment

   4. Photosensitivity

D. **Nursing Interventions and Client Education**

   1. Administer with food and full glass of water.

   2. Avoid lying down for 30 min after administration.

   3. Instruct client to use only as needed for symptoms to reduce risk of GI ulceration.

   4. Instruct client to use sunscreen.

VI Antigout

ANTIGOUT MEDICATIONS

Allopurinol

ACTION	Inhibits uric acid production
THERAPEUTIC USE	Chronic gouty arthritis

Colchicine

ACTION	Inhibits processes to prevent leukocytes from invading joints
THERAPEUTIC USE	Acute gouty arthritis

A. **Precautions/Interactions**

   1. Use caution in clients who have renal, cardiac, or gastrointestinal dysfunction.

   2. Should not be combined with theophylline.

B. **Side/Adverse Effects**

   1. GI distress

   2. Rash and fever (discontinue immediately)

   3. Decreases the metabolism of warfarin

C. **Nursing Interventions and Client Education**

   1. Instruct client to avoid foods high in purines to reduce uric acid.

   2. Monitor CBC and uric acid levels.

   3. Instruct clients to avoid aspirin.

   4. Administer with meals.

Medications for the Nervous System

I Anti-anxiety Medications

A. **Action:** Increase the efficacy of GABA to reduce anxiety

B. **Medications**

1. Benzodiazepines
   a. Alprazolam
   b. Chlordiazepoxide
   c. Diazepam
   d. Lorazepam
2. Buspirone
3. Antidepressants
   a. Venlafaxine
   b. Duloxetine
   c. Paroxetine
   d. Escitalopram

C. **Therapeutic Use**

1. Generalized anxiety disorder and panic disorder
2. Insomnia
3. Alcohol withdrawal
4. Induction of anesthesia

D. **Precautions/Interactions**

1. Benzodiazepines are used with caution in clients who have substance use disorder and liver disease.
2. Venlafaxine, an SNRI, is contraindicated for clients taking MAOIs.

E. **Side/Adverse Effects**

1. CNS depression
2. Paradoxical response (insomnia, excitation, euphoria)
3. Withdrawal symptoms (not with buspirone)
4. Risk of abuse and potential for overdose (benzodiazepines)

F. **Nursing Interventions and Client Education**

1. Monitor vital signs.
2. Instruct clients to never abruptly discontinue medication.
3. Monitor clients for side/adverse effects.
4. Instruct clients to avoid alcohol.

II Antidepressants

A. **Action**

1. SSRI inhibits serotonin reuptake.
2. SNRIs block reuptake of norepinephrine, as well as serotonin with effects similar to the SSRIs.
3. Tricyclic blocks reuptake of norepinephrine and serotonin.
4. MAOI increases norepinephrine, dopamine, and serotonin by blocking MAO-A.

ANTIDEPRESSANT CLASSES

SSRI and SNRI

	SSRI	SNRI
MEDICATIONS	› Citalopram › Fluoxetine › Paroxetine › Sertraline	› Duloxetine › Venlafaxine
PRECAUTIONS/ INTERACTIONS	Avoid alcohol Do not discontinue abruptly Monitor for serotonin syndrome (agitation, confusion, hallucinations) within first 72 hr	
SIDE/ADVERSE EFFECTS	Weight gain Sexual dysfunction Fatigue Drowsiness	

Tricyclic

MEDICATIONS	Amitriptyline Imipramine
PRECAUTIONS/ INTERACTIONS	Do not administer with MAOIs or St. John's wort Must avoid alcohol Contraindicated for clients with seizure disorder
SIDE/ADVERSE EFFECTS	Anticholinergic effects Orthostatic hypotension Cardiac dysrhythmias Decreased seizure threshold

MAOI

MEDICATIONS	Isocarboxazid Tranylcypromine Phenelzine
PRECAUTIONS/ INTERACTIONS	Avoid foods containing tyramine Antihypertensives have additive hypotensive effect Contraindicated with SSRIs, tricyclics, heart failure, CVA, renal insufficiency
SIDE/ADVERSE EFFECTS	CNS stimulation Orthostatic hypotension Hypertensive crisis with intake of tyramine, SSRIs, and tricyclics

B. **Nursing Interventions and Client Education**

1. Assess client for suicide risk.

2. Instruct client to take on daily basis and never miss a dose.

3. Instruct client about therapeutic effects and time of onset.

4. Instruct client to avoid discontinuing drug abruptly.

5. Instruct client to take SSRIs in the morning to minimize sleep disturbances.

6. Provide clients taking MAOIs a list of foods containing tyramine.

7. Advise clients to avoid taking other medications without consulting provider.

III Bipolar Disorder Medications

A. **Action:** Produce neurochemical changes in the brain to control acute mania, depression, and incidence of suicide

B. **Medication**

1. Lithium carbonate

C. **Therapeutic Uses**

1. Bipolar disorder

2. Alcohol use disorder

3. Bulimia

4. Schizophrenia

D. **Precautions/Interactions**

1. Use cautiously in clients who have renal dysfunction, heart disease, hyponatremia, and dehydration.

   a. NSAIDs will increase lithium levels.

   b. Monitor serum sodium levels.

E. **Side/Adverse Effects**

1. GI distress

2. Fine hand tremors

3. Polyuria

4. Hypothyroidism

5. Renal toxicity

F. **Nursing Interventions and Client Education**

1. Monitor therapeutic levels.

2. Monitor serum sodium levels.

3. Instruct clients that therapeutic effects begin in 7 to 14 days.

4. Doses must be administered 1 to 3 times daily per provider prescription.

5. Provide nutritional counseling to include food sources for sodium.

6. Administer with food to decrease GI distress.

IV Antipsychotic Medications

A. **Action:** Block dopamine, acetylcholine, histamine, and norepinephrine receptors in the brain and periphery

B. **Medications**

1. Typical

   a. Chlorpromazine

   b. Fluphenazine

   c. Haloperidol

   d. Thiothixene

2. Atypical (less severe side/adverse effects)

   a. Aripiprazole

   b. Clozapine

   c. Olanzapine

   d. Paliperidone

   e. Quetiapine

   f. Ziprasidone

C. **Therapeutic Use**

1. Acute and chronic psychosis

2. Schizophrenia

3. Manic phase of bipolar disorders

4. Tourette syndrome

5. Delusional and schizoaffective disorders

6. Dementia

D. **Precautions/Interactions**

1. Contraindicated for clients who have severe depression, Parkinson's disease, prolactin-dependent cancer, and severe hypotension.

2. Use with caution in clients who have glaucoma, paralytic ileus, prostate enlargement, or seizure disorder.

E. **Side/Adverse Effects**

1. Typical

   a. Sedation

   b. Extrapyramidal effects

   c. Anticholinergic effects

   d. Tardive dyskinesia

   e. Agranulocytosis

   f. Neuroleptic malignant syndrome

   g. Seizures

2. Atypical

   a. Agranulocytosis

   b. Weight gain

   c. Diabetes

   d. Dyslipidemia

   e. Orthostatic hypotension

   f. Extrapyramidal effects

F. **Nursing Interventions and Client Education**

1. Monitor for side effects within 5 hr to 5 days of administration.

2. Advise client of potential side effects.

3. Monitor CBC.

4. Encourage fluids.

5. Stop medication for signs of neuroleptic malignant syndrome.

v Attention-Deficit/Hyperactivity Disorder Medications

A. **Action:** Increase attention span; reduce impulsive behavior and hyperactivity

1. Stimulants increase levels of norepinephrine, serotonin, and dopamine into the CNS.

2. Nonstimulants increase levels of norepinephrine into the CNS.

ADHD CLASSES

Stimulants

MEDICATION	Dextroamphetamine and amphetamine
	Methylphenidate
SIDE EFFECTS	Insomnia
	Headache
	Suppressed appetite
	Abdominal pain
NURSING INTERVENTIONS AND CLIENT EDUCATION	Administer in early morning; give with or after meals.
	Do not abruptly discontinue.
	Monitor for signs of abuse.
	Monitor for signs of agitation.

Nonstimulants

MEDICATION	Atomoxetine
	Guanfacine: may be used in treatment of Asperger's syndrome
SIDE EFFECTS	GI upset
	Insomnia
	Mood swings
NURSING INTERVENTIONS AND CLIENT EDUCATION	Take medication daily.
	Do not crush or chew.
	Instruct client to immediately report worsening of anxiety, agitation.
	Do not take with MAOIs.

vi Sedative/Hypnotic Medications

A. **Action:** Slow neuronal activity in the brain to induce sedation/sleep

B. **Medications**

1. Benzodiazepines
   a. Lorazepam
   b. Temazepam

2. Benzodiazepine-like medications
   a. Zolpidem
   b. Eszopiclone

C. **Therapeutic Use**

1. Short-term insomnia

2. Difficulty falling or staying asleep

D. **Precautions/Interactions**

1. Use cautiously in clients who have severe mental depression.

2. Avoid combined use with alcohol and medications that depress CNS function.

E. **Side/Adverse Effects**

1. Amnesia

2. Respiratory depression

3. Daytime drowsiness and dizziness

F. **Nursing Interventions and Client Education**

1. Instruct client to take immediately before bedtime because medication has abrupt onset of sleep.

2. Instruct client to avoid alcohol.

3. Warn client and caregivers of potential for sleep activities without recall; notify prescriber immediately.

vii Abstinence Maintenance Medications

A. **Disulfiram**

1. **Action:** Interferes with hepatic oxidation of alcohol, resulting in elevation of blood acetaldehyde levels

2. **Therapeutic Use**
   a. Adjunct to maintain sobriety in treatment of alcohol use disorder

3. **Precautions/Interactions**
   a. INH will increase risk of adverse CNS effects for clients taking disulfiram.
   b. Ingestion of large amounts of alcohol may cause respiratory depression, dysrhythmias, and cardiac arrest.
   c. Adjust medication doses of warfarin and phenytoin.

4. **Side/Adverse Effects**
   a. Drowsiness
   b. Headache
   c. Metallic taste
   d. Hepatotoxicity

5. **Nursing Interventions and Client Education**
   a. Must wait 12 hr between time of last alcohol intake and starting medication.
   b. Instruct client that consumption of alcohol while taking disulfiram will result in flushing, throbbing in head and neck, respiratory difficulty, nausea, copious vomiting, sweating, thirst, chest pain, palpitation, dyspnea, hyperventilation, tachycardia, hypotension, syncope, marked uneasiness, weakness, vertigo, blurred vision, and confusion.
   c. Instruct client that undesirable effects last 30 min to several hours when alcohol is consumed.
   d. Instruct client the effects of disulfiram may stay in the body for weeks after therapy is discontinued.
   e. Instruct client that therapy may last months to years.

B. **Methadone**

1. **Action:** Binds with opiate receptors in CNS to produce analgesic and euphoric effects

2. **Therapeutic Use**
   a. Prevents withdrawal symptoms in clients who were addicted to opiate drugs.

3. **Precautions/Interactions**
   a. Do not use in clients who have severe asthma, chronic respiratory disease, or history of head injury.
   b. Avoid in clients with QT syndrome.
4. **Side/Adverse Effects**
   a. Sedation
   b. Respiratory depression
   c. Paradoxical CNS excitation
5. **Nursing Interventions and Client Education**
   a. Monitor clients for signs of drug tolerance and psychological dependence.
   b. Monitor for respiratory depression.
   c. Instruct client that methadone must be slowly reduced to produce detoxification.
   d. Client must be monitored through treatment center.

VIII Chronic Neurological Disorders

A. **Cholinesterase Inhibitors**
   1. **Action:** Prevent cholinesterase from inactivating acetylcholine, resulting in improved transmission of nerve impulses
   2. **Medications**
      a. Neostigmine
      b. Ambenonium
      c. Edrophonium
   3. **Therapeutic Use**
      a. Myasthenia gravis
   4. **Precautions/Interactions**
      a. Do not administer if heart rate is less than 60/min.
   5. **Side/Adverse Effects**
      a. Slow heart rate
      b. Chest pain, weak pulse, increased sweating, and dizziness
      c. Client feeling like he or she might pass out
      d. Weak or shallow breathing
      e. Urinating more than usual
      f. Seizures
      g. Trouble swallowing
   6. **Nursing Interventions and Client Education**
      a. Dose must be individualized.
      b. Instruct client to keep individual diary to record side effects.
      c. Advise client to wear medical alert bracelet.
      d. Monitor for cholinergic crisis.
B. **Anti-Parkinson's**
   1. **Action:** Increase dopamine to minimize tremors and rigidity
   2. **Medications**
      a. Benztropine
      b. Carbidopa/levodopa
      c. Levodopa

3. **Therapeutic Use**
   a. Parkinson's disease
4. **Precautions/Interactions**
   a. Do not use levodopa within 2 weeks of MAOI use.
   b. Pyridoxine (vitamin B_6) decreases effects of levodopa.
   c. Benztropine is contraindicated in clients who have narrow-angle glaucoma.
   d. Must discontinue 6 to 8 hr before anesthesia.
5. **Side/Adverse Effects**
   a. Muscle twitching (especially eyelid spasms)
   b. Headache
   c. Dizziness
   d. Dark urine
   e. Orthostatic hypotension
6. **Nursing Interventions and Client Education**
   a. Instruct family members to assist with medication regimen.
   b. Instruct client to notify prescriber if sudden loss of the medication effects occurs.
   c. Instruct client that maximum therapeutic effects may take 4 to 6 weeks.
   d. Monitor closely for signs of adverse reactions.
   e. Instruct client to avoid high-protein meals and snacks.
   f. Keep medication away from heat, light, and moisture. If pills become darkened, they have lost potency and must be discarded.

C. **Antiseizure**
   1. **Action:** Slows rates of neuronal activity in the brain by blocking specific channels responsible for neuron firing, which results in an elevation of the seizure threshold
   2. **Medications**
      a. Carbamazepine
      b. Gabapentin
      c. Phenobarbital
      d. Phenytoin
      e. Valproic acid
   3. **Therapeutic Use**
      a. Prevent and/or control seizure activity

ANTISEIZURE MEDICATIONS

Carbamazepine

PRECAUTIONS/ INTERACTIONS	Contraindicated in clients who have bone marrow suppression or bleeding disorders
	Decreases the effectiveness of oral contraceptives and warfarin
SIDE/ADVERSE EFFECTS	Anemia, leukopenia, Stevens-Johnson syndrome

Gabapentin

PRECAUTIONS/ INTERACTIONS	Do not abruptly discontinue
SIDE/ADVERSE EFFECTS	Headaches, weight gain, nausea
	Report CNS depression, seizures, visual changes, and unusual bruising

Phenobarbital

PRECAUTIONS/ INTERACTIONS	Contraindicated in history of substance use disorder
SIDE/ADVERSE EFFECTS	Drowsiness, hypotension, respiratory depression

Phenytoin

PRECAUTIONS/ INTERACTIONS	Causes increased excretion of digoxin, warfarin, oral contraceptives
SIDE/ADVERSE EFFECTS	Gingival hypertrophy, diplopia, drowsiness, hirsutism

Valproic acid

PRECAUTIONS/ INTERACTIONS	Contraindicated in liver disease, pregnancy
SIDE/ADVERSE EFFECTS	Hepatotoxicity, teratogenic effects, pancreatitis

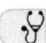

4. **Nursing Interventions and Client Education**
   a. Monitor for therapeutic effects.
   b. Monitor clients taking phenytoin for toxic effects, including serum levels for toxicity.
   c. Instruct clients regarding the importance of compliance; medication is treatment, not a cure.
   d. Individualize treatment regimen.
   e. Instruct client regarding side/adverse effects.
   f. For status epilepticus: diazepam or lorazepam IV push followed by IV phenytoin or fosphenytoin.

D. **Ophthalmologic Medications (Antiglaucoma)**
   1. **Action:** Reduction of aqueous humor
   2. **Medications**
      a. Levobunolol
      b. Timolol
      c. Pilocarpine
      d. Latanoprost
   3. **Precautions/Interactions**
      a. Use caution in clients taking oral beta blocker or calcium channel blocker.

4. **Side/Adverse Effects**
   a. Systemic effect of beta blockers: bradycardia, heart failure, bronchospasm
   b. Brown discoloration of the iris (latanoprost)
   c. Retinal detachment (pilocarpine)

5. **Nursing Interventions and Client Education**
   a. Instruct client to use sterile technique when handling applicator portion of the container.
   b. Hold gentle pressure on the nasolacrimal duct for 30 to 60 seconds immediately after instilling drops.
   c. Monitor pulse rate/rhythm for clients taking oral beta or calcium channel blocker.

SECTION 12

Medications for Pain and Inflammation

I NSAIDs

See "Section 10: Medications for the Musculoskeletal System."

II Acetaminophen

A. **Action:** Slows production of prostaglandins in the CNS
B. **Therapeutic Use**
   1. Analgesic
   2. Antipyretic
C. **Precautions/Interactions**
   1. Use caution in clients who consume three or more alcoholic beverages per day.
   2. Concurrent use of rifampin, INH, carbamazepine, and barbiturates may increase hepatotoxic effects.
   3. Slows the metabolism of warfarin.
D. **Side/Adverse Effects**
   1. Nausea and vomiting
   2. Long-term therapy: hemolytic anemia, leukopenia, neutropenia, and thrombocytopenia
E. **Nursing Interventions and Client Education**
   1. Monitor liver function.
   2. Monitor kidney function.
   3. Be aware of OTC sources of acetaminophen.
   4. Instruct client to take as prescribed and do not exceed 3,000 mg/24 hr.
   5. Instruct client about risk of hepatotoxicity.
   6. Administration to children should be based on age, not to exceed five doses per day (read labels carefully).
   7. Treat acetaminophen overdose with acetylcysteine.

III Opioid Analgesics

A. **Action:** Bind with opiate receptors in the CNS to alter the perception of and emotional response to pain

B. **Medications**
1. Fentanyl
2. Hydromorphone
3. Morphine sulfate
4. Meperidine
5. Codeine, oxycodone

C. **Therapeutic Use**
1. Relief of moderate to severe pain
2. Sedation

D. **Precautions/Interactions**
1. Meperidine is preferred for clients with biliary associated pain.
2. Monitor for potentiation of effects when given with barbiturates, benzodiazepines, phenothiazines, hypnotics, and sedatives.

E. **Side/Adverse Effects**
1. Orthostatic hypotension
2. Constipation
3. Urinary retention
4. Blurred vision
5. Respiratory depression
6. Abstinence syndrome

F. **Nursing Interventions and Client Education**
1. Monitor vital signs.
2. Monitor for respiratory depression.
3. Instruct client regarding administration with PCA pump.
4. Administer naloxone for clients who have respiratory depression.
5. Prevent constipation.
6. Monitor for urinary retention.

SECTION 13

Medications for the Reproductive System

I Contraception

A. **Consider the following when providing client education and support regarding contraception.** Factors that influence choice of a contraceptive include:
1. Age and health status, including risk for STI
2. Religion and culture
3. Plans for future conception
4. Frequency of intercourse
5. Number of sexual partners
6. Personal concerns about availability, spontaneity, ease of use

CONTRACEPTION METHODS

Rhythm method

CONSIDERATIONS FOR USE	Develop "fertile awareness" by noting:
	Cervical mucus changes
	Menstrual cycle pattern
	Basal temperature
CLIENT EDUCATION	Do not have sexual intercourse during "fertile periods"
	Low reliability for preventing pregnancy

Oral contraceptives

CONSIDERATIONS FOR USE	Pill is taken daily
	Adverse effects: breast tenderness, bleeding, nausea/vomiting
CLIENT EDUCATION	Antibiotic therapy, phenytoin and rifampin, reduce effectiveness
	Avoid smoking

Ethinyl estradiol and norelgestromin (contraceptive patch)

CONSIDERATIONS FOR USE	Replace patch each week for 3 weeks
CLIENT EDUCATION	Apply patch to buttocks, abdomen, upper torso, upper/outer arm
	Period will begin on week 4 (no patch)

Medroxyprogesterone

CONSIDERATIONS FOR USE	Injection is administered every 3 months during menstrual cycle
CLIENT EDUCATION	Use backup form of birth control for 7 days after first injection
	Fertility returns approximately 1 year after stopping

Emergency contraception

CONSIDERATIONS FOR USE	A larger-than-normal dose of oral contraceptive
	Taken no later than 72 hr after unprotected sex
	Second dose is repeated 12 hr later
	Antiemetics may be needed
CLIENT EDUCATION	Should discuss options with provider
	Should never be used as the primary method of birth control

Etonogestrel, ethinyl estradiol vaginal ring

CONSIDERATIONS FOR USE	Placed deep into the vagina once every 3 weeks
CLIENT EDUCATION	One size fits most women
	If falls out, rinse in warm water and replace within 3 hr
	Remove ring during week 4; menses should begin

Intrauterine device (IUD)

CONSIDERATIONS FOR USE	Contraindicated for women with diabetes or history of PID
	Risk of infection
	May have cramping and heavier periods

CONTRACEPTION METHODS (CONTINUED)

CLIENT EDUCATION	Hormonal IUD effective for up to 5 years
	Copper IUD effective for up to 10 years
	Must monitor for signs of infection
	Verify string is present

Cervical diaphragm

CONSIDERATIONS FOR USE	Use with spermicide
	Fit by prescriber
	Refitted after childbirth or weight gain/loss
CLIENT EDUCATION	Insert 6 hr prior to and leave in for 6 hr after intercourse
	May be inserted up to 6 hr prior to intercourse; must be left in 6 hr after intercourse
	Refit size with 10 lb or more weight change and following childbirth

Condom

CONSIDERATIONS FOR USE	Use with spermicide
CLIENT EDUCATION	Protects against STIs
	Apply and remove correctly
	Use only water-soluble lubricants

Spermicides

CONSIDERATIONS FOR USE	Available as: › Cream › Gel › Film › Foam › Suppository
CLIENT EDUCATION	Should use with barrier method
	Can insert up to 1 hr before intercourse

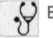

B. **Nursing Interventions and Client Education**

1. Discuss conception and contraceptive plans with client to include reliability, benefits, and risks.
2. Instruct client to maintain regular health screening visits.
3. Instruct client about measures to prevent PID, STIs.
4. Explain that contraceptive decisions may change over the life span.
5. Teach clients unreliable forms of birth control, including coitus interruptus (withdrawal), douching, and breastfeeding.

II Oxytocic

A. **Cervical "Ripening"**

1. **Action:** Prostaglandins cause cervical softening in preparation for cervical dilation and effacement

2. **Medication**
   a. Dinoprostone cervical gel
   b. Misoprostol (unlabeled use)

3. **Precautions/Interactions**
   a. Contraindicated in clients who have acute PID, history of pelvic surgery, abnormal fetal position.

4. **Side/Adverse Effects**
   a. Nausea
   b. Headache
   c. Tremor, tension
   d. Feeling of warmth in the vaginal area
   e. Elevated temperature

5. **Nursing Interventions and Client Education**
   a. Maintain client on bed rest for at least 2 hr (30 min for the gel) after insertion.
   b. Monitor and record maternal vital signs and fetal heart rate.
   c. Monitor for uterine contractions.
   d. Oxytocin augmentation may be initiated as needed.
   e. Major adverse effect is tachysystole.

B. **Oxytocin**

1. **Action:** Stimulates uterine contractions for the purpose of induction or augmentation of labor and prevents postpartum hemorrhage

2. **Therapeutic Use**
   a. Antepartum for contraction stress test (CST)
   b. Intrapartum for induction or augmentation of labor
   c. Postpartum to promote uterine tone

3. **Precautions/Interactions**
   a. Contraindicated with placental abnormalities, fetal malpresentation, previous uterine surgery, and fetal distress.
   b. Bishop Score of 6 and greater when planning induction.

4. **Side/Adverse Effects**
   a. Intense uterine contractions
   b. Uterine hyperstimulation
   c. Uterine rupture
   d. Water intoxication

5. **Nursing Interventions and Client Education**
   a. Administer as secondary infusion via infusion pump for induction or augmentation.
   b. Continuously monitor uterine contractions and fetal heart rate.
   c. Discontinue oxytocin with any signs of uterine hyperstimulation or signs of maternal or fetal distress.
   d. Administer oxygen via face mask 10 L for signs of hyperstimulation.
   e. When used in postpartum, monitor client for uterine bleeding.

III Methylergonovine

A. **Action:** Acts directly on the uterine muscle to stimulate forceful contractions

B. **Therapeutic Use**

1. Postpartum hemorrhage

C. **Precautions/Interactions**

1. Use with extreme caution in clients with hypertension, preeclampsia, heart disease, venoatrial shunts, mitral valve stenosis, sepsis, cardiovascular, hepatic or renal impairment.

D. **Side/Adverse Effects**

1. Potent vasoconstriction

2. Hypertension

3. Headache

E. **Nursing Interventions and Client Education**

1. Continuously monitor blood pressure.

2. Assess uterine bleeding and uterine tone.

IV Tocolytics

A. **Action:** Act on uterine muscle to cease contractions

B. **Therapeutic Use**

1. Stop preterm labor

TOCOLYTIC MEDICATIONS

Terbutaline sulfate

SIDE/ADVERSE EFFECTS	Nervousness	Hyperglycemia
	Tremulousness	Severe palpitations
	Headache	Chest pain
	Nausea and vomiting	Pulmonary edema
NURSING INTERVENTIONS	Monitor contractions and FHT	
	Monitor vital signs	
	Do not administer if pulse rate greater than 130/min or client has chest pain	
	Administer beta blocking agent as antidote	

Nifedipine

SIDE/ADVERSE EFFECTS	Hypotension	Nausea
	Headache	Flushing
NURSING INTERVENTIONS	Monitor BP	
	Avoid concurrent use with magnesium sulfate	
	Monitor contractions and FHT	
	Prevent complication with hypotension	

Magnesium sulfate

SIDE/ADVERSE EFFECTS	Warmth	Diminished DTRs
	Flushing	Decreased urine output
	Respiratory depression	Pulmonary edema
NURSING INTERVENTIONS	Monitor vital signs and DTRs	
	Monitor magnesium levels (therapeutic range 4 to 8 mg/dL)	
	Administer via infusion pump in diluted form	
	Use indwelling catheter to monitor urinary elimination	
	Administer calcium gluconate 10% for signs of toxicity	

V Antenatal Steroids—Betamethasone

A. **Action:** Stimulate production of surfactant in fetus between 24 and 34 weeks gestation

B. **Therapeutic Use**

1. Promote fetal lung maturity in preterm labor when delivery is likely

C. **Side/Adverse Effects**

1. Fluid retention

2. Elevated blood pressure

3. Maternal hyperglycemia and transient increase in WBC

D. **Nursing Interventions and Client Education**

1. Administer two doses (usually IM) 24 hr apart (repeat doses not recommended).

2. Provide emotional support to family.

VI Medications for the Postpartum Client

A. **Rho(D) Immune Globulin (RhoGAM)**

1. **Action:** Suppresses the stimulation of active immunity by Rh-positive foreign red blood cells that enter the maternal circulation at the time of delivery

2. **Therapeutic Use**

a. Rh factor incompatibility to prevent sensitization for subsequent pregnancies

3. **Precautions**

a. Confirm that the mother is Rh-negative.

b. Never administer the IGIM full-dose or microdose products intravenously.

c. Never administer to a neonate.

4. **Nursing Interventions and Client Education**

a. RhoGAM is administered within 72 hr after birth, if indicated (woman is Rh negative, newborn is Rh positive, and Coombs test is negative).

b. RhoGAM is also administered as an injection prophylactically at 28 weeks gestation and after any event where fetal cells can mix with maternal blood.

1) Miscarriage

2) Ectopic pregnancy

3) Induced abortion

4) Amniocentesis

5) Chorionic villus sampling (CVS)

6) Abdominal trauma

B. **Varicella Vaccine**

1. Women who are not immune to varicella should be immunized in the postpartum period.

2. Instruct client to use reliable form of contraception and avoid pregnancy for 3 months.

Complementary and Alternative Therapies

I Safety and Efficacy

A. **The Dietary Supplement Health and Education Act limits the U.S. Food and Drug Administration's (FDA) control over dietary supplements.**

1. Many herbal drug companies make claims based on their own studies, indicating health benefits from using herbal drugs.

   a. These studies are not approved by the FDA.

   b. Labels on the herbal medications must include a disclaimer stating that the FDA has not approved the product for safety and effectiveness.

2. Herbal medications may interact with other medicines and produce serious adverse effects.

II Saw palmetto (*Serenoa repens*)

A. **Purported Use**

1. Treats and prevents benign prostatic hypertrophy (BPH)

B. **Side/Adverse Effects**

1. Headache

2. Altered platelet function

C. **Herb/Medication Interactions**

1. Additive effect with anticoagulants

D. **Studies**

1. Several well-conducted studies support the use of saw palmetto for reducing symptoms of BPH.

E. **Nursing Considerations**

1. Allow 4 to 6 weeks to see effects.

2. Discontinue use prior to surgery.

III Valerian root

A. **Purported Uses**

1. Insomnia

2. Migraines

3. Menstrual cramps

B. **Side/Adverse Effects**

1. Drowsiness

2. Headache, nervousness with prolonged use

C. **Herb/Medication Interactions**

1. Additive effect with barbiturates and benzodiazepines

D. **Studies**

1. Several studies support the use of valerian for mild to moderate sleep disorders and mild anxiety.

E. **Nursing Considerations**

1. Advise client against driving or operating machinery.

2. Advise client against long-term use.

3. Discontinue valerian at least 1 week prior to surgery.

IV St. John's wort (*Hypericum perforatum*)

A. **Purported Uses**

1. Depression

2. Seasonal affective disorder

3. Anxiety

B. **Side/Adverse Effects**

1. Headache

2. Sleep disturbances

3. Phototoxicity (long-term use)

4. Constipation

C. **Herb/Medication Interactions**

1. Many interactions with other medications

   a. Oral contraceptives

   b. Cyclosporine

   c. Warfarin

   d. Reduced antiretroviral effects

   e. Digoxin

   f. Calcium channel blockers

   g. Antidepressants

D. **Studies**

1. Several well-conducted studies support the use of St. John's wort for mild to moderate depression.

E. **Nursing Considerations**

1. St. John's wort has many medication interactions and should not be taken with other medications.

2. Should not be used to treat severe depression.

3. Should only be used with medical guidance.

V Echinacea (*Echinacea purpurea*)

A. **Purported Uses**

1. Prevents and treats the common cold

2. Stimulates the immune system

3. Promotes wound healing

B. **Side/Adverse Effects**

1. Fever and nausea (rare)

2. Anaphylaxis in susceptible individuals

C. **Herb/Medication Interactions**

1. May reduce the effects of immunosuppressants

2. May increase serum levels of alprazolam, calcium channel blockers, and protease inhibitors

D. **Studies**

1. Well-conducted studies have conflicted as to the effectiveness of echinacea in the treatment of the common cold.

E. **Nursing Considerations**

1. Long-term use may cause immunosuppression.

VI Garlic

A. Purported Uses

1. Blocks LDL cholesterol and raises HDL cholesterol; lowers triglycerides
2. Suppresses platelet aggregation and disrupts coagulation
3. Acts as a vasodilator (can lower blood pressure)

B. Herb/Medication Interactions

1. An increased risk of bleeding in clients taking NSAIDs, warfarin, and heparin
2. Decreases levels of saquinavir (a medication for HIV treatment) and cyclosporine

C. Nursing Considerations

1. Question clients about concurrent use of NSAIDs, heparin, and warfarin.
2. Have clients who are taking antiplatelet or anticoagulant medication, cyclosporine, or saquinavir contact their provider prior to taking garlic as a supplement.

VII Ginger root

A. Purported Uses

1. Relieves vertigo and nausea
2. Increases intestinal motility
3. Increases gastric mucus production
4. Decreases GI spasms
5. Produces an anti-inflammatory effect
6. Suppresses platelet aggregation
7. Used to treat morning sickness, motion sickness, nausea from surgery
8. Can decrease pain and stiffness of rheumatoid arthritis

B. Herb/Medication Interactions

1. Use cautiously in clients who are pregnant because high doses can cause uterine contractions
2. Interacts with medications that interfere with coagulation (NSAIDs, warfarin, and heparin)
3. Can increase hypoglycemic effects of diabetes

C. Nursing Considerations

1. Question clients about concurrent use with NSAIDs, heparin, and warfarin.
2. Monitor for hypoglycemia if the client takes insulin or other medication for diabetes.

VIII Ginkgo (*Ginkgo biloba*)

A. Purported Uses

1. Improves cerebral circulation to treat dementia and memory loss
2. Decreases pain with walking in clients who have PAD

B. Side/Adverse Effects

1. Dizziness
2. Stomach upset
3. Vertigo

C. Herb/Medication Interactions

1. May increase the effects of MAOIs, anticoagulants, and antiplatelet aggregates
2. May reduce the effectiveness of insulin

D. Studies

1. Studies conflict as to the effectiveness of ginkgo in all purported uses.

E. Nursing Considerations

1. Discontinue 2 weeks prior to surgery.
2. May cause seizures with overdose.
3. Keep out of the reach of children.

IX Glucosamine (2-Amino-2-deoxyglucose)

A. Purported Uses

1. Relieves osteoarthritis
2. Promotes joint health

B. Side/Adverse Effects

1. Nausea
2. Heartburn

C. Herb/Medication Interactions

1. May increase resistance to antidiabetic agents and insulin
2. May increase risk of bleeding. Use cautiously with clients on anticoagulants

D. Studies

1. Several studies support the use of glucosamine in reducing the symptoms of osteoarthritis in the knees.

E. Nursing Considerations

1. Use glucosamine with caution in clients who have a shellfish allergy.
2. Monitor glucose frequently in clients who have diabetes mellitus.
3. Allow extended time to see the effects of glucosamine.
4. Used often in combination with chondroitin.

X Omega-3 fatty acids

A. **Purported Uses**

  1. Improves hypertriglyceridemia

  2. Helps maintain cardiac health

B. **Side/Adverse Effects**

  1. Nausea

  2. Diarrhea

C. **Herb/Medication Interactions**

  1. May increase risk of vitamin A or D overdose

D. **Studies**

  1. Several well-conducted studies support the use of omega-3 fatty acids in reducing blood triglyceride levels, preventing cardiovascular disease in clients who have a history of a heart attack, and slightly reducing blood pressure.

  2. Studies support improvement in symptoms of bipolar disorder.

E. **Nursing Considerations**

  1. Omega-3 fatty acids are found in fish oils, nuts, and vegetable oils.

  2. Some fish contain methylmercury and polychlorinated biphenyls (PCBs) that can be harmful in large amounts, especially in women who are pregnant or nursing.

XI Melatonin

A. **Purported Use**

  1. Treats insomnia and jet lag

B. **Side/Adverse Effects**

  1. Morning grogginess

  2. Lower body temperature

  3. Vivid dreams

C. **Herb/Medication Interactions**

  1. Beta blockers

  2. Warfarin

  3. Steroids

D. **Studies**

  1. Several studies support antioxidant effects.

E. **Nursing Considerations**

  1. Pregnant or nursing women should not take melatonin.

XII Nursing Assessments for Herbal Medications

A. **Ask the client specifically about herbal medications, vitamins, or other supplements during the client interview.**

B. **Over-the-counter medications are often not considered medications by the client.**

C. **Nursing Interventions**

  1. Instruct the client that herbal medications and supplements are not regulated by the FDA, often interact with other medications, and may cause serious adverse effects.

  2. Instruct the client that it is important to use herbal medications and supplements cautiously and with medical supervision.

  3. Discourage use in pregnant and nursing mothers, infants, young children, and older adults who have cardiovascular or liver disease.

HERBS AND PURPORTED USES

Match the following herbs with their purported use.

1. Treat and prevent benign prostatic hypertrophy
2. Manage migraines, insomnia, and menstrual cramps
3. Treat depression, seasonal affective disorder, and anxiety
4. Prevent and treat the common cold, stimulate immune system
5. Improve cerebral circulation
6. Relieve osteoarthritis and promote joint health
7. Improve hypertriglyceridemia and maintain cardiac health
8. Manage insomnia and jet lag
9. Relieves vertigo and nausea

A. Glucosamine
B. Echinacea
C. Ginkgo
D. Omega-3 fatty acids
E. Ginger root
F. Saw palmetto
G. St. John's wort
H. Valerian root
I. Melatonin

Answer Key: 1. F; 2. H; 3. G; 4. B; 5. C; 6. A; 7. D; 8. I; 9. E

UNIT FIVE

Fundamentals for Nursing

Client Safety

I Falls

A significant number of reported facility accidents are related to falls. The nurse is accountable for implementation of essential actions to reduce the risk associated with falls.

A. **Contributing Factors**

  1. Identify characteristics that increase risk for falls:
     a. Older age
     b. Impaired mobility
     c. Cognitive and/or sensory impairment
     d. Bowel and bladder dysfunction
     e. Adverse effects of medications
     f. History of falls

B. **Nursing Interventions**

  1. Complete a fall risk assessment upon admission and update as needed. An individualized plan of care should be completed based on the fall-risk assessment. (See the worksheet at the end of the Fundamentals section to complete a fall risk assessment.)
  2. Communicate identified risks with the health care team.
  3. Assign clients at risk for falls to a room close to the nurses' station and assess frequently.
  4. Provide the client with nonskid footwear.
  5. Keep the floor free of clutter and maintain an unobstructed path to the bathroom.
  6. Orient the client to the setting (grab bars, call light), including how to locate and use all necessary items.
  7. Maintain the bed in a low position.
  8. Instruct a client who is unsteady to use the call light for assistance before ambulating.
  9. Answer call lights promptly to prevent clients who are at risk from trying to ambulate independently.
  10. Provide adequate lighting (such as a nightlight for necessary trips to the bathroom).
  11. Determine the client's ability to use assistive devices (e.g., walkers, canes). Keep all items within reach.
  12. Use chair or bed sensors for clients who are at risk of getting up unattended.
  13. Lock wheels on beds, wheelchairs, and gurneys to prevent rolling during transfers or stops.
  14. Report and document all incidents per the facility's policy.

II Restraints

A. **Current client safety standards focus on reducing the need for client restraints.** The type or technique of restraint or seclusion used must be the least restrictive intervention that will be effective to protect the client, staff members, or others from harm.

B. **Definition:** Restraints include human, mechanical, chemical, or physical devices that restrict freedom of movement or diminish the client's access to parts of the body.

C. **Nursing Interventions**

  1. Implement nonpharmacologic measures such as distraction, frequent observation, or diversion activities.
  2. Prior to application, review manufacturer's instructions for correct application.
  3. Notify the provider immediately when restraints are implemented.
  4. Remove the restraints and assess client every 2 hr.
  5. Assess neurovascular and neurosensory status every 2 hr.
  6. Leave the restraint loose enough to prevent injury.
  7. Always tie the restraint to the bed frame (using loose knots that are easily removed).
  8. Reassess the need for continued use. Providers may renew the prescription with a maximum of 24 hr of consecutive use.
  9. Document:
     a. Behaviors making restraint necessary.
     b. Alternatives attempted and the client's behavior while in restraints.
     c. Type and location of the restraint and time applied.
     d. Frequency and type of care (e.g., range of motion, removal, assessment of skin, and neurovascular status).
  10. Restraints and/or seclusion should **never**:
     a. Interfere with treatment.
     b. Be used for staff convenience, client punishment, or for clients who are physically or emotionally unstable.

III Seizure Precautions

Seizures may have a sudden onset and include loss of consciousness, violent tonic-clonic movements, or risk of injury to the client (head injury, aspiration, and falls).

A. **Nursing Interventions**

  1. Assess seizure history, noting frequency, presence of auras, and sequence of events.
  2. Identify precipitating factors that may exacerbate or lead to seizures.
  3. Review medication history. If routine lab work is required (such as phenytoin), when was last level drawn?
  4. Place rescue equipment at the client's bedside, including oxygen, an oral airway, and suction equipment.
  5. Establish IV or saline lock access for high-risk clients.
  6. Inspect the client's environment for items that may cause injury in the event of a seizure. Remove any unnecessary items from the immediate environment.
  7. At the onset of a seizure, position the client for safety, and remain with the client.
  8. If sitting or standing, ease the client to the floor. Protect the client's head. If the client is in bed, raise the side rails and pad for safety.
  9. Roll the client to the side with the head flexed slightly forward.
  10. Do not put anything in the client's mouth.
  11. Loosen restrictive clothing.
  12. Administer medications as prescribed.

13. Document precipitating behaviors or events and a description of the event (e.g., movements, loss of consciousness, loss of continence, injuries, mention of aura, postictal state).

14. Report the seizure to the provider.

Environmental Safety

I Fire

All staff must be instructed in fire response procedures.

A. **Nursing Interventions**

1. Know the facility's fire drill and evacuation plan.
2. Keep emergency numbers near or on the phone at all times.
3. Know the location of all fire alarms, extinguishers, and exits, including oxygen shut-off valves.
4. Follow the fire response sequence in the facility (**RACE**):
   a. **R** – Rescue: Protect and evacuate clients in immediate danger.
   b. **A** – Alarm: Activate the alarm and report the fire.
   c. **C** – Contain: Close doors or windows.
   d. **E** – Extinguish: Use correct fire extinguisher to eliminate the fire.
      1) **Class A:** paper, wood, cloth, or trash
      2) **Class B:** flammable liquids and gases
      3) **Class C:** electrical fires
5. Extinguish properly (**PASS**):
   a. **P** – Pull
   b. **A** – Aim
   c. **S** – Squeeze
   d. **S** – Sweep
6. Considerations for home health setting
   a. Post "No Smoking" signs.
   b. Assess for risk (e.g., oxygen therapy, smoking, electrical equipment).
   c. Teach client to develop a plan of action in the event of a fire, including a route of exit and a location where family members will meet.
   d. Instruct client to keep fire extinguisher accessible.
   e. Review "Stop, Drop, and Roll."

II Equipment

All staff should be alert for potential safety hazards.

A. **Nursing Interventions**

1. Electrical equipment must be grounded.
2. Do not overcrowd outlets.
3. The use of extension cords is not permitted in any client care areas.
4. Only use equipment for its intended purpose.
5. Regularly inspect equipment for frayed cords.
6. Disconnect all equipment prior to cleaning.

III Chemical Agents and Radiation

Nurses must review institutional guidelines and follow all safety guidelines.

A. **Nursing Interventions**

1. Determine type and amount of radiation used.
2. Place a sign on door: "Caution: Radioactive Material."
3. Wear monitoring badge to record amount of exposure.
4. Wear appropriate protective equipment.
5. Dispose of items removed from the room in appropriate containers.
6. Never handle any type of radioactive agent with bare hands.

Ergonomics and Client Positioning

I Lifting and Transfer of Clients

Implement safe care using proper body mechanics when lifting, positioning, transporting, or assisting a client to reduce the risk of injury. Obtain proper training before using any mechanical lift device, and always follow manufacturers' recommendations for use.

A. **Nursing Interventions**

1. Assess mobility and strength.
2. Instruct client to assist when possible.
3. Use mechanical lift and assistive devices.
4. Avoid twisting the thoracic spine or bending at the waist.
5. Use major muscle groups, and tighten abdominal muscles.

II Client Transfer and Positioning

Maintain safe practices with client transfer and ensure proper positioning of clients to maintain good body alignment.

A. **Nursing Interventions**

1. Transferring clients from bed to chair or chair to bed
   a. Instruct the client on how to assist when possible.
   b. Lower the bed to the lowest setting.
   c. Position the bed or chair so that the client is moving toward the strong side.
   d. Assist the client to stand, then pivot.
2. Repositioning clients in bed
   a. Raise the bed to waist level.
   b. Lower side rails.
   c. Use slide boards or draw sheets.
   d. Have the client fold his arms across his chest while lifting the head off of the bed.
   e. Proceed in one smooth movement.
   f. Collaborate with other staff members for assistance.

Position: Semi-Fowler's

DESCRIPTION	Head of bed elevated to 30°
INDICATIONS	Gastric feedings, head injury, postoperative cranial surgery, increased intracranial pressure, respiratory illness, postoperative cataract removal

Position: Fowler's

DESCRIPTION	Head of bed elevated to 45° to 60°
INDICATIONS	Postoperative abdominal surgery, respiratory illness or cardiac problems with dyspnea, bleeding esophageal varices, postoperative thyroidectomy, cataract removal

Position: High-Fowler's

DESCRIPTION	Head of bed elevated to 90°
INDICATIONS	Respiratory illness with dyspnea, emphysema, status asthmaticus, pneumothorax, cardiac problems with dyspnea, feeding, hiatal hernia, during and after meals, insertion of nasogastric tube

Position: Supine

DESCRIPTION	Lying on back, head, and shoulders; slightly elevated with a small pillow
INDICATIONS	Spinal cord injury (no pillow)

Position: Prone

DESCRIPTION	Lying on abdomen, legs extended, and head turned to the side
INDICATIONS	Client who is immobilized or unconscious, post lumbar puncture 6 to 12 hr, post myelogram 12 to 24 hr (oil-based dye), postoperative tonsillectomy and adenoidectomy

Position: Lateral (side-lying)

DESCRIPTION	Lying on side with most of the body weight borne by the lateral aspect of the lower ilium
INDICATIONS	Post abdominal surgery, client who is unconscious, seizures (head to side), postoperative tonsillectomy and adenoidectomy, postoperative pyloric stenosis of the lower scapula and the lateral (right side), post liver biopsy (right side), rectal irrigations

Position: Sims' (semi-prone)

DESCRIPTION	Lying on left side with most of the body weight borne by the anterior aspect of the ilium, humerus, and clavicle
INDICATIONS	Client who is unconscious, enema administration

Position: Lithotomy

DESCRIPTION	Lying on the back with hips and knees flexed at right angles and feet in stirrups
INDICATIONS	Perineal, rectal, and vaginal procedures

Position: Trendelenburg

DESCRIPTION	Head and body lowered while feet are elevated
INDICATIONS	Some surgeries; during labor if umbilical cord pressure is trying to be relieved

Position: Modified Trendelenburg

DESCRIPTION	Supine with the legs elevated
INDICATIONS	Shock

Position: Reverse Trendelenburg

DESCRIPTION	Head elevated while feet are lowered
INDICATIONS	Cervical traction; to feed clients restricted to supine position, such as post cardiac catheterization

Position: Elevate one or more extremities

DESCRIPTION	Elevate legs/feet or arms/hands by adjusting or supporting with pillows
INDICATIONS	Thrombophlebitis, application of cast, edema, postoperative surgical procedure on extremity

Position: Dorsal Recumbent

DESCRIPTION	Supine with knees flexed
INDICATIONS	Urinary catheterization of female, abdominal assessment, abdominal wound evisceration

SECTION 4

Assistive Devices for Ambulation

Definition: Used to provide an extension of the upper extremities to help transmit body weight and provide support for the client (e.g., canes, crutches, walkers)

A. **Collaborative Care**
1. Nursing Interventions
   a. Determine mobility status and ability to bear weight per provider's prescription.
   b. Assess for the need of a safety belt.
   c. Instruct client to wear shoes with nonslip soles.
   d. Assess for risk of orthostatic hypotension.
   e. Provide safe environment free of clutter.

B. **Client Education and Referral**
1. Avoid rapid position changes to prevent orthostatic hypotension.
2. Inspect rubber tips on the device for wear and replace as needed.
3. Physical therapy consult.

C. **Crutches**
1. Assess client for correct fit of crutches: approximately 3 finger widths between the axilla and top of the crutch.
2. Position hands on hand grips with elbows flexed at 30°. (Do not bear weight on axilla.)

D. **Crutches: Non-weight bearing**
1. Begin in the tripod position, maintain weight on the "unaffected" (weight bearing) extremity.
2. Advance both crutches and the affected extremity.
3. Move the unaffected weight-bearing foot/leg forward (beyond the crutches).
4. Advance both crutches, and then the affected extremity.
5. Continue sequence, making steps of equal length.

E. **Crutches: Weight bearing**
1. Move crutches forward about one step's length.
2. Move "affected" leg forward, level with the crutch tips.
3. Move the "unaffected" leg forward.
4. Continue sequence, making steps of equal length.

BASIC TRIPOD POSITION

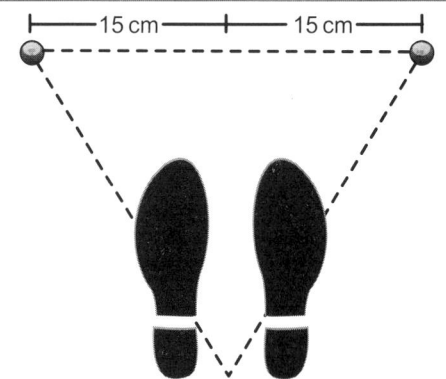

A. FOUR-POINT ALTERNATING GATE	B. THREE-POINT GAIT	C. TWO-POINT GAIT
Order of foot/crutch movement is shown with solid foot and crutch tips.	Unaffected leg bears weight. Weight bearing indicated with solid foot and crutch tips.	Weight partially distributed on each foot. Weight bearing indicated with solid foot and crutch tips.

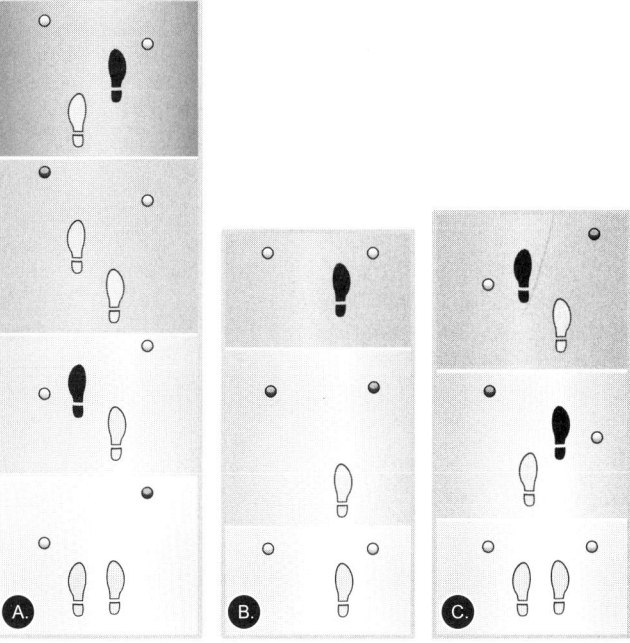

F. **Walking up stairs**
1. Hold onto rail with one hand and crutches with the other hand.
2. Push down on the stair rail and the crutches and step up with the unaffected leg.
3. If not allowed to place weight on the affected leg, hop up with the unaffected leg.
4. Bring the affected leg and the crutches up beside the unaffected leg.
5. Remember, the unaffected leg goes up first and the crutches move with the affected leg.

G. **Walking down stairs**
1. Place the affected leg and the crutches down on the step below; support weight by leaning on the crutches and the stair rail.
2. Bring the unaffected leg down.
3. Remember the affected leg goes down first and the crutches move with the affected leg.

H. **Cane**
1. For correct size, have the client wear shoes. The correct length is measured from the greater trochanter to the floor.
2. Cane is used on the unaffected (stronger) side to provide support to the opposite lower limb.
3. Move the cane forward 6 to 10 in, then move the weaker leg forward. Finally, advance the stronger leg past the cane.
4. Another method of cane walking includes having the client move the affected extremity and cane at the same time.

I. **Walker**
1. For correct size, have the client wear shoes. The client's wrists are even with the hand grips on the walker when arms are dangling downward.
2. Advance the walker approximately 12 inches.
3. Advance with the affected lower limb.
4. Move unaffected limb forward.
5. Assess appropriateness of a rolling walker if walker is being used for support due to overall weakness. A rolling walker is not appropriate for a client with Parkinson's disease due to shuffling gait.

Infection Control

All members of the health care team are accountable for adhering to measures to reduce the growth and transmission of infectious agents. According to the Centers for Disease Control and Prevention (CDC), hand hygiene is the single most important practice in preventing health care associated infections (HAIs).

CHAIN OF INFECTION

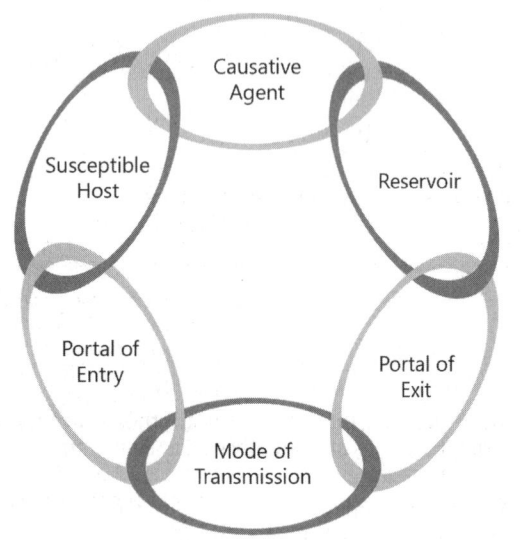

I Medical Asepsis (Clean Technique)

Precise practices to reduce the number, growth, and spread of microorganisms

 A. **Nursing Interventions**

1. Perform hand hygiene frequently.
2. Use personal protective equipment (PPE) as indicated.
3. Do not place items on the floor of client's room.
4. Do not shake linens.
5. Clean least soiled area first.
6. Place moist items in plastic bags.
7. Educate client and caregivers.

II Surgical Asepsis (Sterile Technique)

Precise practices to eliminate all microorganisms from an object or area (surgical technique)

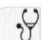 A. **Nursing Interventions**

1. Avoid coughing, sneezing, and talking directly over field.
2. Only dry, sterile items touch the field (1-inch border is nonsterile).
3. Keep all objects above the waist and within vision (do not turn back to sterile field).
4. Wash hands and don sterile gloves to perform procedure.

III Isolation Guidelines

A group of actions that include hand hygiene and the use of barrier precautions intended to reduce the transmission of infectious organisms

IV Standard Precautions (Tier One)

Applies to all body fluids, non-intact skin, and mucous membranes. Standard Precautions should be implemented for all clients.

A. **PPE:** As needed to prevent contact with body fluids: gloves, mask, gown, and goggles

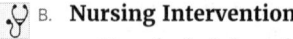 B. **Nursing Interventions**

1. Use alcohol-based waterless product after contact with client. Hand hygiene using soap is recommended when hands are visibly soiled or contaminated with blood or body fluids.
2. Determine need for client-specific, disease-specific precautions.
3. Provide education to health care team, clients, and visitors.
4. Report communicable diseases per CDC policy.
5. Handle all blood and body fluids as if contaminated.
6. Use PPE to reduce risk of transmission.
   a. Gown and gloves when touching blood or body fluids, non-intact skin, mucous membranes, or contaminated materials.
   b. Masks and face and eye protection when anticipating splashing of body fluids.
   c. PPE is disposed of in the client's room.
7. Consider room placement for client safety.
   a. Private room is needed only if client is unable to maintain hygiene.
   b. Cohort (client must have same organism).
      1) Avoid placing clients on isolation precautions in the same room with clients who are immunocompromised, have open wounds, or have anticipated prolonged lengths of stay.
      2) Ensure clients are located more than 3 ft from each other. (Use privacy curtain between beds to minimize opportunities for direct contact.)
      3) Change protective attire and perform hand hygiene between contact with clients in the same room, regardless of disease status.
8. Clean equipment according to facility policy.
9. Discard all needles and sharps in the appropriate containers; do not recap.
10. Place contaminated linens in the appropriate receptacle per the facility's policy.
11. Clean spills with a solution of bleach and water (1:10 dilution).

v *Transmission-Based Precautions (Tier Two)*

Transmission–based precautions are used in addition to standard precautions for clients who are known or suspected to be infected or colonized with infectious organisms.

A. **Airborne Precautions**

1. Diseases known to be transmitted by air for infectious agents smaller than 5 mcg (e.g., measles, varicella, pulmonary or laryngeal tuberculosis)

2. **PPE: Mask** (N95 respirator for known or suspected TB)

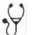

   a. **Nursing Interventions** (in addition to standard precautions)

   1) Provide private room with monitored negative airflow (i.e., air exchange and air discharge through HEPA filter).

   2) Keep door closed.

   3) Respiratory protection:

      a) The nurse must be FIT tested for N95 respirator.

      b) Apply a small, particulate mask (surgical mask) to the client if leaving room for medical necessity.

B. **Droplet Precautions**

1. Prevent the transmission of pathogens spread through close contact with mucous membranes or respiratory secretions.

2. Protect against droplets larger than 5 mcg (e.g., streptococcal pharyngitis, pneumonia, scarlet fever, rubella, pertussis, mumps, mycoplasma pneumonia, meningococcal pneumonia/sepsis, pneumonic plague).

3. **PPE: Mask**

   a. **Nursing Interventions** (in addition to standard precautions)

   1) Private room preferred, may cohort with client who has infection with same organism.

   2) Keep door closed.

   3) Mask is required when personnel is within 3 ft of the client.

C. **Contact Precautions** (includes enteric precautions)

1. Prevent transmission of infectious agents that are spread by direct or indirect contact with the client or the client's environment. These precautions are applied in the presence of wound drainage, fecal incontinence, or other bodily discharges that suggest an increased potential for environmental contamination and risk of transmission.

2. **PPE: Gloves, gown; as-needed use of mask and goggles**

   a. **Nursing Interventions** (in addition to standard precautions)

   1) Private room preferred; may cohort with client who has infection with same organism

   2) Gloves and gown worn by caregivers and visitors

   3) Disposal of infectious dressing material into nonporous bag

   4) Dedicated equipment for the client or disinfect after each use

   5) Client to leave room only for essential clinical reasons

3. **Protective Isolation**

   a. Used to protect clients who have an increased susceptibility to infections, are receiving chemotherapy, or are immunosuppressed or neutropenic

   b. **Nursing Interventions**

   1) Follow standard precautions.

   2) Institute maximum protection, which may include the use of sterile linens, food, and other supplies.

   3) Minimize exposure to microorganisms found on the outer layers of fresh flowers, fruits, and vegetables.

   4) Wear sterile gloves and gown/mask when in contact with client.

   5) Maximum protection will require ventilated/positive pressure room.

ORDER OF PPE APPLICATION / ORDER OF PPE REMOVAL

ORDER OF PPE APPLICATION	ORDER OF PPE REMOVAL
GOES UP THE BODY, THEN TO HANDS	REMOVAL IS IN ALPHABETICAL ORDER
Gown: Cover body from the bottom of the neck to the knees and wrists. Fasten securely behind the neck and at waist.	**Gloves:** Extend arms and slowly peel one glove downward, turning it inside out. With the ungloved hand, slide a finger under the inside portion of the remaining glove, turning inside out, and discard.
Mask: Secure with ties or elastic. Pinch the flexible bridge to secure at nose. Must extend below and under the chin.	**Goggles/face shield:** Grasp the ear pieces or headband only to remove.
Goggles/face shield: Verify fit is secure to prevent slipping.	**Gown:** Unfasten neck, then waist ties; pull gown forward away from the body, folding it inside out and rolling it into a bundle for disposal.
Gloves: Use correct size for a snug fit. Must extend upward to completely cover the wrist portion of the gown.	**Mask:** Remove by only touching ties. Take care not to touch the front of the mask.

PRECAUTIONS REQUIRED FOR SPECIFIC DISEASE PROCESS

AIDS/HIV*

PRECAUTIONS	Standard
DURATION OF PRECAUTIONS	Duration of illness
RESERVOIR	Blood and body fluids, including breast milk
NURSING CONSIDERATIONS	PPE if in contact with potentially contaminated materials; transmission in health care setting is rare with adherence to proper sterilization and disinfection guidelines

Chickenpox (varicella)*

PRECAUTIONS	Standard/airborne/contact
DURATION OF PRECAUTIONS	Until lesions crust over
RESERVOIR	Lesions, respiratory secretions
NURSING CONSIDERATIONS	Persons who are pregnant or have not had chickenpox or the vaccine should not care for the client.

*Disease that must be reported to the CDC

Clostridium difficile

PRECAUTIONS	Standard/contact (enteric precautions)
DURATION OF PRECAUTIONS	Duration of illness
RESERVOIR	Feces
NURSING CONSIDERATIONS	Staff and visitors must don PPE upon entry to the room. Private room preferred. May cohort; must provide a dedicated toilet for each client. Maintain precautions for duration of diarrhea.

Hepatitis A*

PRECAUTIONS	Standard/contact if client has fecal incontinence
DURATION OF PRECAUTIONS	Until 7 days after onset of jaundice
RESERVOIR	Feces
NURSING CONSIDERATIONS	Contact precautions used, particularly for clients wearing diapers or who are incontinent; can be spread up to 2 weeks before symptomatic.

Hepatitis B*

PRECAUTIONS	Standard
DURATION OF PRECAUTIONS	Duration of illness
RESERVOIR	Blood and body fluids infected with hepatitis B virus
NURSING CONSIDERATIONS	Contact precautions for blood and body fluids; follow disinfection and sterilization guidelines for reusable equipment.

Hepatitis C*

PRECAUTIONS	Standard – additional precautions specific to hemodialysis unit
DURATION OF PRECAUTIONS	Duration of illness
RESERVOIR	Blood and body fluids infected with hepatitis C virus
NURSING CONSIDERATIONS	Contact precautions for blood and body fluids; follow disinfection and sterilization guidelines for reusable equipment.

Herpes simplex (recurrent oral, skin, genital)

PRECAUTIONS	Standard/contact
DURATION OF PRECAUTIONS	Until lesions crust over
RESERVOIR	Fluid from lesions
NURSING CONSIDERATIONS	Horizontal transmission from contact with skin and secretions; vertical transmission from mother to child in utero or childbirth.

*Disease that must be reported to the CDC

Herpes zoster (shingles) – disseminated or localized in clients who are immunocompromised

PRECAUTIONS	Standard/airborne/contact
DURATION OF PRECAUTIONS	Duration of illness or with visible lesions
RESERVOIR	Lesions
NURSING CONSIDERATIONS	Persons who have not had chickenpox or the vaccine should not provide care.

Measles (Rubeola virus)*

PRECAUTIONS	Standard/airborne
DURATION OF PRECAUTIONS	Duration of illness
RESERVOIR	Respiratory secretions
NURSING CONSIDERATIONS	Virus can live on infected surfaces for up to 2 hr. Contagious from 4 days before to 4 days after the rash appears; nonimmune individuals must be excluded from areas of outbreak (e.g., school, hospital, childcare) until 21 days after onset of rash in diagnosed case of measles, unless they receive post-exposure prophylaxis.

Meningococcal disease*

PRECAUTIONS	Standard/droplet
DURATION OF PRECAUTIONS	Until 24 hr therapy; continuous
RESERVOIR	Respiratory secretions
NURSING CONSIDERATIONS	Post-exposure prophylaxis is recommended to control outbreaks.

Methicillin-resistant Staphylococcus aureus (MRSA)

PRECAUTIONS	Standard/contact
DURATION OF PRECAUTIONS	Duration of illness
RESERVOIR	Body fluids and sites contaminated with MRSA
NURSING CONSIDERATIONS	Spread by direct contact with wound; can lead to complicated infections, sepsis, and pneumonia.

Pneumonia

PRECAUTIONS	Standard/droplet
DURATION OF PRECAUTIONS	Until culture is negative
RESERVOIR	Respiratory secretions
NURSING CONSIDERATIONS	Consider organism-specific precautions as indicated; Streptococcus pneumoniae, invasive disease must be reported to CDC.

Respiratory syncytial virus

PRECAUTIONS	Standard/contact/droplet
DURATION OF PRECAUTIONS	Duration of illness
RESERVOIR	Respiratory secretions

*Disease that must be reported to the CDC

PRECAUTIONS REQUIRED FOR SPECIFIC DISEASE PROCESS (CONTINUED)

NURSING CONSIDERATIONS	Contact/droplet precautions; palivizumab for high risk infants; follow established guidelines for administration of ribavirin.

Rotavirus

PRECAUTIONS	Standard/contact
DURATION OF PRECAUTIONS	Duration of illness
RESERVOIR	Feces
NURSING CONSIDERATIONS	Rotavirus vaccine effective in preventing severe disease in infants and young children; continue enteric precautions for 3 days after illness subsides.

Rubella*

PRECAUTIONS	Standard/droplet
DURATION OF PRECAUTIONS	7 days after onset of rash
RESERVOIR	Respiratory secretions
NURSING CONSIDERATIONS	Nonimmune pregnant women should not care for these clients.

Salmonellosis*

PRECAUTIONS	Standard/contact precautions
DURATION OF PRECAUTIONS	Duration of illness
RESERVOIR	Feces
NURSING CONSIDERATIONS	Increased risk of contamination while caring for children who are wearing diapers or incontinent.

Shigellosis (dysentery)*

PRECAUTIONS	Standard/contact precautions
DURATION OF PRECAUTIONS	Duration of illness
RESERVOIR	Feces
NURSING CONSIDERATIONS	Contact precautions used, particularly for children who are wearing diapers or incontinent.

Staphylococcus aureus (infection or colonization)

PRECAUTIONS	Standard/contact precautions
DURATION OF PRECAUTIONS	Duration of illness
RESERVOIR	Body fluids and sites contaminated with MRSA
NURSING CONSIDERATIONS	High-risk clients: immunocompromised, chronic disease, recent surgery, IV or indwelling catheter; risk for antibiotic resistance.

Tuberculosis (TB) (pulmonary)*

PRECAUTIONS	Standard/airborne precautions
DURATION OF PRECAUTIONS	Until three sputum smears are negative on consecutive days or TB is ruled out
RESERVOIR	Airborne respiratory droplet nuclei
NURSING CONSIDERATIONS	N95 mask; client wears surgical mask when transported outside of negative-airflow room.

*Disease that must be reported to the CDC

PRECAUTIONS REQUIRED FOR SPECIFIC DISEASE PROCESS (CONTINUED)

Vancomycin-resistant enterococci (VRE) (infection or colonization)*

PRECAUTIONS	Standard/contact precautions
DURATION OF PRECAUTIONS	Until three negative cultures from infectious site (1 week apart)
RESERVOIR	Intestines, female genital tract, and environment (normal flora)
NURSING CONSIDERATIONS	Most infections occur in hospital; can be spread by touching surfaces, such as equipment that contains VRE.

*Disease that must be reported to the CDC

Point to Remember

If moving clients to other areas of the facility, have the client wear a surgical mask if they have an airborne or droplet infection. Assure all draining wounds are covered.

SECTION 6

Health Promotion and Disease Prevention

Nurses contribute greatly to the health of clients and population groups using health promotion and disease prevention strategies. Nursing care of the client incorporates knowledge of early detection of disease and actions to promote optimal health.

Health Promotion

Includes client education, health risk assessment, wellness assessment, lifestyle and behavior changes, and environmental control programs

HEALTH PROMOTION AND DISEASE PREVENTION

PREVENTIVE CARE	EXAMPLES OF PREVENTION ACTIVITIES
Primary prevention: Focus is on promoting health and preventing disease.	Immunization programs Child car seat education Nutrition and fitness activities Health education programs
Secondary prevention: Focus is on early identification of illness, providing treatment, and conducting activities geared to prevent a worsening health status.	Communicable disease screening and case finding Early detection and treatment of hypertension Exercise programs for older adults who are frail
Tertiary prevention: Focus is on preventing long-term consequences of chronic illness or disability and supporting optimal functioning.	Prevention of pressure ulcers as a complication of spinal cord injury Promoting independence for a client following stroke

II Disease Prevention

A. Nursing Interventions

1. Conduct a risk factor assessment.
2. Educate clients to follow standards for recommended screenings.
3. Identify lifestyle risk behaviors requiring modification.
4. Encourage client to continue health–promoting behaviors.
5. Instruct client about preventive immunizations.

SCREENING GUIDELINES*

TEST	FEMALE	MALE
Routine physical	20 to 40 years Annually	20 to 40 years Every 3 to 5 years Annually at age 40
Dental assessments	Every 6 months	Every 6 months
Blood pressure	Begin age 20 Minimum every 2 years Annually if higher than 120/80 mm Hg	Begin age 20 Minimum every 2 years Annually if higher than 120/80 mm Hg
Body mass index (BMI)	Begin age 20 Each health care visit	Begin age 20 Each health care visit
Blood cholesterol	Begin age 20 Minimum every 5 years (if no risk factors)	Begin age 20 Minimum every 5 years (if no risk factors)
Blood glucose	Begin age 45 Minimum every 3 years	Begin age 45 Minimum every 3 years
Colorectal screening	Fecal occult blood annually begin age 50 AND Flexible sigmoidoscopy every 5 years*, or Colonoscopy every 10 years, or Double-contrast barium enema every 5 years*, or CT colonography (virtual colonoscopy) every 5 years **NOTE:** Frequency may increase based upon results.	Fecal occult blood annually begin age 50 AND Flexible sigmoidoscopy every 5 years*, or Colonoscopy every 10 years, or Double-contrast barium enema every 5 years*, or CT colonography (virtual colonoscopy) every 5 years **NOTE:** Frequency may increase based upon results.
Pap test	Ages 21 to 65 years: Papanicolaou test (Pap smear) every 3 years; at age 30, may decrease Pap screening to every 5 years if human papilloma virus screening performed, as well. No testing is needed after age 65 if previous testing was normal and not high risk for cervical cancer.	n/a
Clinical breast exam	Begin at age 20, every 3 years Begin at age 40, yearly	n/a
Mammogram	Begin age 40, yearly Ages 55 and older may choose to have mammogram every 1 to 2 years.	n/a
Prostate-specific antigen test and digital rectal exam	n/a	Annual digital rectal examination (DRE) and prostate specific antigen (PSA) blood test.
Testicular exam	n/a	Begin age 15 Monthly testicular self-exam, clinical testicular exam at each routine visit.

*American Diabetes Association, American Heart Association, American Cancer Society, and National Institutes of Health, CDC

FALL ASSESSMENT ACTIVITY

A 70-year-old client is admitted with infected diabetic ulceration of the right foot and possible fracture of the left arm after a fall at home. History reveals 36 pack-year history of smoking (stopped after MI), IDDM for 22 years, MI with CABG x three 2 years ago, and HTN. Current medications: insulin isophane, clopidogrel, metoprolol, furosemide, potassium chloride, zolpidem, and hydrocodone/acetaminophen PRN. **Based on the scenario, perform a fall assessment using the Morse Fall Scale below.**

Morse Fall Scale

		SCORE
1. History of falling; immediate or within 3 months	No = 0 Yes = 25	
2. Secondary diagnosis	No = 0 Yes = 15	
3. Ambulatory aid	None, bed rest, nurse = 0 Crutches, cane, walker = 15 Furniture = 30	
4. IV/heparin lock	No = 0 Yes = 20	
5. Gait/transferring	Normal, bed rest, immobile = 0 Weak = 10 Impaired = 20	
6. Mental status	Oriented to own ability = 0 Forgets limitations = 15	
	TOTAL:	

Risk Level:

According to the score, look at the risk level on chart below. Before viewing the interventions as instructed on the chart, identify five nursing actions you should implement for the client to minimize risk of falls.

	RISK LEVEL	MFS SCORE	ACTION
1.	No Risk	0 to 24	None
2.	Low Risk	25 to 50	See *Standard Fall Prevention Interventions on following page*
3.			
4.	High Risk	51 or greater	See *High-Risk Fall Prevention Interventions on following page*
5.			

http://www.ahrq.gov/sites/default/files/publications/files/fallpxtoolkit.pdf

Answer key on next page.

STANDARD FALL PREVENTION INTERVENTIONS

Clients who are scored "low-risk" on the **Morse Fall Scale** (score of 25 to 50) will have the following interventions implemented by the nursing staff.

› Direct Care
  » Assess fall risk upon admission, change in status, transfer to another unit, and discharge.
  » Assign client to a bed that enables client to exit the bed toward client's stronger side whenever possible.
  » Assess coordination and balance before assisting with transfer and mobility activities.
  » Implement bowel and bladder programs to decrease urgency and incontinence.
  » Use treaded socks for all clients.

› All Staff
  » Approach client toward unaffected side to maximize participation in care.
  » Transfer client toward stronger side.

› Education
  » Actively engage client and family in all aspects of fall prevention program.
  » Instruct client in all activities prior to initiating assistive devices.
  » Teach client use of grab bars.
  » Instruct client in medication time/dose, side/adverse effects, and interactions with food/medications.

› Equipment
  » Lock all movable equipment before transferring clients.
  » Individualize equipment specific to client needs.

› Environment
  » Place client care articles within reach.
  » Provide physically safe environment (eliminate spills, clutter, electrical cords, and unnecessary equipment).
  » Provide adequate lighting.

HIGH-RISK FALL PREVENTION INTERVENTIONS

These interventions are designed to be implemented for clients with multiple fall risk factors and those who have fallen. These interventions are designed to reduce severity of injuries due to falls, as well as to prevent falls from reoccurring, supplementing standard fall prevention interventions.

› Equipment
  » Bed and/or chair alarms
  » Alarms at exits
  » Nurse call and communication systems
  » Low beds
  » Raised edge mattress
  » Video camera surveillance
  » Nonskid floor mat

› Environment
  » Clear client environment of all hazards

› Education
  » Exercise
  » Nutrition
  » Home safety
  » Plan for emergency fall notification procedure.

A 70-year-old client is admitted with infected diabetic ulceration of right foot. History reveals 36 pack-year history of smoking (stopped after MI), IDDM for 22 years, MI with CABG x three 2 years ago, and HTN. Current medications: insulin isophane, clopidogrel, metoprolol, furosemide, potassium chloride, zolpidem, and hydrocodone/acetaminophen PRN. Based on the scenario, perform a fall assessment using the Morse Fall Scale below.

Answers to Fall Assessment Activity Answers

1. 25; 2. 15; 3. 0; 4. 0; 5. 0; Total: 40

Risk Level: Low Risk (answers may be any of the options below)

  1. Call light in reach
  2. Bed in low position
  3. Use nonskid footwear
  4. Assist client with transfers/ambulation
  5. Assess for need of ambulation devices
  6. Adequate lighting including night lights
  7. Promptly enter to assist client when called
  8. Monitor blood sugars before meals and at bedtime
  9. Monitor for possible orthostatic BP after pain medications
  10. Assess sensations in lower extremities due to impaired circulation

UNIT SIX

Adult Medical Surgical Nursing

Fluids and Electrolytes

Fluids and Electrolytes

Nurses should review the client's health history and laboratory data and perform a clinical assessment. Many health problems can cause changes in balance of fluids and electrolytes. The nurse should be prepared to manage the client with imbalances.

A. **Body Fluids**

1. Adults: 50% to 60% of total body weight is water
2. Infants: 75% to 80% of total body weight is water
3. Two-thirds of body fluid is intracellular (ICF)
4. One-third of body fluid is extracellular (ECF)

NOTE: 1 kg (2.2 lb) of body weight is approximate to 1 L of fluid.

Fluid Imbalance

A. **Fluid Volume Deficit (FVD)**

1. Fluid intake is less than needed to meet body requirements. The most common type is isotonic dehydration.
2. Contributing Factors
   a. Excess GI and/or renal loss
   b. Diaphoresis
   c. Fever
   d. Long-term NPO
   e. Hemorrhage
   f. Insufficient intake
   g. Burns
   h. Diuretic therapy
   i. Aging: Older adults have less body water and decreased thirst sensation.
3. Manifestations
   a. Weight loss
   b. Dry mucous membranes
   c. Increased heart rate and respirations
   d. Thready pulse
   e. Capillary refill less than 3 seconds
   f. Weakness, fatigue
   g. Orthostatic hypotension
   h. Poor skin turgor
   i. LATE SIGNS: Oliguria, decreased CVP, flattened neck veins
4. Diagnostic Procedures
   a. Serum electrolytes, BUN, creatinine, Hct (Hct may be high due to hemoconcentration.)
   b. Urine: specific gravity and osmolarity

5. **Collaborative Care and Nursing Int.**
   a. Monitor vital signs, pulse quality, a..
   b. Monitor skin turgor. In older adults, che over sternum or forehead.
   c. Maintain strict I&O. Output should be at least 0.5 mL/kg/hr.
   d. Weigh client daily.
   e. Monitor laboratory data.
   f. Correct underlying cause.
   g. Fluid replacement:
      1) Increase oral fluid intake; initiate oral rehydration solution.
      2) IV fluids for severe dehydration/maintain as prescribed.
      3) Monitor response to therapy.
   h. Initiate fall precautions.
6. Medications
   a. Electrolyte replacement
   b. Intravenous fluids

INTRAVENOUS FLUIDS

Isotonic

INDICATION	Treatment of vascular system fluid deficit
CHARACTERISTICS	Concentration equal to plasma Prevent fluid shift between compartments
SOLUTIONS	Normal saline (0.9% NS) Lactated Ringer's (LR) 5% dextrose in water (D_5W)

Hypotonic

INDICATION	Treatment of intracellular dehydration
CHARACTERISTICS	Lower osmolality than the ECF Shift fluid from ECF to ICF
SOLUTIONS	0.45% normal saline (0.45% NS) 2.5% dextrose in 0.45% saline ($D_{2.5}45\%$ NS)

Hypertonic

INDICATION	Used only when serum osmolality is critically low
CHARACTERISTICS	Osmolality higher than the ECF Shift fluid from ICF to ECF
SOLUTIONS	10% dextrose in water ($D_{10}W$) 50% dextrose in water ($D_{50}W$) 5% dextrose in 0.9% saline (D_5NS) 5% dextrose in 0.45% saline (D_5W in 0.45% NaCl) 5% dextrose in lactated Ringer's (D_5LR)

Fluid Volume Excess (FVE)

1. Fluid intake or retention is greater than the body's needs.
2. Contributing Factors
   a. Kidney failure (late phase)
   b. Heart failure
   c. Cirrhosis
   d. Interstitial to plasma fluid shifts (e.g., hypertonic fluids, burns)
   e. Excessive water intake
   f. Long-term corticosteroid therapy
3. Manifestations
   a. Cough, dyspnea, crackles
   b. Increased blood pressure
   c. Tachypnea and tachycardia
   d. Bounding pulse
   e. Weight gain (1 L water = 1 kg of weight)
   f. Jugular vein distention
   g. Increased central venous pressure
   h. Pitting edema
4. Diagnostic Procedures (may be decreased due to hemodilution)
   a. Serum: electrolytes, BUN, creatinine, Hct
   b. Urine: specific gravity and osmolarity
   c. Chest x-ray if respiratory complications present

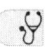

5. **Collaborative Care and Nursing Interventions**
   a. Monitor respiratory rate, symmetry, and effort.
   b. Monitor breath sounds for signs of pulmonary edema.
   c. Monitor for edema; measure pitting edema on scale of 1+ (minimal) to 4+ (severe); monitor dependent edema by measuring circumference of extremities.
   d. Monitor for ascites, and measure abdominal girth.
   e. Weigh the client daily.
   f. Maintain strict I&O.
   g. Monitor vital signs.
   h. Administer diuretics (osmotic, loop) as prescribed.
   i. Limit fluid intake.
   j. Maintain skin integrity.
   k. Use semi-Fowler's position; reposition every 2 hr.
   l. Restrict sodium intake.

III Electrolyte Imbalances

A. **Normal Electrolyte Ranges**
   1. Major Intracellular Electrolytes
      a. Potassium
      b. Phosphorus
      c. Magnesium
   2. Major Extracellular Electrolytes
      a. Sodium
      b. Calcium
      c. Chloride
      d. Bicarbonate

B. **Function**
   1. Maintain homeostasis.
   2. Promote neuromuscular excitability.
   3. Maintain fluid volume.
   4. Distribute water between fluid compartments.
   5. Maintain cardiac stability.
   6. Regulate acid–base balance.

MAJOR ELECTROLYTES: IMBALANCE/INTERVENTIONS

Potassium (K+): Hypokalemia

RISK FACTORS	Adverse effects of medications › Corticosteroids › Diuretics › Digitalis › Laxatives (abuse of)	Body fluid loss › Vomiting › Diarrhea › Wound drainage › NG suction	Excessive diaphoresis Kidney disease Dietary deficiency Alkalosis
MANIFESTATIONS	Muscle weakness, cramping Fatigue Nausea, vomiting	Irritability, confusion Decreased bowel motility Paresthesia	Dysrhythmias Flat and/or inverted T waves (ECG)
INTERVENTIONS	Monitor respiratory status. Initiate fall precautions. Initiate and monitor potassium replacement (oral, IV).	Monitor ECG. Monitor I&O. Monitor arterial HCO_3 and pH.	Provide client education. Dietary sources Medications
	NOTE: NEVER give K+ IV bolus; MUST dilute. NOTE: "No P = No K." If the client is not urinating, do NOT administer potassium.		

Potassium (K+): Hyperkalemia

RISK FACTORS	Renal failure Adrenal insufficiency	Acidosis Excessive potassium intake	Medications › Potassium-sparing diuretics › ACE inhibitors
MANIFESTATIONS	Peaked T-waves (ECG) Ventricular dysrhythmias	Muscle twitching and paresthesia (early) Ascending muscle weakness (late)	Increased bowel motility
INTERVENTIONS	Monitor ECG. Monitor bowel sounds. Initiate dialysis. Dietary restriction and teaching.	Administer medications. › Kayexalate (monitor bowel sounds) › 50% glucose with insulin › Calcium gluconate	› Bicarbonate › Loop diuretics

Sodium (Na+): Hyponatremia

RISK FACTORS	GI loss SIADH Adrenal insufficiency NPO status	Restricted sodium diet Water intoxication Excessive diaphoresis	Medications › Diuretics › Anticonvulsants › SSRIs › Lithium › Demeclocycline
MANIFESTATIONS	Weakness Lethargy Confusion Seizures	Headache Anorexia, nausea, vomiting Muscle cramps, twitching Hypotension	Tachycardia Weight gain, edema
INTERVENTIONS	Sodium replacement (oral, GI tube, IV) Restrict oral fluid intake.	Daily weight I&O	Medication: conivaptan hydrochloride Seizure precautions
	NOTE: Risk with hypertonic solutions—cerebral edema		

Sodium (Na+): Hypernatremia

RISK FACTORS	Dehydration GI loss Hyperaldosteronism	Hypertonic tube feedings Diabetes insipidus Kidney failure	Burns Heatstroke Corticosteroids
MANIFESTATIONS	Fever Swollen, dry tongue Sticky mucous membranes Hallucinations	Lethargy, restlessness, irritability Seizures Tachycardia Hypertension	Hyperreflexia, twitching Pulmonary edema
INTERVENTIONS	Daily weight I&O Seizure precautions	IV infusion of hypotonic or isotonic fluid Diuretics	Dietary sodium restriction and education Increased oral fluid intake

MAJOR ELECTROLYTES: IMBALANCE/INTERVENTIONS (CONTINUED)

Calcium (Ca⁺⁺): Hypocalcemia

RISK FACTORS	Hypoparathyroidism Hypomagnesemia Kidney failure	Vitamin D deficiency Inadequate intake GI loss (wound drainage, diarrhea)	Disease process › Celiac disease › Lactose intolerance › Crohn's disease › Alcohol use disorder
MANIFESTATIONS	Tetany, cramps Paresthesia Dysrhythmias	Trousseau's sign Chvostek's sign Seizures	Hyperreflexia Impaired clotting time
INTERVENTIONS	Seizure precautions IV calcium replacement	Daily calcium supplements Vitamin D therapy	Monitor for orthostatic hypotension. Dietary increase and education
	NOTE: IV calcium must be administered slowly and the site monitored for extravasation. It is diluted in D₅W, NEVER in NS.		

Calcium has an inverse relationship with phosphorus.

Calcium (Ca⁺⁺): Hypercalcemia

RISK FACTORS	Hyperparathyroidism Malignant disease Prolonged immobilization Dehydration	Vitamin D excess Thiazide diuretics Lithium Glucocorticoids	Digoxin toxicity Overuse of calcium supplements Hyperthyroidism
MANIFESTATIONS	Muscle weakness Hypercalciuria/kidney stones Dysrhythmias Lethargy/coma	Hyporeflexia Pathologic fractures Flank pain Deep bone pain	Polyuria, polydipsia, dehydration Hypertension Nausea, vomiting
INTERVENTIONS	Increase mobility Isotonic IVF Dialysis Cardiac monitoring	Medications › Furosemide › Calcitonin › Glucocorticoids	› Bisphosphonates › Calcium chelators

Calcium has an inverse relationship with phosphorus.

Magnesium (Mg⁺⁺): Hypomagnesemia

RISK FACTORS	GI loss Alcoholism Hypocalcemia Hypokalemia DKA	Hyperparathyroidism Malabsorption TPN Laxative abuse Acute MI	Medications › Cisplatin › Cyclosporine › Aminoglycoside antibiotics › Diuretics › Amphotericin B
MANIFESTATIONS	Paresthesias Dysrhythmias Trousseau's sign Chvostek's sign	Agitation, confusion Hyperreflexia Hypertension	Insomnia, irritability Anorexia, nausea, vomiting Dysphagia
INTERVENTIONS	Seizure precautions Monitor swallowing. Dietary measures and education	Administer medications. › IV magnesium sulfate › PO magnesium salts	Monitor urine output. Monitor respirations.
	NOTE: Monitor for signs of magnesium toxicity with IV replacement, and treat with calcium gluconate.		

Magnesium (Mg^{++}): Hypermagnesemia

RISK FACTORS	Renal failure	Adrenal insufficiency	Lithium toxicity
	Excessive Mg^{++} therapy	Laxative overuse	Extensive soft tissue injury or necrosis
MANIFESTATIONS	Hypotension	Bradypnea	Hyporeflexia
	Drowsiness	Coma	Nausea, vomiting
	Bradycardia	Cardiac arrest	Facial flushing
INTERVENTIONS	Mechanical ventilation	Administer medications.	Monitor respirations and blood pressure.
	IV fluids: lactated Ringer's or NS	› IV calcium gluconate	Monitor deep-tendon reflexes.
		› Loop diuretics	
	NOTE: Magnesium should not be administered to clients in renal failure.		

Phosphorus: Hypophosphatemia

RISK FACTORS	Vitamin D deficiency	Hypomagnesemia	TPN
	Refeeding after starvation	Hypokalemia	Overuse of antacids
	Alcohol use disorder	Excessive loss of body fluids: sweat, diarrhea, vomiting, hyperventilation	
	DKA		
	Alkalosis	Burns	
MANIFESTATIONS	Paresthesia	Chest pain	Seizures
	Muscle weakness	Confusion	Nystagmus
	Bone pain and deformities		
INTERVENTIONS	Oral phosphate replacement	Gradual introduction of solution for clients on TPN	Dietary management and education
	Careful IV administration of phosphorus (for severe cases)	Protect from infection.	Seizure precautions

Phosphorus has an inverse relationship with calcium.

Phosphorus: Hyperphosphatemia

RISK FACTORS	Renal failure	High vitamin D	Excessive enema use
	Chemotherapy	High phosphorus intake	Acidosis
	Acute pancreatitis	Hypoparathyroidism	
MANIFESTATIONS	Tetany, cramps	Trousseau's sign	Anorexia, nausea, vomiting
	Paresthesias	Chvostek's sign	Soft tissue calcifications
	Dysrhythmias	Hyperreflexia	
INTERVENTIONS	Medications	IV NS	
	› Vitamin D	Dialysis	
	› Aluminum hydroxide	Dietary management and education	
	› Diuretics		

Phosphorus has an inverse relationship with calcium.

IV Acid-Base Balance

A. **Definition:** Acid–base imbalances range from simple to complex. The four basic imbalances include the following.

ACID-BASE IMBALANCES

	PH	PCO$_2$	HCO$_3$
Normal value	7.35 to 7.45	35 to 45 mm Hg	21 to 28 mEq/L
Metabolic acidosis	↓	Normal	↓
Metabolic alkalosis	↑	Normal	↑
Respiratory acidosis	↓	↑	Normal
Respiratory alkalosis	↑	↓	Normal

B. **ROME:** "**R**espiratory **O**pposite, **M**etabolic **E**qual"

ROME

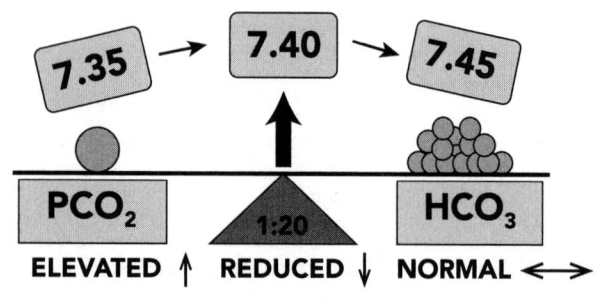

1. Remember the normal	2. Remember the possibilities	3. Use arrows
pH 7.35 to 7.45 PCO$_2$ 35 to 45 HCO$_3$ 21 to 28	Normal Abnormal (uncompensated) Partially compensated Fully compensated	Normal Elevated Reduced

Abnormals

Respiratory acidosis	Metabolic acidosis
Respiratory alkalosis	Metabolic alkalosis

Tips

If all three are normal, ABGs are NORMAL.

If two are abnormal, ABGs are fully compensated when pH has returned to normal and uncompensated when two values are abnormal.

If three are abnormal, ABGs are partially compensated or combined disorder.

C. **Regulation of acid–base balance is primarily controlled by:**

1. Lungs (regulate carbonic acid through respiration)
2. Kidneys (regulate bicarbonate by retention or excretion)

ACID-BASED IMBALANCE INTERVENTIONS

Metabolic Acidosis

RISK FACTORS	Diarrhea Fever Hypoxia Starvation Seizure	Overdose: salicylates or ethanol Renal failure DKA Dehydration
MANIFESTATIONS	Vital signs: bradycardia, weak pulses, hypotension, tachypnea Flaccid paralysis Confusion	Hyporeflexia Lethargy Warm, flushed, dry skin Kussmaul respirations
INTERVENTIONS	Treat underlying cause. Administer fluids, electrolytes.	

Metabolic Alkalosis

RISK FACTORS	Ingestion of antacids GI suction Hypokalemia	TPN Blood transfusion Prolonged vomiting
MANIFESTATIONS	Dizziness Paresthesia	Hypertonic muscles Decreased respirations
INTERVENTIONS	Treat underlying cause. Administer fluids, electrolytes.	

Respiratory Acidosis

RISK FACTORS	Respiratory depression Pneumothorax	Airway obstruction Inadequate ventilation
MANIFESTATIONS	Dizziness Palpitations	Muscle twitching Convulsions
INTERVENTIONS	Maintain patent airway. Reversal agents for narcotics	Regulation ventilation therapy Bronchodilators Mucolytics

Respiratory Alkalosis

RISK FACTORS	Hyperventilation Hypoxemia Altitude sickness	Asphyxiation Asthma Pneumonia
MANIFESTATIONS	Tachypnea Anxiety, tetany Paresthesia	Palpitations Chest pain
INTERVENTIONS	Regulate oxygen therapy. Reduce anxiety. Rebreathing techniques	

ACID-BASE WORKSHEET

	PH	PCO₂	HCO₃	ACID-BASE IMBALANCE	COMPENSATION
1.	7.24	83	24		
2.	7.58	48	36		
3.	7.47	29	22		
4.	7.30	59	29		
5.	7.48	39	32		
6.	7.27	37	16		

Answer Key: 1. respiratory acidosis, uncompensated; 2. metabolic alkalosis, partially compensated; 3. respiratory alkalosis, uncompensated; 4. respiratory acidosis, partially compensated; 5. metabolic alkalosis, uncompensated; 6. metabolic acidosis, uncompensated

SECTION 2

Respiratory System Alterations

The respiratory system includes upper airways, lungs, lower airways, and alveolar air sacs (base of lungs). The lungs aid the body in oxygenation and tissue perfusion.

I Diagnostic Tests for Respiratory Disorders

A. Noninvasive Procedures

1. Chest x-ray (CXR): Use lead shield for adults of childbearing age.
2. Pulse oximetry
3. Pulmonary function tests
4. Sputum culture
5. Computed tomography (CT)
6. Magnetic resonance imaging (MRI)

B. Invasive Procedures

1. **Arterial blood gas** (ABGs via arterial puncture or arterial line): allows the most accurate method of assessing respiratory function
   a. Perform Allen test if no arterial line.
   b. Sample is drawn into heparinized syringe
   c. Keep on ice and transport to laboratory immediately.
   d. Document amount and method of oxygen delivered for accurate results.
   e. Apply direct pressure to puncture site at least 5 min (longer for clients at risk for bleeding).
   f. Monitor for hematoma.
2. **Bronchoscopy**: Visualize larynx, trachea, bronchi; obtain tissue biopsy; foreign body removal.
   a. Obtain informed consent.
   b. Maintain NPO 8 to 12 hr.
   c. Provide local anesthetic throat spray.
   d. Position upright.
   e. Administer medications as prescribed (e.g., atropine [to reduce oral secretions], sedation, and/or anti-anxiety).
   f. Label specimens.
   g. Observe post-procedure:
      1) Gag reflex
      2) Bleeding
      3) Respiratory status, vital signs, and level of consciousness
3. **Mantoux test**: Positive test indicates exposure to tuberculosis. Diagnosis must be confirmed with sputum culture for presence of acid-fast bacillus (AFB).
   a. Administer 0.1 mL of purified protein derivative intradermal to upper half inner surface of forearm (insert needle bevel up).
   b. Assess for reaction in 48 to 72 hr following injection; induration (hardening) of 10 mm or greater is considered a positive test; 5 mm may be considered significant if immunocompromised.
4. **QuantiFERON-TB Gold test (QFT-GT) and T-SPOT.TB**: Identify the presence of *Mycobacterium tuberculosis* infection by measuring the immune response to the TB bacteria in whole blood.
5. **Thoracentesis**: surgical perforation of the pleural space to obtain specimen, to remove fluid or air, or to instill medication
   a. Obtain informed consent.
   b. Educate client: remain still, feeling of pressure, positioning.
   c. Position upright.
   d. Monitor respiratory status and vital signs.
   e. Label specimens.
   f. Document client response, amount, color, and viscosity of fluid (maximum amount of fluid to be removed at one time is 1 L).
   g. Chest tube at bedside.
   h. Obtain CXR before and after procedure.

II Disorders of the Respiratory System: Airflow Problems

A. Asthma: chronic inflammatory disorder of the airways resulting in intermittent and reversible airflow obstruction of the bronchioles

1. Contributing Factors
   a. Extrinsic: antigen-antibody reaction triggered by food, medications, or inhaled substances
   b. Intrinsic: pathophysiological abnormalities within the respiratory tract
   c. Older clients: beta receptors are less responsive to agonist and trigger bronchospasms
2. Manifestations
   a. Sudden, severe dyspnea with use of accessory muscles
   b. Sitting up, leaning forward
   c. Diaphoresis and anxiety
   d. Wheezing, gasping

e. Coughing

f. Cyanosis (late sign)

g. Barrel chest

3. Diagnostic Procedures

   a. ABGs

   b. Sputum cultures

   c. Pulmonary function tests

4. Collaborative Care

   a. **Nursing Interventions**

     1) Remain with the client during the attack.

     2) Position in high-Fowler's.

     3) Assess lung sounds and pulse oximetry.

     4) Administer oxygen therapy.

     5) Maintain IV access.

   b. Medications

     1) Bronchodilators

       a) Short-acting inhaled: albuterol for rapid relief

       b) Methylxanthines: theophylline; monitor therapeutic range for toxicity

     2) Anti-inflammatory

       a) Corticosteroids: fluticasone and prednisone

       b) Leukotriene antagonists: montelukast

     3) Combination Agents

       a) Ipratropium and albuterol

       b) Fluticasone and salmeterol

> **NOTE:** With inhaled agents, administer bronchodilators BEFORE anti-inflammatory medication.

   c. Therapeutic Measures

     1) Respiratory treatments

     2) Oxygen administration

   d. Client Education and Referral

     1) Avoidance of allergens and triggers

     2) Proper use of inhaler and peak flow monitoring

B. **Status asthmaticus** is a life-threatening episode of airway obstruction that is often unresponsive to treatment.

1. Manifestations

   a. Extreme wheezing

   b. Labored breathing

   c. Use of accessory muscles

   d. Distended neck veins

   e. High risk for cardiac and/or respiratory arrest

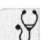

2. **Nursing Interventions**

   a. Place in high-Fowler's.

   b. Prepare for emergency intubation.

   c. Administer oxygen, epinephrine, and systemic steroid as prescribed.

   d. Provide emotional support.

C. **Chronic obstructive pulmonary disease (COPD)** encompasses pulmonary emphysema and chronic bronchitis. COPD is not reversible.

1. **Pulmonary emphysema**: destruction of alveoli, narrowing of bronchioles, and trapping of air resulting in loss of lung elasticity

   a. Contributing Factors

     1) Cigarette smoking (main causative factor); passive smoke inhalation

     2) Advanced age

     3) Exposure to air pollution

     4) Alpha-antitrypsin deficiency (inability to break down pollutants)

     5) Occupational dust and chemical exposure

   b. Manifestations

     1) Dyspnea with productive cough

     2) Difficult exhalation, use of pursed-lip breathing

     3) Wheezing, crackles

     4) Barrel chest

     5) Shallow, rapid respirations

     6) Respiratory acidosis with hypoxia

     7) Weight loss

     8) Clubbed fingernails

     9) Fatigue

2. **Chronic bronchitis**: inflammation and hypersecretion of mucus in the bronchi and bronchioles caused by chronic exposure to irritants

   a. Contributing Factors

     1) Cigarette smoking (main causative factor)

     2) Exposure to air pollution and other environmental irritants

   b. Manifestations

     1) Productive cough

     2) Thick, tenacious sputum

     3) Hypoxemia

     4) Respiratory acidosis

   c. Diagnostic Procedures for COPD

     1) Chest x-ray

     2) Pulmonary function tests: air remains trapped in lungs

     3) Pulse oximetry: often less than 90%

     4) ABGs: chronic respiratory acidosis

     5) Computed tomography (CT)

d. Collaborative Care

   1) **Nursing Interventions**

     a) Assess respiratory status.

     b) Assess cardiac status for signs of right-sided failure.

     c) Position upright and leaning forward.

     d) Schedule activities to allow for frequent rest periods.

     e) Administer oxygen therapy as prescribed.

     f) Use incentive spirometry, breathing techniques, effective coughing.

     g) Encourage fluids 2 to 3 L per day unless contraindicated.

     h) Encourage high-calorie diet.

     i) Provide emotional support.

   2) Medications

     a) Bronchodilators

     b) Beta adrenergic agents

     c) Cholinergic antagonists

     d) Corticosteroids

     e) Methylxanthines

     f) Anti-inflammatory agents

     g) Mucolytic agents

   3) Therapeutic Measures

     a) Chest physiotherapy/pulmonary drainage

     b) Lung reduction surgery

   4) Client Education and Referral

     a) Breathing techniques

     b) Oxygen therapy

     c) Medications

     d) Nutrition

     e) Promote smoking cessation

     f) Infection prevention measures

     g) Encourage immunizations for pneumonia and influenza

     h) Pulmonary rehabilitation

     i) Activity pacing

3. Complications of COPD

  a. **Cor pulmonale:** right-sided heart failure caused by pulmonary disease

   1) Manifestations

     a) Hypoxia and hypoxemia

     b) Extreme dyspnea

     c) Cyanotic lips

     d) JVD

     e) Dependent edema

     f) Hepatomegaly

     g) Pulmonary hypertension

  2) Collaborative Care

   a) **Nursing Interventions**

     (1) Monitor respiratory status.

     (2) Monitor cardiac status and assess for indications of right-sided heart failure.

     (3) Administer oxygen therapy as prescribed.

     (4) Ensure adequate rest periods.

     (5) Encourage low-sodium diet.

     (6) Maintain fluid balance; possible fluid restriction.

     (7) Administer medications as prescribed.

   b) Medications

     (1) Diuretics

     (2) Digoxin

   c) Therapeutic Measures

     (1) Mechanical ventilation

D. **Carbon dioxide toxicity:** stuporous secondary to increased CO_2 retention

  1. Contributing Factors

   a. Carbon dioxide retention

   b. Excessive oxygen delivery

  2. Manifestations

   a. Alteration in level of consciousness

   b. Tachypnea

   c. Increased blood pressure

   d. Tachycardia with dysrhythmias

  3. Collaborative Care

   a. Monitor pulse oximetry and ABGs.

   b. Avoid excessive concentrations of oxygen.

   c. Provide pulmonary hygiene.

   d. Provide ventilatory support with CPAP, BiPAP, or mechanical ventilation.

E. **Pneumonia** is an inflammatory process in the lungs that produces excess fluid and exudate that fill the alveoli; classified as bacterial, viral, fungal, or chemical.

  1. Contributing Factors

   a. Advanced age

   b. No pneumococcal vaccination within the last 5 years

   c. No influenza vaccine within the last year

   d. Chronic lung disease

   e. Immunocompromised

   f. Mechanical ventilation

   g. Postoperative

   h. Sedation and opioid use

   i. Prolonged immobility

   j. Tobacco use

   k. Enteral tube feeding

2. Manifestations
   a. Tachypnea and tachycardia
   b. Sudden onset of chills, fever, flushing, diaphoresis
   c. Productive cough
   d. Dyspnea with pleuritic pain
   e. Crackles
   f. Elevated WBC
   g. Decreased O_2 saturation
3. Diagnostic Procedures
   a. Chest x-ray
   b. Pulse oximetry
   c. Sputum culture and sensitivity
4. Collaborative Care
   a. **Nursing Interventions**
      1) Assess respiratory status.
      2) Administer oxygen.
      3) Assess sputum.
      4) Monitor vital signs.
      5) Encourage 3 L of fluid per day.
      6) Provide pulmonary hygiene.
      7) Encourage mouth care.
      8) Promote nutrition.
   b. Medications
      1) Anti-infectives
      2) Antipyretics
      3) Bronchodilators
      4) Anti-inflammatories
   c. Client Education
      1) Medication administration
      2) Preventive measures
      3) Pneumonia and influenza vaccine
F. **Tuberculosis** is an infectious disease caused by *Mycobacterium tuberculosis* and transmitted through aerosolization (i.e., an airborne route).
   1. Contributing Factors
      a. Older and homeless populations
      b. Lower socioeconomic status
      c. Foreign immigrants
      d. Those in frequent contact with untreated persons
      e. Overcrowded living conditions
   2. Manifestations
      a. Cough, hemoptysis
      b. Positive sputum culture for acid-fast bacillus (AFB)
      c. Low-grade fever with night sweats
      d. Anorexia, weight loss
      e. Malaise, fatigue
   3. Diagnostic Procedures
      a. Mantoux
      b. Sputum culture and smear for AFB to confirm diagnosis
      c. Serum analysis, QFT-G
      d. Chest x-ray

4. Collaborative Care
   a. **Nursing Interventions**
      1) Initiate airborne isolation precautions.
      2) Obtain sputum sample before administering medications.
      3) Maintain adequate nutritional status.
      4) Teach the client to avoid foods containing tyramine when taking INH.
      5) Inform the client that rifampin can alter the metabolism of certain other medications.
      6) Monitor laboratory findings for liver and kidney function.
   b. Medications: combination drug therapy
      1) Administer medications on an empty stomach at the same time every day.
      2) Medications should be taken for 6 to 12 months, as directed.
      3) Instruct the client to watch for indications of hepatotoxicity, nephrotoxicity, and/or visual changes, and to notify a provider if any of these are noted.
      4) Medications to treat TB
         a) Isoniazid (INH)
         b) Rifampin
         c) Pyrazinamide
         d) Ethambutol
         e) Fluoroquinolones and aminoglycosides (if TB is resistant to anti-TB drugs)
   c. Client Education and Referral
      1) Instruct client to follow infection control measures.
      2) Ensure medication compliance and follow-up care.
5. Cases of diagnosed TB are reported to local or state health department.
   a. Refer all high-risk clients to local health department for testing and prophylactic treatment regimen.
G. **Laryngeal cancer:** malignant cells occurring in the mucosal tissue of the larynx; more common in men between the ages of 55 and 70
   1. Contributing Factors
      a. Smoking
      b. Radiation exposure
      c. Chronic laryngitis and/or straining of vocal cords
   2. Manifestations
      a. Hoarseness extending longer than 2 weeks
      b. Dysphagia
      c. Dyspnea
      d. Cough
      e. Persistent sore throat
      f. Hard, immobile lymph nodes in neck
      g. Weight loss, anorexia

3. Diagnostic Procedures
   a. MRI
   b. Direct laryngoscopy with biopsy
   c. X-ray and CT
   d. Bone scan and positron emission tomography (PET) scan
4. Collaborative Care
   a. **Nursing Interventions**
      1) Maintain patent airway.
      2) Swallowing precautions
      3) Emotional support
      4) Nutrition
      5) Pain management
      6) Administer medications as elixir when possible.
   b. Therapeutic Measures
      1) Partial or total laryngectomy
      2) Radiation therapy
   c. Client Education and Referral
      1) Communication method
      2) Stoma care
      3) Swallowing maneuvers
      4) Speech therapy

H. **Lung cancer:** leading cause of cancer-related deaths for both men and women in the U.S.; primary or metastatic disease; most commonly occurs between the ages of 45 and 70 years
   1. Contributing Factors
      a. Smoking (first- and second-hand smoke)
      b. Radiation exposure
      c. Chronic exposure to inhaled irritants
      d. Older adult
   2. Manifestations
      a. Chronic cough
      b. Chronic dyspnea
      c. Hemoptysis
      d. Hoarseness
      e. Fatigue, weight loss, anorexia
      f. Clubbing of fingers
      g. Chest wall pain
   3. Diagnostic Procedures
      a. Chest x-ray and CT scan
      b. CT-guided needle aspiration
      c. Bronchoscopy with biopsy
      d. TNM system for staging
         1) T – Tumor
         2) N – Nodes
         3) M – Metastasis

4. Collaborative Care
   a. **Nursing Interventions**
      1) Maintain patent airway.
      2) Suction as indicated by assessment.
      3) Monitor vital signs and pulse oximetry.
      4) Monitor nutritional status.
      5) Position in high-Fowler's.
      6) Provide emotional support.
      7) Assess and treat stomatitis.
      8) Ensure protection for immunocompromised client.
   b. Medications
      1) Chemotherapeutic agents
      2) Opioid narcotics
   c. Therapeutic Measures
      1) Palliative Care
         a) Medication
         b) Thoracentesis
      2) Surgical
         a) Tumor excision
         b) Pneumonectomy, lobectomy, wedge resection
         c) Radiation
   d. Client Education and Referral
      1) Medications
      2) Constipation prevention and management
      3) Mouth and skin care
      4) Nutrition
5. Respiratory services
6. Radiology
7. Rehabilitation
8. Nutrition
9. Hospice

III Respiratory Emergencies

A. **Pulmonary embolism:** a life-threatening hypoxic condition caused by a collection of particulate matter (solid, gas, or liquid) that enters venous circulation and lodges in the pulmonary vessels causing pulmonary blood flow obstruction
   1. Contributing Factors
      a. Chronic atrial fibrillation
      b. Hypercoagulability
      c. Long bone fracture
      d. Long-term immobility
      e. Oral contraceptive or estrogen therapy
      f. Obesity
      g. Postoperative
      h. PVD, DVT
      i. Sickle cell anemia
      j. Central venous catheters

2. Manifestations
   a. Dyspnea, tachypnea
   b. Sharp, stabbing pain on inspiration
   c. Tachycardia, hypotension
   d. Sense of impending doom
   e. Diaphoresis
   f. Decreased SaO_2
   g. Pleural effusion
   h. Crackles and cough

NOTE: Petechiae over chest and axilla are present with fat emboli.

3. Diagnostic Procedures
   a. ABGs
   b. D-dimer
   c. Chest x-ray
   d. V/Q scan
   e. Pulmonary angiography
4. Collaborative Care
   a. **Nursing Interventions**
      1) Assess respiratory status and vital signs.
      2) Provide respiratory support.
      3) Provide oxygen therapy.
      4) Position in high-Fowler's.
      5) Initiate IV access.
      6) Provide emotional support.
   b. Medications
      1) Thrombolytics
      2) Anticoagulants
   c. Therapeutic Measures
      1) Embolectomy
      2) Vena cava filter
   d. Client Education and Referral
      1) Preventive measures
      2) Dietary precautions with vitamin K
      3) Follow-up for PT or INR
      4) Bleeding precautions
      5) Home oxygen therapy
5. Cardiology and Pulmonary Services
   a. Respiratory care

B. **Pneumothorax:** a collection of air or gas in the chest or pleural space that causes part or all of a lung to collapse due to a loss of negative pressure

C. **Tension pneumothorax:** occurs when air enters the pleural space during inspiration through a one-way valve and is not able to exit upon expiration. The trapped air causes pressure on the heart and the lung. As a result, the increase in pressure compresses blood vessels and limits venous return, leading to a decrease in cardiac output. Death can result if not treated immediately.

D. **Hemothorax:** accumulation of blood in the pleural cavity
   1. Contributing Factors
      a. Blunt chest trauma
      b. COPD
      c. Closed/occluded chest tube
      d. Advanced age
      e. Penetrating chest wounds
   2. Manifestations
      a. Respiratory distress
      b. Tracheal deviation to unaffected side (tension pneumothorax)
      c. Reduced or absent breath sound (affected side)
      d. Asymmetrical chest wall movement
      e. Hyperresonance on percussion due to trapped air (pneumothorax)
      f. Subcutaneous emphysema
      g. Chest pain
   3. Diagnostic Procedures
      a. Chest x-ray
      b. Thoracentesis (hemothorax)
   4. Collaborative Care
      a. **Nursing Interventions**
         1) Monitor respiratory status.
         2) Administer oxygen.
         3) Position in high-Fowler's.
         4) Monitor chest tube and dressing.
         5) Provide emotional support.
      b. Therapeutic Measures
         1) Chest Tube Insertion
            a) Chest tube: inserted to pleural space for draining fluid, blood, or air; re-establishes a negative pressure; facilitates lung expansion
               (1) Position supine or semi-Fowler's.
               (2) Verify informed consent is signed.
               (3) Prepare chest drainage system prior to insertion.
               (4) Administer pain and sedation medication as prescribed.
               (5) Assist provider as needed during insertion.
               (6) Apply dressing to insertion site.
               (7) Maintain chest tube system.
               (8) Monitor respiratory status, pulse oximetry, vital signs, and client response.
               (9) Monitor for complications.

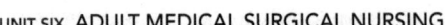

CHEST TUBE COMPLICATIONS

COMPLICATION	NURSING INTERVENTIONS
Air leak (continuous rapid bubbling in the water seal chamber)	Start at the chest and move down tubing to locate leak; tighten connection or replace drainage system. Keep connection taped securely.
No tidaling in water seal chamber	Check for kinks in the tubing. Check breath sounds (lungs re-expanded).
No bubbling in suction control chamber	Verify tubing is attached. Verify water is filled to prescribed level. Check wall suction regulator.
Chest tube is disconnected from system	Insert open end of the chest tube into sterile water until system can be replaced.
Chest tube accidentally pulled from client	Cover insertion site with sterile dressing, taped on three sides. Contact provider. Prepare for reinsertion.

IV Airway Management

A. **Oxygen therapy** is used in many acute and chronic respiratory problems to improve cellular oxygenation and prevent hypoxia or hypoxemia.

1. Clinical Manifestations (hypoxia and hypoxemia)

MANIFESTATIONS OF HYPOXIA AND HYPOXEMIA

EARLY	LATE
Tachypnea	Bradypnea
Tachycardia	Bradycardia
Restlessness	Confusion and stupor
Pale skin and mucous membranes	Cyanotic skin and mucous membranes
Elevated blood pressure	Hypotension
Use of accessory muscles, nasal flaring, adventitious lung sounds	Cardiac dysrhythmias

2. Collaborative Care

OXYGEN DELIVERY DEVICES

DEVICE	FIO₂/FLOW RATE
Nasal cannula	24% to 44% at 1 to 6 L/min
Simple face mask	40% to 60% at 6 to 8 L/min
Partial rebreather mask	50% to 75% at 8 to 11 L/min
Nonrebreather mask	80% to 100% at 12 L/min
Venturi mask	24% to 40% at 4 to 8 L/min
Aerosol mask, face tent	30% to 100% at 8 to 10 L/min
T-piece	30% to 100% at 8 to 10 L/min

3. Client Education

   a. Assess for electrical hazards.

   b. Post "oxygen in use" sign.

   c. Wear cotton gown.

   d. No smoking.

B. **Suctioning:** use of a suction machine and catheter to remove secretions from the airway

1. Clinical Manifestations (indicating a need for suctioning)

   a. Restlessness

   b. Tachypnea

   c. Tachycardia

   d. Decreased SaO₂

   e. Adventitious breath sounds

   f. Visualization of secretions

   g. Absence of spontaneous cough

2. Collaborative Care

   a. Perform hand hygiene.

   b. Explain procedure.

   c. Don required PPE.

   d. Position client to semi- or high-Fowler's.

   e. Obtain baseline breath sounds, vital signs, and SaO₂.

   f. Use medical aseptic technique (oral suction).

   g. Use surgical aseptic technique for all other types.

   h. Hyperoxygenate client.

   i. Suction 10 to 15 seconds (rotating motion); limit to 2 to 3 attempts.

   j. Allow recovery between attempts (20 to 30 seconds).

   k. Document amount, color, and consistency of secretions, as well as client response.

C. **Tracheostomy care:** care of a tracheostomy to maintain a patent airway and optimal ventilation

1. Collaborative Care

   a. Explain the procedure.

   b. Position client in semi- or high-Fowler's.

   c. At all times, keep two extra tracheostomy tubes (one the client's size and one a smaller size) at the bedside in the event of accidental decannulation.

   d. Suction client only as clinically indicated (never on routine schedule). Surgical asepsis is used for tracheal suctioning.

   e. Assess for respiratory distress.

   f. Provide tracheostomy care every 8 hr and as needed.

   g. Change tracheostomy tubes as prescribed.

2. Client Education and Referral

   a. Tracheostomy care

   b. Prevention of respiratory infections

   c. Nutrition

   d. Home health care agency

   e. Community support group

D. **Mechanical ventilation** provides respiratory support through the controlled delivery of ventilation and oxygenation via an endotracheal tube, tracheostomy tube, or noninvasive ventilation via mask through continuous positive airway pressure (CPAP) or bi-level positive airway pressure (BiPAP).

1. Indication

   a. During surgery

   b. Acute respiratory distress

   c. Respiratory failure

2. **Nursing Interventions**

   a. Explain procedure to client.

   b. Establish means of communication, such as asking yes/no questions, providing writing materials, using a dry erase board and/or a picture communication board, or lip reading.

   c. Maintain Patent Airway:

      1) Ensure advanced airway device is secured (endotracheal tube or tracheostomy tube).

      2) Assess position and placement of tube, document in centimeters at the client's lips or teeth.

      3) Prevent accidental extubation; wrist restraints may be required.

      4) Suction oral and tracheal secretions as indicated by assessment.

      5) Assess respiratory status every 1 to 2 hr and as needed.

      6) Monitor ventilator settings and alarms. Never turn off ventilator alarms. If the cause of an alarm cannot be identified and corrected, and the client's respiratory status begins to decline, the nurse should ventilate the client using a manual resuscitation bag until the issue is resolved.

         a) Low-pressure alarm—indicates low volume and is usually associated with tube disconnection, cuff leak, or tube dislodgement

         b) High-pressure alarm—indicates increased pressure, which may be caused by secretions, kinking of tube, pulmonary edema, or the client coughing or biting the tube

         c) Apnea alarm—indicates there has been no spontaneous breath within a preset time period

      7) Maintain adequate but not excessive cuff pressure (less than 20 mm Hg is recommended to reduce risk of tracheal necrosis).

      8) Administer medications as prescribed:

         a) Analgesics

         b) Sedation

         c) Neuromuscular blocking agents

      9) Reposition endotracheal tube every 24 hr or by protocol. Monitor skin for breakdown.

   d. Prevent complications:

      1) Pneumonia

         a) Hand hygiene

         b) Elevate head of bed.

         c) Oral hygiene

      2) Pneumothorax

         a) Caused by high ventilation pressures

         b) Auscultate lung sounds frequently.

         c) Consider if sudden respiratory distress

         d) Requires immediate action (chest tube)

RESPIRATORY END-OF-SECTION REVIEW

1. The client who is experiencing respiratory distress should be placed in _____ position unless contraindicated.

2. The first inhaled medication to be given to a client experiencing an acute asthma attack is a _____.

3. The client with a history of COPD should receive _____ concentrations of oxygen to prevent a decrease in his hypoxic drive to breathe.

4. The nurse teaches the client with a diagnosis of COPD to use _____ breathing to facilitate the exhalation of trapped air from the lungs.

5. A client is considered to have a positive Mantoux test when induration is _____ or greater in the nonimmunocompromised client. The Mantoux test indicates exposure to TB not _____ disease. The diagnosis of tuberculosis is confirmed with a _____ acid-fast bacillus (AFB) sputum culture.

6. The client with a suspected diagnosis of TB should be placed on _____ precautions.

7. _____ should be obtained prior to administering antibiotics to a client with the diagnosis of pneumonia.

8. The most precise noninvasive oxygen delivery system is the _____ mask.

9. The most common cause of a low-pressure ventilator alarm is a _____; the most common cause of a high-pressure ventilator alarm is _____. If the nurse cannot quickly resolve the issue causing the ventilator alarm and the client's respiratory status begins to decline, the nurse should _____ the client.

10. The client who has had a laryngectomy needs to be placed on _____ precautions to prevent aspiration.

WORD BANK

10 mm

Active

Airborne

Blood cultures

High-Fowler's

Leak

Low

Manually ventilate

Occlusion

Positive

Pursed-lip

Short-acting bronchodilator

Swallowing

Venturi

Answer Key: 1. High-Fowler's; 2. Short-acting bronchodilator; 3. Low; 4. Pursed-lip; 5. 10 mm, active, positive; 6. Airborne; 7. Blood cultures; 8. Venturi; 9. Leak, occlusion, manually ventilate; 10. Swallowing

Perioperative Care

A. **Preoperative phase:** Procedures or teaching completed prior to a surgical procedure reduce potential complications and postoperative discomfort, relieve anxiety, and increase participation in care.

1. Care of the Client Before Surgery

   a. **Nursing Interventions**

      1) Take client history.

      2) Identify risk factors: infants, elderly, chronic illness, malnutrition, respiratory conditions, obesity, emergent procedures.

      3) Check for informed consent (a nurse may witness only).

      4) Perform baseline assessment.

      5) Assess allergies.

      6) Verify NPO status.

   b. Medications

      1) Anesthesia

         a) Inhalation

         b) Intravenous

         c) Regional

         d) Topical

      2) Antibiotics

      3) Anticholinergics

      4) Narcotics

      5) Sedatives

   c. Diagnostic Tests

      1) Laboratory profile

      2) Chest x-ray

      3) ECG

      4) Pregnancy test for females

   d. Client Education

      1) Fears and anxiety

      2) Medications

         a) Hold anticoagulants for 7 to 10 days prior to surgery (e.g., warfarin or aspirin).

      3) Invasive procedures

      4) Incentive spirometry

      5) Turn, position, and perform early ambulation, including leg exercises.

      6) Analgesics and pain control methods

      7) Routine and expected postoperative care

      8) Pre-, intra-, and postoperative routines

B. **Intraoperative phase:** begins when client enters the surgical suite and ends with transfer to postanesthesia recovery area. Nursing focus is on safety, client advocacy, and health team collaboration.

1. The Universal Protocol (safety initiative from Joint Commission)

   a. Conduct a preprocedure verification process.

   b. Mark the procedure site.

   c. Perform a "time out" before starting the procedure.

2. Collaborative Care

   a. Perioperative Nursing Staff

      1) Holding

      2) Circulator

      3) Scrub

      4) Specialty

   b. **Nursing Interventions**

      1) Implement role according to established standards.

      2) Maintain safe environment.

      3) Ensure strict asepsis.

      4) Apply grounding devices.

      5) Ensure correct sponge, needle, and instrument count.

      6) Position client.

      7) Remain alert to complications.

      8) Communicate with surgical team.

   c. Therapeutic Measures

      1) Blood transfusion

      2) Radiology

      3) Biopsy

      4) Laboratory profiles

C. **Postoperative phase:** begins when client enters the postanesthesia recovery area and continues until discharge from the health care facility

1. Collaborative Care

   a. **Nursing Interventions**: immediate recovery period

      1) Ongoing Assessment

         a) Pulmonary

            (1) Verify airway and check gag reflex.

            (2) Assess for bilateral breath sounds.

            (3) Encourage coughing and deep breathing.

         b) Circulatory

            (1) Compare vital signs to baseline.

            (2) Assess tissue perfusion.

         c) Neurological

            (1) Evaluate the level of consciousness.

            (2) Assess reflexes and movement.

         d) Genitourinary

            (1) Monitor I&O.

            (2) Assess urinary output (color, clarity, and amount).

e) Gastrointestinal

   (1) Assess for bowel sounds.

   (2) Assess for abdominal distention.

f) Integument

   (1) Assess color.

   (2) Assess wound.

   (3) Assess drainage insertion sites.

g) **Nursing Interventions**

   (1) Verify IV fluid type, rate, and site.

   (2) Check dressings for type and amount of drainage.

   (3) Identify drainage, including color and amount.

   (4) If NG tube, determine type and amount of suction ordered.

   (5) Position in semi-Fowler's to facilitate maximum oxygenation.

   (6) Monitor O_2 saturation.

   (7) Ensure thermoregulation.

   (8) Provide pain management.

   (9) Maintain NPO until the client is alert and a gag reflex returns.

   (10) Prevent complications (see table).

   (11) Transfer or discharge client to unit or home.

COMMON POSTOPERATIVE COMPLICATIONS

Atelectasis

OCCURRENCE	First 48 hr	
MANIFESTATIONS	Tachycardia Tachypnea	Shallow respirations
INTERVENTIONS	Incentive spirometer T,C,DB q 2 hr Early ambulation	Hydration Monitor respiratory rate and rhythm.

Hypostatic pneumonia

OCCURRENCE	After 48 hr	
MANIFESTATIONS	Febrile Tachycardia	Tachypnea Crackles, rhonchi
INTERVENTIONS	Incentive spirometer T,C,DB q 2 hr Early ambulation	Hydration Mucolytics

Respiratory depression

OCCURRENCE	Immediate to 48 hr	
MANIFESTATIONS	Bradypnea Shallow respirations	Decreased LOC
INTERVENTIONS	Monitor respiratory rate and rhythm. Monitor client's LOC. Regulate narcotics.	Oxygen therapy Narcotic antagonist: naloxone

COMMON POSTOPERATIVE COMPLICATIONS (CONTINUED)

Hypoxia

OCCURRENCE	Immediate to 48 hr	
MANIFESTATIONS	Confusion Increased BP, pulse	Tachypnea
INTERVENTIONS	Monitor vital signs. Oxygen therapy	Resolve underlying problem.

Nausea

OCCURRENCE	Immediate to 48 hr	
MANIFESTATIONS	Nausea	
INTERVENTIONS	Comfort measures Relaxation Mouth care	Antiemetic NG tube to decompress stomach

Shock

OCCURRENCE	Immediate to 48 hr	
MANIFESTATIONS	Decreased BP, pulse, urinary output Cold, clammy, pale skin	Lethargy Stupor
INTERVENTIONS	Monitor vital signs. Replace fluids. Position in modified Trendelenburg.	I&O Monitor LOC. Administer vasopressors as prescribed.

Urinary retention/hesitancy

OCCURRENCE	Immediate to 3 days	
MANIFESTATIONS	Inability to void Bladder distention	Restlessness Increased BP
INTERVENTIONS	Privacy Bladder scan	Offer bedpan. I&O

Decreased peristalsis/paralytic ileus

OCCURRENCE	2 to 4 days
MANIFESTATIONS	Hypoactive/absent bowel sounds No flatus
INTERVENTIONS	NG to decompress stomach Limit narcotics. Ambulation Prokinetic agents: metoclopramide as prescribed

Wound hemorrhage

OCCURRENCE	Immediate to discharge
MANIFESTATIONS	Bleeding from drainage tubes or surgical site Signs of shock
INTERVENTIONS	Assess site. Identify early signs. Monitor drainage device, keep patent. Avoid tension at surgical site.

COMMON POSTOPERATIVE COMPLICATIONS (CONTINUED)

Thrombophlebitis

OCCURRENCE	7 to 14 days
MANIFESTATIONS	Redness, warmth, calf tenderness/pain, edema at site
INTERVENTIONS	Early ambulation Apply antiembolic stockings or sequential compression devices as prescribed. Avoid actions that decrease venous flow. Anticoagulant prophylaxis

Delayed wound healing

OCCURRENCE	5 to 6 days
MANIFESTATIONS	Edema, redness, pallor, separation at edges, absence of granulation tissue
INTERVENTIONS	Splint incision as needed. Use incision support devices (abdominal binder). Promote high-protein diet.

Wound infection

OCCURRENCE	3 to 5 days
MANIFESTATIONS	Signs of delayed healing with purulent/discolored drainage, pain in incisional area
INTERVENTIONS	Promote healthy diet, adequate fluid intake, adequate rest, and exercise. Wound care Antibiotics as prescribed

Wound dehiscence/evisceration

OCCURRENCE	4 to 15 days
MANIFESTATIONS	Open wound revealing underlying tissue (dehiscence) or organs (evisceration)
INTERVENTIONS	Position client to decrease tension at suture line. Apply sterile saline-soaked gauze. Notify surgeon. Instruct client not to cough or strain. Provide emotional support.

Urinary tract infection

OCCURRENCE	5 to 8 days
MANIFESTATIONS	Frequency, urgency, dysuria Malodorous, cloudy urine
INTERVENTIONS	Wipe front to back after urination. Limit use of indwelling catheters. Encourage voiding. Increase fluids 3 L/day. Cranberry juice Antibiotics as prescribed Uroanalgesics as prescribed

---

Gastrointestinal, Hepatic, and Pancreatic Disorders

A. **Impaired function of the GI tract, pancreas, and liver resulting from structural, mechanical, motility, infection, or cancerous conditions**

B. **Contributing Factors**
   1. History of autoimmune disorder
   2. Alcohol use disorder
   3. Dietary patterns
   4. NSAID use
   5. Age
   6. Family history
   7. Previous abdominal surgery
   8. Allergies
   9. Musculoskeletal impairment (e.g., CVA, MS)
   10. Obesity
   11. Smoking
   12. Sedentary lifestyle
   13. Stress

Diagnostic Procedures

A. **Laboratory Profiles: gastric aspirate**
   1. Hydrochloric Acid and Pepsin (evaluate Zollinger–Ellison syndrome)
      a. NPO 12 hr.
      b. Avoid alcohol, tobacco, medications that change gastric pH for 24 hr.
      c. Insert NG tube.
      d. Aspirate gastric contents.
      e. Obtain pH.

B. **Laboratory Profiles: hepatic or pancreatic disease**
   1. Albumin
   2. Ammonia: liver's ability to break down protein by-products
   3. Bilirubin: measured directly in the blood
   4. Cholesterol
      a. Total cholesterol
      b. LDL ("bad")
      c. HDL ("good")
      d. Triglycerides
   5. Liver Enzymes
      a. ALT/SGPT
      b. AST/SGOT
      c. ALP
   6. Pancreatic Enzymes
      a. Amylase
      b. Lipase
      c. Prothrombin time

C. **Laboratory Profiles: GI parasites, bacteria, or bleeding**

1. Stool Sample

   a. Inspect for color, consistency.

   b. Tests

      1) Ova and parasites

      2) *Clostridium difficile (C. diff)*

      3) Urobilinogen

      4) Fecal fat (steatorrhea)

      5) Fecal nitrogen

      6) Food residues

      7) Cytotoxic assay (preferred over stool culture)

   KEY POINT: When obtaining a stool sample, have the client defecate into a bedpan or bedside commode. Use an approved specimen container. It must be uncontaminated by urine or toilet paper and sent promptly to the lab.

2. Fecal Screening Tests (may be obtained at home and mailed in)

   a. Fecal Occult Blood Test

      1) Recommended annually to detect colon cancer.

      2) Instruct to avoid red meat, aspirin, turnips, and horseradish at least 72 hr prior to testing to avoid false positive results. Ingestion of vitamin C–rich foods or supplements may result in a false negative.

      3) NSAIDs and anticoagulants should be discontinued 7 days prior to testing.

   b. Fecal immunochemical test (e.g., Hemosure, Hematest II SENSA, HemoQuant)

   c. Stool DNA

D. **Breath Tests**

1. Hydrogen Breath Test

   a. To evaluate carbohydrate absorption

   b. Aids in the detection of bacterial overgrowth in intestine

2. Urea Breath Test

   a. To detect presence of *H. pylori*

   b. Instruct to avoid antibiotics and bismuth subsalicylate 1 month before the test; proton pump inhibitors and sucralfate 1 week before testing; and H_2 inhibitors for 24 hr before testing.

E. **Endoscopy:** allows direct visualization of tissues, cavities, and organs using a flexible fiber-optic tube

1. Colonoscopy: exam of the entire large intestine

   a. Bowel prep to clear fecal contents (1 to 3 day prep)

   b. Clear liquid diet 12 to 24 hr before procedure

   c. NPO except water 6 to 8 hr before procedure

   d. IV sedation

   e. Monitor post-procedure for excessive bleeding or severe pain.

2. Virtual Colonoscopy

   a. Bowel prep as for traditional colonoscopy

   b. Performed using MRI or CT

   c. Small tube is placed in the rectum

   d. Images viewed on screen

3. Sigmoidoscopy: exam of rectum and sigmoid colon

   a. Clear liquid diet 24 hr before procedure

   b. Laxative the evening before the procedure

   c. Enema the morning of the procedure

   d. Sedation is not required.

   e. Tissue biopsy may be performed.

   f. Report excessive bleeding.

4. Small bowel capsule endoscopy: video exam of small bowel, including distal ileum

   a. Only water is allowed 8 to 10 hr before test.

   b. NPO 2 hr before test.

   c. Client's abdomen is marked for location of placement for sensors.

   d. Client wears abdominal belt housing data recorder.

   e. Administer video capsule with full glass of water.

   f. Resume normal diet 4 hr after swallowing pill.

   g. Return to the facility with capsule equipment for download of data.

   h. Procedure takes approximately 8 hr.

   i. Capsule will be excreted via stool (may or may not be seen); no action needed.

5. Esophagogastroduodenoscopy (EGD): exam of esophagus, stomach, and duodenum (identify bleeding, Crohn's disease, colitis)

   a. NPO 6 to 8 hr before procedure.

   b. Avoid anticoagulants, aspirin, or NSAIDs for several days before test.

   c. IV sedation.

   d. Atropine to dry secretions.

   e. Local anesthetic is sprayed to inactivate gag reflex.

   f. Prevent aspiration.

   g. Monitor for signs of perforation, pain, bleeding, or fever.

   h. Comfort measures for hoarseness or sore throat (several days).

6. Endoscopic retrograde cholangiopancreatography (ERCP): exam of liver, gallbladder, bile ducts, and pancreas

   a. NPO 6 to 8 hr before procedure.

   b. Avoid anticoagulants, aspirin, or NSAIDs for several days before test.

   c. Assess for allergies to x-ray dye.

   d. IV sedation.

   e. May have colicky abdominal discomfort.

   f. Monitor for severe pain, fever, nausea, or vomiting (indicates perforation).

F. **Radiographic Studies (with or without contrast)**

1. Barium series: x-ray visualization from the mouth to the duodenojejunal junction; may include a small bowel follow-through

2. Preprocedure

    a. NPO 8 hr before procedure.

    b. Avoid opioid analgesics and anticholinergic medications for 24 hr before the test.

    c. Avoid smoking or chewing gum.

    d. Have client drink 16 ounces of barium liquid.

    e. Client will assume multiple positions during the x-ray exam.

    f. Postprocedure

        1) Teach client to include additional fiber and fluids to promote barium elimination.

        2) Visualize stool for barium contents next 24 to 72 hr (will be chalky white).

        3) Brown stool should return when barium is evacuated.

        4) Mild laxative or stool softener as needed to promote bowel elimination.

G. **Liver biopsy:** needle inserted through abdominal wall to obtain sample for biopsy or tissue examination; performed under fluoroscopy

1. Preparation

    a. Obtain informed consent.

    b. Assess coagulation studies (PT, aPTT, INR, platelet count).

    c. NPO 8 to 10 hr before procedure.

    d. Position on affected side to promote hemostasis.

    e. Monitor for bleeding complications.

H. **Paracentesis:** needle inserted through abdominal wall into peritoneal cavity, withdrawing fluid accumulated due to ascites

1. Have client void.

2. Obtain baseline vital signs.

3. Position upright.

4. Administer mild sedation.

5. Administer prescribed IV fluids or albumin to restore fluid balance (as much as 4 L to 6 L of fluid is slowly drained from the abdomen).

6. Monitor vital signs.

7. Record weight before and after procedure.

8. Measure abdominal girth before and after procedure.

9. Assess laboratory profile before and after procedure: albumin, amylase, protein, BUN, creatinine.

II Gastrointestinal Therapeutic Procedures

GASTROINTESTINAL TUBES

TUBE	PURPOSE	🩺 NURSING INTERVENTIONS

Nasogastric
› **Levin**: single lumen
› **Salem sump**: double lumen
  » Suction, aspiration
  » Vent
	Decompress stomach (ileus, gastric atony, or intestinal obstruction).
	Obtain specimens for analysis (pH of gastric fluid and the presence of blood).
		Elevate head of bed.
		Verify placement.
		Provide frequent mouth care.
		Maintain NPO.

Miller-Abbott: double lumen › Aspiration › Inflate balloon at tip.	Small bowel suction	Reposition every 1 hr. Do NOT tape tube to nose. Monitor advancement of tube. Assess color of gastric contents.
Sengstaken-Blakemore: triple lumen › Esophageal balloon › Gastric balloon › Suction, irrigation	For treatment of esophageal varices Can cause potential trauma and complications for the client, such as rebleeding, pneumonia, and respiratory obstruction	Monitor for respiratory distress (most clients have ETT). Keep scissors at bedside. Monitor signs of shock.

A. **Enteral feeding tubes:** delivery of a nutritionally complete feeding directly into the stomach, duodenum, or jejunum

❗ Point to Remember

The auscultatory method of checking placement is NOT considered reliable. Initial placement of the nasogastric or nasointestinal tube should be checked by x-ray. Subsequent placement should be checked by aspirating stomach or intestinal contents and measuring pH. Gastric pH should be between 1.5 and 4; intestinal aspirate pH is around 6; respiratory aspirate pH is 7 or higher.

1. Small-Bore Nasogastric Feeding Tubes

    a. Obtain x-ray to determine placement.

    b. Assess gastric pH before each feeding; every 4 hr for continuous feeding.

    c. Maintain a semi-Fowler's position while feeding is infusing.

    d. Assess residual in the stomach and refeed the residual, unless it exceeds the maximum.

    e. Provide nose and mouth care.

    f. Replace tube every 4 weeks.

❗ Point to Remember

If residual exceeds 100 mL for intermittent feedings, or 2 hr worth of a continuous feeding, hold or stop the feeding; do NOT refeed aspirate; notify the provider.

2. Small-bore nasointestinal/jejunostomy tubes: inserted through the skin and occasionally sutured in place for long-term feeding

   a. Obtain x-ray to determine placement (prior to initial feeding).

   b. Assess length of exposed tubing (tube migration).

   c. Assess placement prior to feeding using intestinal pH.

   d. Maintain a semi-Fowler's position.

   e. Assess residual (greater volume indicates upward migration).

3. Monitor for Complications

   a. Refeeding syndrome can be life-threatening.

   b. Bleeding

   c. Infection

   d. Tube misplacement/dislodgement, aspiration: Immediately remove any tube suspected of being dislodged or misplaced.

   e. Abdominal distention, nausea, vomiting, diarrhea, constipation

   f. Fluid imbalance: Hyperosmolar preparations can lead to dehydration.

   g. Electrolyte imbalance: the most common are hyponatremia and hyperkalemia

4. Percutaneous Endoscopic Gastrostomy (PEG)

   a. Assess skin integrity.

   b. Assess residual volume.

   c. Allow feeding to infuse slowly (raise/lower syringe).

   d. Flush with 30 mL warm water before and after feeding.

   e. Maintain semi-Fowler's position 1 to 2 hr after feeding.

B. **Parenteral nutrition:** IV administration of a hypertonic intravenous solution made up of glucose, insulin, minerals, lipids, electrolytes, and other essential nutrients. Used when the client cannot effectively use the GI tract for nutrition.

   1. Partial or Peripheral Parenteral Nutrition (PPN)

      a. Used when client can eat, but cannot take in enough nutrients to meet needs

      b. Administered through a large distal arm vein or PICC line

   2. Total Parenteral Nutrition (TPN)

      a. Used when the client requires intensive nutritional support for an extended time period

      b. Delivered through a central vein

   3. Contributing Factors

      a. Gastrointestinal mobility disorders

      b. Inability to achieve or maintain adequate nutrition for body requirements

      c. Short bowel syndrome

      d. Chronic pancreatitis

      e. Severe burns

      f. Malabsorption disorders

4. Collaborative Care

   a. **Nursing Interventions**

      1) Confirm placement by chest x-ray.

      2) Monitor central line insertion site for local infection.

      3) Maintain strict surgical asepsis for dressing change (every 72 hr).

      4) Change tubing and remaining TPN every 24 hr.

      5) Monitor for signs of systemic infection.

      6) Monitor glucose, electrolytes, and fluid balance.

      7) Prevent air embolism.

      8) Use infusion pump.

      9) Keep 10% dextrose/water available.

      10) For clients receiving fat emulsions, monitor for fat overload syndrome: fever, increased triglycerides, clotting problems, and multi-system organ failure; discontinue infusion and notify provider immediately.

III Oral and Esophageal Disorders

A. **Dental Caries**

   1. An erosive process of the tooth that occurs when acid is formed by the action of bacteria on fermentable carbohydrates

   2. Contributing Factors

      a. Dental plaque

      b. Poor oral hygiene

      c. Lack of fluoridated water

      d. High intake of refined carbohydrates

      e. Decrease in saliva

   3. Manifestations

      a. Halitosis

      b. Tooth pain

      c. Tooth erosion, discoloring

   4. Collaborative Care

      a. **Nursing Interventions**

         1) Teach to regularly use preventive measures.

            a) Brush teeth after eating.

            b) Floss.

            c) Increase intake of fresh fruits and vegetables, nuts, cheese, plain yogurt.

            d) If water is not fluoridated, obtain from other source.

            e) Dental sealants

            f) Twice-yearly dental cleaning and screening

B. **Salivary Gland, Oral Mucosa, and Pharyngeal Disorders**

1. Salivary glands consist of the parotid, submandibular, sublingual, and buccal glands. Disorders may affect lubrication, protection from harmful bacteria, and digestion. Disorders include candidiasis (thrush), parotitis, sialoadenitis, salivary calculus, stomatitis, and cancer.

2. Contributing Factors

   a. Tobacco use

   b. Alcohol use disorder

   c. Aging

   d. Dehydration

   e. Radiation

   f. Stress

   g. Malnutrition

   h. Poor oral hygiene

   i. Immunosuppression

3. Manifestations

   a. Pain

   b. Cheesy white plaque (candidiasis)

   c. Inflammation and redness

   d. Persistent, painless oral lesion that does not heal (cancer)

   e. Xerostomia

4. Collaborative Care

   a. **Nursing Interventions**

      1) Monitor nutritional status: refer to dietitian PRN.

      2) Monitor swallowing ability.

      3) Implement alternatives to oral communication PRN.

      4) Ensure adequate food and fluid intake.

      5) Perform and teach regular and thorough oral hygiene.

      6) Minimize pain.

      7) Monitor for indications of infection.

      8) Promote a positive self–image.

C. **Gastroesophageal Reflux Disease**

1. A condition in which the lower esophageal sphincter (LES) does not close properly, allowing stomach contents to back up into the esophagus.

2. Contributing Factors

   a. Older adults

   b. Obesity

   c. Smoking

   d. Heavy alcohol use

   e. Ingestion of very large meals

   f. Obstructive sleep apnea

3. Manifestations

   a. Dyspepsia

   b. Regurgitation

   c. Eructation

   d. Flatulence

   e. Coughing, hoarseness, wheezing

   f. Water brash

   g. Dysphagia

   h. Odynophagia

4. Collaborative Care

   a. **Nursing Interventions**

      1) Teach client dietary management.

         a) Limit or eliminate foods that decrease LES pressure: chocolate, caffeine, fried and/or fatty foods, alcohol, carbonated beverages, spicy and acidic foods.

         b) 4 to 6 small meals per day

         c) Eat slowly and chew thoroughly.

         d) Eating nothing for at least 3 hr before going to bed

      2) Teach to elevate the head of bed 6 to 12 inches.

      3) Teach to sleep on right side.

      4) Refer to smoking, alcohol cessation programs PRN.

      5) Encourage maintenance of proper weight.

      6) Teach to wear loose clothing.

      7) Medications

         a) Histamine blockers: famotidine, ranitidine

         b) Antacids

         c) Proton pump inhibitors: omeprazole, esomeprazole, or pantoprazole may be administered IV short term.

      8) Endoscopic procedures

D. **Hiatal Hernia**

1. A portion of the stomach protrudes through the esophageal hiatus of the diaphragm into the chest.

HIATAL HERNIA

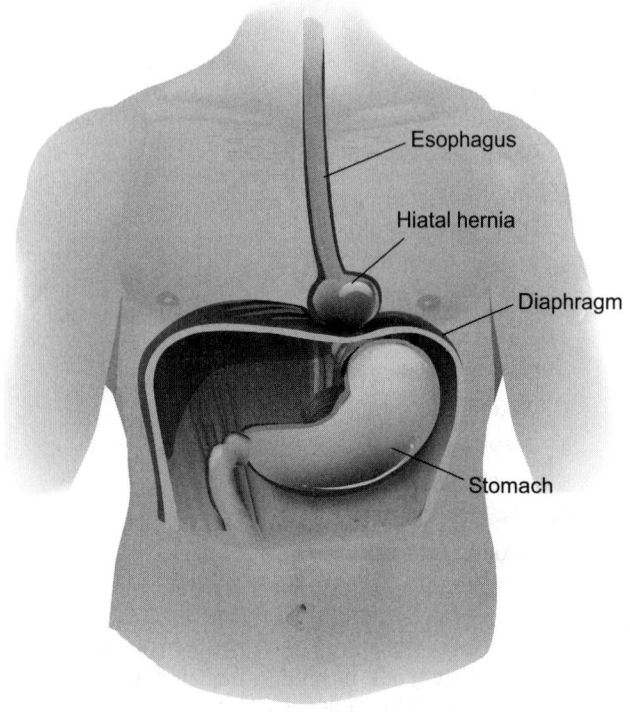

ALLEN CROSWHITE
ASSESSMENT TECHNOLOGIES INSTITUTE

2. Contributing Factors
   a. High-fat diet
   b. Caffeinated beverages
   c. Tobacco products
   d. Medications: Ca^{++} channel blockers, anticholinergics, nitrates
   e. Obesity
3. Manifestations
   a. Regurgitation
   b. Persistent heartburn and dysphagia
   c. Belching
   d. Epigastric pain
   e. Dysphagia
   f. Breathlessness or feeling of suffocation after eating
   g. Chest pain that mimics angina
   h. Symptoms worsen after a meal or when supine
4. Collaborative Care

   a. **Nursing Interventions**
      1) Prepare for barium swallow with fluoroscopy.
      2) Assess diet history.
      3) Encourage small frequent meals.
      4) Avoid eating 3 hr prior to bedtime.
      5) Sit upright 1 to 2 hr after meals.

      6) Elevate head of bed.
      7) Encourage weight reduction for clients with BMI greater than 25.
      8) Avoid straining or vigorous exercise.
      9) Wear loose clothing around abdomen.
      10) Monitor for complications.
         a) Bleeding or esophageal ulcers
         b) Barrett's esophagus
         c) Aggravation of asthma, chronic cough, and pulmonary fibrosis
   b. Medications
      1) Antacids
      2) Histamine$_2$ receptor antagonists
      3) Prokinetic agents
      4) Proton pump inhibitors
   c. Client Education
      1) Dietary medication regimen
      2) Precautions to prevent aspiration
   d. Therapeutic Measures
      1) Hiatal hernia—fundoplication if other measures ineffective

IV Gastrointestinal Disorders

A. **Peptic Ulcer Disease (PUD)**

1. Ulcerations in the stomach or duodenum as a result of mucosal tissue destruction; high risk of perforation and bleeding. May be referred to as gastric, duodenal, or esophageal ulcer, depending on location.
2. Contributing Factors
   a. NSAIDs
   b. Corticosteroids
   c. *H. pylori* infection
   d. Uncontrolled stress
   e. Smoking
   f. Caffeine
   g. Alcohol
   h. Type O blood
   i. Age between 40 and 60 years
3. Manifestations
   a. Dyspepsia
   b. Dull, gnawing, burning, midepigastric and/or back pain with localized tenderness
   c. Symptoms worsen with empty stomach
   d. Relief noted with antacids
   e. Belching
   f. Bloating
   g. Vomiting of undigested food that may or may not be proceeded by nausea
   h. Melena
   i. Decreased hematocrit and hemoglobin

4. Collaborative Care
   a. **Nursing Interventions**
      1) Refer to smoking and/or alcohol cessation programs PRN.
      2) Encourage stress-relieving techniques such as biofeedback, meditation, relaxation exercises.
      3) Teach dietary modifications.
         a) Avoid very cold and very hot foods.
         b) Eat three regular meals per day (small, frequent feedings are not necessary if an antacid or histamine blocker is taken).
         c) Avoid caffeine, alcohol, decaffeinated coffee, milk, and cream (diet is very individual— some may be able to tolerate these foods better than others).
      4) If other methods are not effective, prepare client for surgery (e.g., pyloroplasty, antrectomy).
   b. Medications
      1) Triple therapy for 10 to 14 days: two antibiotics— metronidazole or amoxicillin and clarithromycin— plus a proton pump inhibitor (preferred treatment)
      2) Quadruple therapy that adds bismuth salts to the previous
      3) Mucosal healing agents
      4) Stool softeners
      5) Antacids
      6) Histamine$_2$ receptor antagonists
      7) Prokinetic agents
      8) Proton pump inhibitors
   c. Diagnostic Tests
      1) EGD
      2) Chest and abdominal x-ray
      3) Hematocrit and hemoglobin
      4) Stool specimen
   d. Client Education
      1) Symptom management
      2) Medication therapy
      3) Nutrition therapy
      4) Stress reduction

B. **Irritable Bowel Syndrome (IBS)**
   1. Chronic disorder with recurrent diarrhea, constipation, and/or abdominal pain and bloating (most common digestive disorder seen in clinical practice)
   2. Contributing Factors
      a. Smoking
      b. Caffeine
      c. NSAIDs
      d. Stress
      e. Mental or behavioral illness
      f. High-fat diet
      g. Female gender
      h. Family history
      i. Dairy products
      j. Alcohol

3. Manifestations
   a. Weight loss
   b. Fatigue and malaise
   c. Erratic bowel patterns
   d. Abdominal pain relieved by defecation
   e. Abdominal distention
   f. Mucus with passage of stool
   g. Colicky abdomen with diffuse tenderness
4. Collaborative Care
   a. **Nursing Interventions**
      1) Encourage a diet high in fiber.
      2) Encourage regular exercise such as walking and yoga.
      3) Teach stress-reduction techniques.
      4) Teach to eat at regular times.
      5) Teach to eat slowly and chew thoroughly.
      6) Teach importance of adequate fluid intake, but discourage fluids with meals.
      7) Encourage a food diary to identify triggers.
   b. Medications
      1) Bulk agents (such as psyllium)
      2) Antidiarrheals
      3) Antidepressants
      4) Anticholinergics
      5) Antispasmodics
      6) Probiotics
      7) Complementary Agents
         a) Peppermint oil
         b) Artichoke leaf extract
         c) Caraway oil
   c. Diagnostic Tests
      1) Endoscopy
      2) Chest and abdominal x-ray
      3) Test for *H. pylori*
   d. Client Education
      1) Keeping diary to identify triggers
      2) Avoidance of causative agents
      3) Symptom management
      4) Medication therapy
      5) Nutrition therapy
      6) Stress reduction

c. **Inflammatory Bowel Disease**

! Point to Remember

Do not confuse inflammatory bowel disease with irritable bowel syndrome, which is much less severe. Inflammatory bowel disease is an autoimmune disorder and includes Crohn's disease and ulcerative colitis.

1. **Crohn's Disease**

   a. Inflammation of the GI tract that extends through all layers. It can occur anywhere in the intestinal tract, but most commonly occurs in the distal (terminal) ileum. It is characterized by the "cobblestone" appearance of ulcers that are separated by normal tissue.

CROHN'S DISEASE

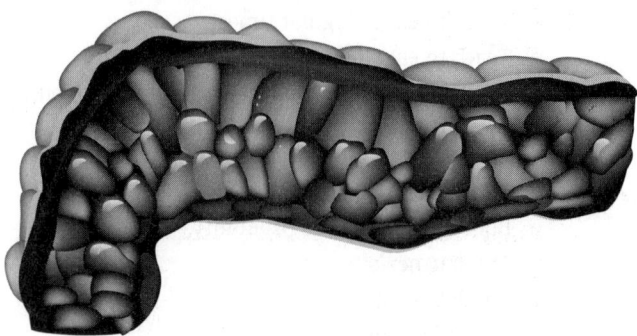

ALLEN CROSWHITE
ASSESSMENT TECHNOLOGIES INSTITUTE

   b. Contributing Factors
      1) Family history
      2) Jewish ancestry
      3) Bacterial infection
      4) Smoking
      5) Adolescents or young adults (ages 15 to 40)
      6) Living in an urban area
   c. Manifestations
      1) Abdominal pain (right lower quadrant); does not resolve with defecation; pain is aggravated by eating
      2) Low-grade fever
      3) Diarrhea, steatorrhea
      4) Weight loss (may become emaciated)
      5) Formation of fistulas (abnormal tracts between bowel and skin/bladder or vagina)
      6) Usually, there is no bleeding (which helps differentiate from ulcerative colitis).
      7) Low-grade fever, leukocytosis
      8) May be accompanied by arthritis, skin lesions, conjunctivitis, and/or oral ulcers
      9) "String sign" on x-ray: indicates constriction in a segment of the terminal ileum
      10) Decreased hematocrit and hemoglobin, elevated ESR

   d. Collaborative Care
      1) **Nursing Interventions**
         a) Promote adequate rest periods.
         b) Record color, volume, frequency, and consistency of stools.
         c) Monitor and prevent fluid deficit.
         d) Nutrition therapy includes high-calorie, protein, low-fiber, no dairy.
         e) Provide supportive care.
         f) Monitor for complications:
            (1) Intestinal obstruction
            (2) Perianal disease
            (3) Fluid electrolyte imbalances
            (4) Malnutrition
            (5) Fistula, abscess
         g) If the above measures are not effective, prepare for surgery: bowel resection with possible ileostomy or stricturoplasty.
         h) Refer to support group.
      2) Medications
         a) Steroids
         b) Anti-infective: metronidazole
         c) Aminosalicylates (5-ASAs)
         d) Immune modulators: infliximab, adalimumab, certolizumab, and natalizumab
         e) TPN
      3) Therapeutic Measures
         a) Bowel resection (possible ileostomy)
         b) Stricturoplasty
         c) Laboratory profiles: Hct, hemoglobin, C-reactive protein, WBC, ESR
         d) Abdominal x-ray
      4) Client Education
         a) Refer to support group.
         b) Dietary
         c) Health promotion and relaxation

2. **Ulcerative Colitis**

   a. Recurrent ulcerative and inflammatory disease of the superficial mucosa of the colon. It usually begins in the rectum and spreads proximally through the entire colon. It is characterized by contiguous ulcers.
   b. Contributing Factors
      1) Family history
      2) Jewish ancestry
      3) Isotretinoin (Accutane) use
      4) Young and middle-age adults (females 15 to 25 years; males 55 to 65 years)
      5) Caucasian ethnicity
      6) Low-fiber diet

c. Manifestations
1) Liquid, bloody stool (10 to 20 per day)
2) Low-grade fever
3) Abdominal distention along the colon
4) High-pitched bowel sounds
5) Rebound tenderness indicates perforation/peritonitis
6) Passage of mucus and pus from the bowel
7) Left, lower quadrant abdominal pain
8) Anorexia and weight loss
9) Vomiting and dehydration
10) Sensation of an urgent need to defecate
11) Hypocalcemia, anemia
12) Associated arthritis, conjunctivitis, skin lesions, and/or liver problems

Point to Remember

Bleeding is common with ulcerative colitis. This helps differentiate it from Crohn's disease, in which bleeding is rare.

d. Collaborative Care
1) **Nursing Interventions**
   a) Promote adequate rest periods.
   b) Record color, volume, frequency, and consistency of stools.
   c) Maintain NPO status during acute phase.
   d) Monitor for dehydration; maintain fluid balance.
   e) Monitor electrolytes; IV fluids may be indicated for imbalances.
   f) Provide dietary management and client education.
      (1) Increase oral fluids.
      (2) Low-residue, high-calorie, high-protein diet
   g) Administer multivitamin and supplemental iron.
   h) Refer to support group.
   i) If the above measures are not successful, prepare for surgery: proctocolectomy with ileostomy.
2) Medications
   a) Antidiarrheals (monitor for megacolon)
   b) Aminosalicylates (5-ASAs)
   c) Immune modulators: infliximab, adalimumab, certolizumab, and natalizumab
   d) TPN
   e) Corticosteroids (oral, parenteral, topical)
3) Therapeutic Measures
   a) Surgical management is indicated for bowel perforation, toxic megacolon, hemorrhage, and colon cancer.
      (1) Colectomy and ileostomy
      (2) Total proctocolectomy with permanent ileostomy
      (3) Laboratory profiles: Hct, hemoglobin, C-reactive protein, WBC, ESR
      (4) Abdominal x-ray

4) Client Education
   a) Refer to support group.
   b) Dietary
   c) Health promotion and relaxation

D. **Diverticular Disease**
1. Includes three conditions that involve numerous small sacs or pockets in the wall of the colon
   a. Diverticulosis: the presence of pouchlike herniations (diverticula) along the wall of the intestines; most common in the sigmoid colon
   b. Diverticular bleeding: results from injury of small vessels near the diverticula
   c. Diverticulitis: inflammation of one or more diverticula
2. Contributing Factors
   a. Aging
   b. Constipation
   c. Diet risk: low-fiber, high-fat, and red meat
   d. Connective tissue disorders causing weakness in the colon wall
3. Manifestations (diverticulitis)
   a. Alternating diarrhea with constipation
   b. Painful cramps or tenderness in the lower abdomen (lower left quadrant)
   c. Chills or fever
   d. Tachycardia; nausea and vomiting
4. Collaborative Care
   a. **Nursing Interventions**
      1) Dietary management
         a) Diverticulitis: begin with clear liquids; advance to a low-fiber diet.
         b) Diverticulosis: provide a high-fiber diet.
         c) Educate about fiber sources.
         d) Teach to avoid foods with nuts, seeds, or kernels (such as popcorn).
         e) Increase fluid intake to 3 L/day.
         f) Refer for nutritional counseling.
      2) Manage pain.
      3) Avoid laxatives.
      4) Monitor bowel elimination patterns.
      5) Monitor for complications (obstruction, hemorrhage, infection).
      6) In event of complications, prepare for surgery: colon resection.
   b. Medications
      1) Bulk laxatives (preventive)
      2) Metronidazole
      3) Trimethoprim/sulfamethoxazole
      4) Ciprofloxacin
      5) Antispasmodics (oxyphencyclimine)
      6) Analgesics (meperidine)

Point to Remember

Morphine is contraindicated because it can increase pressure in the colon, exacerbating symptoms.

c. Therapeutic Measures

    1) Emergency colon resection for peritonitis, bowel obstruction, or abscess

d. Client Teaching

    1) High-fiber versus low-fiber diet

    2) Collaborate with nutritionist.

    3) Preventive measures

E. **Abdominal Hernia**

1. Protrusion of bowel through the muscle wall of abdominal cavity (umbilical, ventral, inguinal/femoral). Classified as reducible, irreducible, or strangulated.

! Point to Remember

Absent bowel sounds can indicate strangulation, which cuts off the blood supply to the bowel. This is a medical emergency that can result in ischemia and obstruction, leading to necrosis and perforation. Manifestations are abdominal distention, nausea, vomiting, pain, fever, and tachycardia.

FEMORAL HERNIA

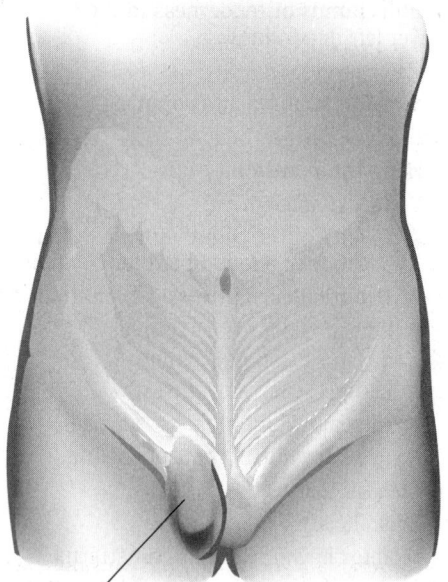

femoral hernia

2. Contributing Factors

a. Aging

b. Male gender

c. Obesity

d. Heavy lifting or straining

e. Abdominal surgery

f. Pregnancy

g. Congenital or acquired muscle weakness

h. Ascites, distension

3. Manifestations

a. Client reports "lump" felt at the involved site.

b. Pain in groin when bending, coughing, or lifting

c. Absent bowel sounds (strangulated)

d. Palpation of mass

4. Collaborative Care

a. **Nursing Interventions**

    1) Wear abdominal binder for support of herniated tissue.

    2) Encourage increased fluid intake.

    3) Monitor for complications: strangulation, perforation.

    4) Prepare for surgery: minimally invasive inguinal hernia repair (i.e., MIIHR or herniorrhaphy) or laparoscopic repair; bowel resection for strangulation.

    5) Postsurgical Care

        a) Allow to stand to void (males).

        b) For inguinal repair: elevate scrotum and apply ice.

        c) Teach to avoid coughing during recovery period.

        d) Teach to avoid lifting or straining for 4 to 6 weeks.

    6) Medications

        a) Analgesics

        b) Stool softeners

b. Therapeutic Procedures

    1) Herniorrhaphy laparoscopic repair

F. **Peritonitis**

1. Inflammation of peritoneum and lining of abdominal cavity; results from infection of the peritoneum due to puncture (surgery or trauma), septicemia, or rupture of part of the gastrointestinal tract; can be life-threatening

2. Manifestations

a. Rigid board-like abdomen (hallmark sign)

b. Nausea and vomiting

c. Tachycardic, febrile

d. Rebound abdominal tenderness

3. **Nursing Interventions**

a. Positioning—Fowler's or semi-Fowler's

b. Nasogastric tube to low intermittent suction

c. Oxygen

d. Monitor fluid and electrolytes.

e. Antibiotics as prescribed

4. Therapeutic Procedures

a. Exploratory surgery as needed based on client condition

G. **Intestinal Obstruction**

1. Partial or complete blockage of intestinal contents; can be the result of mechanical obstruction (e.g., adhesions, tumors, volvulus), neurogenic (such as paralytic ileus), or vascular (such as mesenteric artery occlusion)

2. Etiologies: any disorder that causes a mechanical or functional intestinal obstruction

3. Contributing Factors

   a. Crohn's disease

   b. Radiation therapy

   c. Fecal impaction

   d. Carcinomas

   e. Surgical procedures

   f. Narcotics

   g. Hypokalemia

   h. Diverticulitis

4. Manifestations

   a. Inability to pass flatus or stool for greater than 8 hr

   b. Abdominal distention

   c. Hyperactive bowel sounds above site of obstruction

   d. Hypoactive or active bowel sounds below site of obstruction

COMPARISON OF INTESTINAL OBSTRUCTION MANIFESTATIONS

Small Bowel	Large Intestine
Sporadic, colicky pain	Diffuse and constant pain
Visible peristaltic waves	Significant abdominal distention
Profuse, projectile vomitus with fecal odor (vomiting relieves pain)	Infrequent vomiting, leakage of fecal fluid around impaction

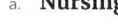

5. Collaborative Care

   a. **Nursing Interventions**

      1) NPO

      2) Assess bowel sounds.

      3) IV fluids

      4) Preoperative care

      5) NG tube for decompression

      6) Prevent fluid and electrolyte deficit.

   b. Therapeutic Measures

      1) Abdominal x-rays

      2) Endoscopy

      3) CT scan

      4) Surgical intervention (remove obstruction, resection)

   c. Client Teaching

      1) Preventive measures based on etiology

      2) Diet

V Gastric Surgical Procedures

A. **Bariatric Surgery for Morbid Obesity**

1. Morbid obesity is more than 2 times ideal body weight, which places clients at high risk for multiple health problems. Bariatric surgery is performed when nonsurgical attempts at weight reduction fail. Methods include: restrictive (gastric banding—reduces volume of the stomach), and malabsorptive (Roux-en-Y gastric bypass—interferes with food and nutrient absorption).

2. Indications for Surgery

   a. BMI greater than 40

   b. BMI greater than 35 with other diseases

   c. Repeated failure of nonsurgical weight reduction

3. Collaborative Care

   a. **Nursing Interventions**

      1) Preoperative Care

         a) Ensure thorough psychological preparation.

         b) Teach what to expect postsurgically: diet of liquids and pureed foods for first 6 weeks.

         c) Reinforce healthy lifestyle changes.

         d) Ensure support systems are available.

      2) Postoperative Care

         a) Immediate priority is airway.

         b) Ensure abdominal binder is in place.

         c) Place in semi-Fowler's position.

         d) Assist client to ambulate as soon as able, the day of surgery.

         e) Measure and compare abdominal girth; listen for bowel sounds.

         f) Collaborate with dietitian to introduce six small feedings per day; begin with 1 oz cups of clear liquids; increase amount as tolerated.

         g) Monitor for manifestations of dumping syndrome: tachycardia, nausea, diarrhea, abdominal cramping, diaphoresis; and anastomotic leak.

! Point to Remember

Anastomotic leaks are the most common complication and can be life-threatening. Monitor for increasing back, shoulder, and/or abdominal pain; restlessness; tachycardia; oliguria. Report to provider immediately.

      3) Medications

         a) Analgesics

         b) Antispasmodics

         c) Multivitamin

      4) Long-Term Management

         a) To prevent dumping syndrome: eat slowly; avoid drinking liquids with meals, after beginning solid foods; consume a high-protein, high-fat, low- to moderate-carbohydrate diet; lie flat with head slightly elevated for 30 to 60 min after eating.

         b) Encourage increase in physical activity.

         c) Provide ongoing psychological support.

B. **Colostomy:** a surgical procedure that brings the end of the colon through the abdominal wall, creating an opening for the evacuation of fecal material. May be temporary or permanent.

1. Indications

   a. Cancer or tumors

   b. Obstructive bowel disease

   c. Colectomy

   d. Severe diverticulitis or Crohn's disease

   e. Trauma

2. Collaborative Care

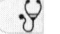

   a. **Nursing Interventions**

      1) Monitor ostomy site.

      2) Monitor output from stoma (the higher an ostomy is placed in the small intestine, the more liquid and acidic the output will be).

      3) Empty ostomy bag when ¼ to ½ full.

      4) Fit appliance to prevent leakage.

      5) Monitor for complications: fluid and electrolyte imbalances, ischemia of ostomy; bleeding, infection, peristomal skin irritation.

      6) Offer emotional support.

      7) Refer to support group.

   b. Client Education

      1) Teach how to fit, care for, and change appliance.

      2) Refer to ostomy nurse for additional teaching.

      3) A breath mint may be placed in bag to reduce odor.

      4) Dietary Management

         a) Teach to avoid hard-to-digest foods such as nuts, popcorn, celery, seeds, and coconut.

         b) Teach to maintain adequate fluid intake.

         c) Teach to reintroduce foods one at a time.

         d) Teach what foods may contribute to odor and gas: cruciferous vegetables, asparagus, fish, eggs, garlic, beans.

VI Hepatic Disorders

A. **Cirrhosis:** a chronic disease characterized by extensive, irreversible scarring of the liver that disrupts structure and function

1. Contributing Factors

   a. Alcohol consumption (Laennec's)

   b. Postnecrotic (hepatitis, chemicals)

   c. Biliary disease

   d. Severe right-sided heart failure

2. Manifestations

   a. Early Stage

      1) Enlarged liver

      2) Jaundice

      3) Gastrointestinal disturbances

      4) Weight loss

   b. Late Stage

      1) Liver becomes smaller and nodular

      2) Splenomegaly

      3) Ascites, distended abdominal veins; increased pressure in the portal system

      4) Bleeding tendencies; decreased vitamin K and prothrombin; anemia

      5) Esophageal varices, internal hemorrhoids; increased pressure in the portal area

      6) Dyspnea from ascites and anemia

      7) Pruritus from dry skin

      8) Clay-colored stools; no bile in stool

      9) Tea-colored urine; bile in urine

   c. End Stage—portal systemic encephalopathy

      1) Prodromal: slurred speech, vacant stare, restlessness, neurological deterioration

      2) Impending: asterixis (flapping tremors), apraxia, lethargy, confusion

      3) Stuporous: marked mental confusion, somnolence

      4) Coma: unarousable, fetor hepaticus, seizures, high mortality rate

3. Collaborative Care

   a. **Nursing Interventions**

      1) Encourage rest.

      2) Weigh the client daily and measure abdominal girth.

      3) Assess skin integrity frequently.

      4) Monitor I&O.

      5) Assess for bleeding and hemorrhoids.

      6) Avoid hepatotoxic medications.

      7) Maintain a high-calorie, low-protein (20 to 40 g/day), low-fat, low-sodium diet.

      8) Limit sodium and fluid intake as prescribed.

      9) Monitor liver enzymes, bilirubin, hematologic testing: CBC, WBC, platelets, PT/INR, and ammonia levels.

   b. Medications

      1) Diuretics: spironolactone, furosemide

      2) Neomycin and metronidazole: reduces intestinal bacteria.

      3) Lactulose: decreases ammonia levels.

      4) Supplemental vitamins (B_1 and B complex, A, C, and K; folic acid; and thiamine) as prescribed

      5) Fat-soluble vitamin supplements and folic acid may need to be given IV.

      6) Proton pump inhibitors and H_2 receptor antagonist

      7) Albumin IV to decrease ascites

c. Therapeutic Measures
   1) Liver biopsy
   2) EGD
   3) Paracentesis
   4) Transjugular intrahepatic portosystemic shunt (TIPS)
d. Client Education
   1) Alcohol abstinence
   2) Dietary guidelines
   3) Bleeding risk and precautions
4. Referral and Follow-up
   a. Alcohol recovery program
   b. Nutrition
   c. Social services

B. **Hepatitis**
1. Inflammation of the liver caused by infectious organisms, chemicals, or toxins. Cases must be reported to the local health department.

CHARACTERISTICS OF HEPATITIS

Mode of transmission

TYPE A (HAV)	Fecal-oral route Person-to-person	Food/water contamination
TYPE B (HBV)	Unprotected sex Sharing needles Needlesticks	Blood products; organ transplant before 1992
TYPE C (HCV)	Blood-to-blood Illicit IV drug sharing Unprotected sex	Blood products; organ transplant before 1992

Manifestations

TYPE A (HAV)	Mild course "Flu-like" Advanced age and chronic disease increase severity.	
TYPE B (HBV)	May be asymptomatic RUQ pain Anorexia, N/V Fatigue	Febrile Dark urine Light-colored stool Jaundice
TYPE C (HCV)	Most are asymptomatic Diagnosis with blood testing Chronic inflammation progresses to cirrhosis.	

Prevention

TYPE A (HAV)	Hand washing Vaccine for ages 2 and older 2 doses 6 to 18 months apart
TYPE B (HBV)	Vaccine infants and high-risk populations 3 doses over 6-month period
TYPE C (HCV)	Avoid high-risk behaviors.

Treatment

TYPE A (HAV)	Symptom-specific May have change in medication regimen to "rest liver"
TYPE B (HBV)	Antiviral drugs
TYPE C (HCV)	Administer peginterferon alfa-2B (PegIntron). Monitor kidney function.

C. **Nonviral Hepatitis**
1. Definition: liver injury and inflammation caused by ingestion of drugs and chemicals (industrial toxins, alcohol, drugs)
2. Contributing Factors
   a. Inhalation of hepatotoxic agents
   b. Drug toxicity
   c. Alcohol
   d. Secondary infection may occur with Epstein-Barr, herpes simplex, varicella-zoster, and cytomegalovirus.
3. Manifestations
   a. Jaundice
   b. Liver enlargement
   c. Liver necrosis
4. Collaborative Care
   a. Monitor signs of liver impairment.
   b. Monitor client for right upper quadrant pain.
   c. Monitor weight.
   d. Treatment is specific to symptoms and causative factors.

D. **Gallbladder Disease**
1. Types
   a. Cholecystitis: inflammation of the gallbladder
   b. Cholelithiasis: presence of stones in the gallbladder
2. Contributing Factors
   a. More common in females
   b. Obesity
   c. High-fat diet
   d. Older adults
   e. Type 2 diabetes
3. Manifestations
   a. Sharp right upper quadrant, epigastric, or shoulder pain
   b. Nausea and vomiting after ingestion of high-fat food
   c. Murphy's sign
   d. Flatulence
   e. Dyspepsia
   f. Dark urine, clay-colored stool

4. Diagnostic Procedures
   a. Ultrasound
   b. Hepatobiliary (HIDA) scan
   c. Endoscopic retrograde cholangiopancreatography (ERCP)
   d. Cholangiography
5. Collaborative Care
   a. **Nursing Interventions**
      1) Administer analgesics as prescribed.
      2) Prevent F&E imbalances.
      3) Maintain low-fat diet.
      4) Provide postoperative care.
      5) Cholecystectomy client may have T-tube 1 to 2 weeks post-op.
         a) Monitor drainage; keep below level of GB.
         b) Empty collection bag every 8 hr.
         c) Report drainage amounts greater than 1,000 mL/day.
         d) Never irrigate without physician order.
      6) Observe color of stool.
      7) Monitor for indications of postcholecystectomy syndrome (manifestations of cholecystitis after surgery) and report to physician.
   b. Medications
      1) Analgesics: morphine or hydromorphone (acute biliary pain); ketorolac (mild to moderate pain)
      2) Antiemetics
      3) Anticholinergics
      4) Ursodeoxycholic acid and chenodiol can be used to nonsurgically dissolve stones.
      5) Antibiotics
   c. Therapeutic Measures
      1) Sphincterotomy with stone removal may be done with ERCP.
      2) Extracorporeal shock wave lithotripsy (ESWL) to break up stones (only for small cholesterol stones)
      3) Cholecystectomy
   d. Client Education
      1) Resume regular low-fat diet.
      2) Prevent dumping syndrome.
      3) Care of T-tube (postdischarge)

VII Pancreatic Disorders

A. **Acute Pancreatitis**
   1. Inflammation of the pancreas caused by autodigestion by exocrine enzymes. It is life-threatening.
B. **Chronic pancreatitis:** progressive disease of the pancreas characterized by remissions and exacerbations resulting in diminished function
   1. Contributing Factors
      a. Alcohol use disorder
      b. Gallstones
      c. Illegal drug use
      d. Infection
      e. Blunt abdominal trauma
      f. Operative manipulation and trauma
   2. Manifestations
      a. Severe midepigastric or left upper quadrant pain
      b. Pain intensifies after meals and when lying down.
      c. Nausea and vomiting
      d. Weight loss
      e. Abdominal tenderness; ascites
      f. Elevated amylase and lipase
      g. Steatorrhea
      h. Turner's sign
      i. Cullen's sign
   3. Diagnostic Procedures
      a. Laboratory profiles: liver enzymes, bilirubin, pancreatic enzymes
      b. CT scan with contrast
   4. Collaborative Care
      a. **Nursing Interventions**
         1) Dietary Management
            a) NPO initially
            b) After 24 to 48 hr, begin jejunal feedings.
            c) When food is tolerated, advance to small, frequent, moderate to high-carbohydrate, high-protein, low-fat meals.
         2) Nasogastric tube for the severely ill, with intractable vomiting or biliary obstruction
         3) Pain management
         4) Position for comfort (e.g. fetal, sitting up, leaning forward).
         5) Monitor bowel sounds.
         6) I&O
         7) Monitor for indications of hypocalcemia and hypomagnesemia.
         8) Monitor respirations.
         9) Reassure clients, and carefully explain procedures to reduce anxiety.

b. Medications

1) Antibiotics

2) Opioid analgesics: morphine or hydromorphone; **meperidine is contraindicated**

3) Anticholinergics

4) Pancreatic enzymes

5) H$_2$ blockers or proton pump inhibitors

c. Therapeutic Measures

1) TPN

2) ERCP to create an opening in sphincter of Oddi if cause is gallstones

3) Cholecystectomy

4) Pancreaticojejunostomy (Roux-en-Y) to "reroute" pancreatic secretions to the jejunum

d. Client Education for Chronic Pancreatitis

1) Take enzymes before meals and snacks.

2) Follow up with all scheduled laboratory testing.

3) Nutrition: high-caloric needs.

4) Abstain from alcohol.

5) Limit fat intake.

5. Referral and Follow-up

a. Alcohol recovery program

b. Home health for clients requiring long-term TPN

c. Refer to a dietitian.

C. **Pancreatic Cancer**

1. Carcinoma has vague symptoms and is usually diagnosed in late stages after liver or gallbladder involvement. High mortality rate.

2. Contributing Factors

a. Older age

b. Tobacco use

c. Chronic pancreatitis

d. Diabetes mellitus

e. Cirrhosis

f. High intake of red meat, processed meat

g. Obesity

h. Small number have an inherited risk

3. Manifestations

a. Fatigue, anorexia, flatulence

b. Pruritus

c. Weight loss, palpable abdominal mass, abdominal pain that may radiate to the back

d. Hepatomegaly, jaundice (late sign when cancer blocks the bile duct)

e. Ascites

f. Clay-colored stools; dark urine

g. Glucose intolerance

4. Diagnostic Procedures

a. Carcinoembryonic Antigen (CEA) Levels

1) Expected findings: less than 2.5 nonsmoker; less than 5 ng/ml smoker

2) Critical findings: greater than 6 ng/ml

b. Elevated serum amylase and lipase

c. Elevated alkaline phosphatase and bilirubin

d. ERCP

e. Ultrasound, CT scan

5. Collaborative Care

a. **Nursing Interventions**

1) Palliative care measures

2) Pain management

3) Monitor blood glucose levels.

4) Provide nutritional support (enteral supplements and TPN).

b. Medications

1) Opioid analgesics: morphine or hydromorphone

c. Therapeutic Measures

1) Chemotherapy may be used to shrink the tumor size. The nurse monitors for myelosuppression and pancytopenia.

2) Radiation therapy

3) Partial pancreatectomy for small tumors

4) **Whipple procedure:** Pancreatoduodenectomy is the most common operation to remove (i.e., resect) pancreatic cancers. Procedure done when cancer is located in the head of the pancreas. Involves removing the head of the pancreas, duodenum, parts of the jejunum and stomach, gallbladder, and possibly spleen. The pancreatic duct is reconnected to the common bile duct, and the stomach is connected to the jejunum. May be done laparoscopically.

a) **Nursing Interventions**

(1) Provide routine postoperative care.

(2) Monitor NG output. Observe for bloody or bile-tinged drainage, which can indicate anastomotic disruption.

(3) Maintain a semi-Fowler's position to prevent stress on suture line.

(4) Facilitate coughing, deep breathing, and use of incentive spirometer.

(5) Monitor blood glucose and administer insulin as needed.

(6) Provide analgesia.

d. Client Education

1) Encourage client to seek palliative care at home, cancer support group, and available community resources.

2) Support measures for pain, anorexia, and weight loss.

Disorders of the Musculoskeletal System

I Diagnostic Tests for Musculoskeletal Disorders

A. **Arthroscopy:** visualizes internal structures of shoulder or knee joints. Cannot be done if infection present; client must be able to bend joint at least 40 degrees.

1. Apply ice and elevate 24 hr post-procedure.
2. Collaborate with physical therapist for exercises.

B. **Bone scan:** Radioactive medium is injected for viewing entire skeleton, primarily to detect tumors, arthritis, osteomyelitis, osteoporosis, vertebral compression fractures, and unexplained bone pain.

1. Technician or physician administers the isotope 4 to 6 hr prior to testing.
2. Client must lie still for 30 to 60 min as imaging is performed.
3. Increase fluids post procedures.

C. **Dual-energy x-ray absorptiometry (DEXA) scan:** most common screening tool for measuring bone mineral density for diagnosis of osteopenia and osteoporosis

1. Baseline for women in their 40s.
2. Client should wear loose clothing without zippers or metal.
3. Client must remove jewelry.
4. Instruct client to stop vitamin D and calcium supplementation 48 hr prior to scan.

D. **Electromyography (EMG) and nerve conduction studies:** used to evaluate muscle weakness by emission of low-frequency electrical stimulation (e.g., ALS, carpal tunnel, myasthenia gravis, Guillain-Barré)

1. Client will be asked to perform activities for measurement of muscle activity.
2. Observe needle insertion sites for hematoma.
3. Support client with anxiety related to testing.

E. **Magnetic resonance imaging (MRI):** imaging produced through interaction of magnetic fields, radio waves, and atomic nuclei to diagnose muscle, tissue, and bone disorders

1. Client must remove all metal objects (inquire about surgically implanted devices, nonvisible piercings). Canes, crutches, and walkers generally must be left outside of the MRI room; assist client as necessary to stretcher.
2. Contraindicated for clients with pacemakers, stents, and surgical clips.
3. Clients with titanium joint replacements may have MRI.
4. Assess client for claustrophobia if closed scanner is used.
5. Assess client for ability to lie still in supine position for 45 to 60 min.

F. **Laboratory**

1. Serum calcium
2. Serum phosphorus
3. Alkaline phosphatase
4. Creatine kinase
5. Lactic dehydrogenase
6. Aspartate aminotransferase
7. Aldolase

II Arthritis

Inflammation of one or more joints, which results in pain, swelling, stiffness, and limited movement

A. **Osteoarthritis:** progressive degenerative deterioration and loss of cartilage in one or more joints

1. Contributing Factors
   a. Aging
   b. Female
   c. Metabolic disease
   d. Obesity
   e. Repetitive use or abuse of joints
   f. Smoking

2. Manifestations
   a. Chronic joint pain and stiffness
   b. Pain diminished after rest and worsens after activity
   c. Crepitus
   d. Limited movement
   e. Heberden's nodes (closest to the end of the fingers and toes)
   f. Bouchard's nodes (middle joints of fingers or toes)
   g. Excess joint fluid (especially with knee involvement)
   h. Skeletal muscle atrophy from disuse

ARTHRITIS MANIFESTATIONS

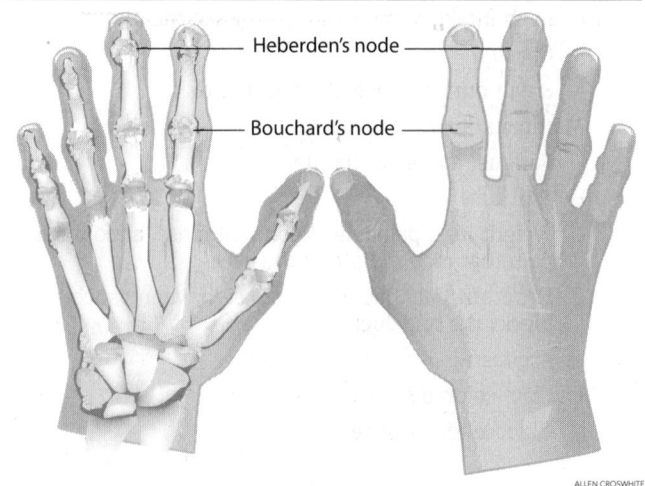

Heberden's node

Bouchard's node

ALLEN CROSWHITE
ASSESSMENT TECHNOLOGIES INSTITUTE

3. Diagnostic Procedures
   a. X-rays
   b. MRI
   c. Erythrocyte sedimentation rate (ESR) and serum C-reactive protein (CRP) show slight elevation.
4. Collaborative Care
   a. **Nursing Interventions**
      1) Assess and manage pain.
      2) Instruct client to use ice or heat for comfort.
      3) Encourage client to perform range of motion and isometric exercises.
      4) Encourage adequate rest and sleep as needed to relieve pain.
      5) Involve physical therapy as appropriate.
      6) Use assistive devices to help increase independence and complete activities of daily living.
   b. Medications
      1) NSAIDs
      2) Corticosteroids
      3) Topical analgesics
      4) Supplements
         a) Glucosamine
         b) Chondroitin sulfate
   c. Therapeutic Measures
      1) Total joint arthroplasty
      2) Total joint replacement
   d. Client Education
      1) Use of mobility devices and safety
      2) Prevention of complications
      3) Perform exercises per treatment plan.
5. Referral and Follow-up
   a. Physical therapy
   b. Rehabilitation therapy

B. **Rheumatoid arthritis:** chronic, progressive autoimmune connective tissue disorder primarily affecting synovial joints
   1. Contributing Factors
      a. Physical and emotional stress
      b. Female gender
      c. Young to middle age
      d. Family history
   2. Manifestations
      a. Morning stiffness; pain at rest or after immobility
      b. Bilateral joint inflammation with decreased range of motion
      c. Joint deformity in late stages
      d. Warmth, redness, and edema of affected areas
      e. Dry eyes and mouth (Sjögren's syndrome)
      f. Numbness, tingling, or burning in the hands and feet

3. Diagnostic Procedures
   a. X-ray
   b. MRI
   c. Positive rheumatoid factor
   d. Synovial fluid analysis
   e. Antinuclear antibody test
   f. Erythrocyte sedimentation rate
   g. C-reactive protein
4. Collaborative Care
   a. **Nursing Interventions**
      1) Instruct client to use ice or heat for comfort.
      2) Encourage physical activity to maintain joint mobility (within client's capacity).
      3) Monitor client for indications of fatigue.
      4) Monitor for complications related to therapy (e.g., secondary osteoporosis, vasculitis).
      5) Complementary Therapies
         a) Hypnosis
         b) Imagery
         c) Acupuncture
         d) Music therapy
         e) Omega-3
         f) Tai chi
   b. Medications
      1) NSAIDs
      2) Corticosteroids
      3) Disease-Modifying Antirheumatic Drugs (DMARDs)
         a) Methotrexate
         b) Leflunomide
         c) Hydroxychloroquine
      4) Biologic-Response Modifiers (administered parenterally)
         a) Etanercept
         b) Adalimumab
   c. Therapeutic Measures
      1) Plasmapheresis for severe, life-threatening exacerbation
      2) Synovectomy
      3) Total joint arthroplasty if unresponsive to medication
   d. Client Education
      1) Use of mobility devices and safety
      2) Prevention of complications
      3) Perform exercises per treatment plan.
5. Referral and Follow-up
   a. Occupational/physical therapy
   b. Rehabilitation therapy
   c. Arthritis support group

C. **Gouty arthritis:** systemic inflammatory disease caused by problems with purine metabolism (primary gout) or hyperuricemia (secondary gout)

1. Contributing Factors
   a. Family history
   b. Excessive alcohol intake
   c. High intake of foods with purines (e.g., organ meats, yeast, sardines, spinach)
   d. Obesity
   e. Comorbid conditions of DM and/or kidney disease

2. Manifestations
   a. Excruciating pain and inflammation in one or more small joints (great toe is most common joint; appears warm and red)
   b. Appearance of tophi (i.e., deposits of sodium urate crystals; generally appear after years of gouty arthritis)
   c. Progressive joint damage and deformity
   d. Increased incidence of uric acid renal stone

3. Diagnostic Procedures
   a. Serum uric acid greater than 7 mg/dL
   b. ESR
   c. Synovial fluid analysis (will show uric acid crystals)

4. Collaborative Care
   a. **Nursing Interventions**
      1) Maintain bed rest during acute attacks.
      2) Use bed cradle to keep linen elevated above affected joint.
      3) Promote fluid intake 3 L daily.
      4) Limit foods high in purine.
   b. Medications
      1) Acute phase: colchicine
      2) Chronic treatment: allopurinol
      3) NSAIDs
      4) Corticosteroids
      5) Injection of corticosteroid into affected joint by provider
   c. Client Education
      1) Foods to avoid (i.e., those high in purine)
      2) Instruct client to keep diary of triggering factors.
      3) Avoid alcohol.
      4) Lose weight slowly (rapid weight loss may precipitate a flare-up or increase the incidence of uric acid renal stones).

III Fractures

A break or disruption in the continuity of bone tissue

A. **Types of Fractures**
   1. Closed
   2. Comminuted (i.e., fragmented)
   3. Compression
   4. Displaced
   5. Greenstick
   6. Impacted
   7. Oblique
   8. Open (i.e., compound)
   9. Pathologic (caused by tumors, infection, bone disease)
   10. Spiral
   11. Stress (i.e., small crack in bone)

TYPES OF BONE FRACTURES

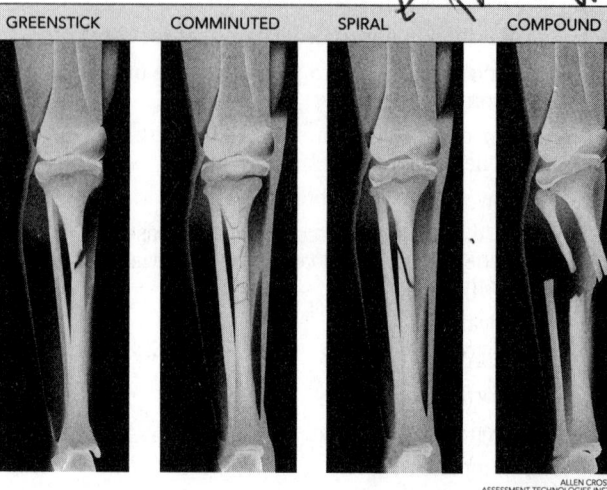

GREENSTICK · COMMINUTED · SPIRAL · COMPOUND

ALLEN CROSWHITE
ASSESSMENT TECHNOLOGIES INSTITUTE

B. **Collaborative Care**
   1. Assess client's neurovascular status (6 P's), noting bilateral comparisons.
      a. Pain
      b. Pressure
      c. Paralysis
      d. Pallor
      e. Pulselessness
      f. Paresthesia
   2. Monitor for changes in skin temperature.
   3. Monitor for complications of fat embolism (most common with long bone fractures):
      a. Confusion, anxiety
      b. Tachycardia
      c. Chest pain
      d. Tachypnea
      e. Hemoptysis
      f. Petechiae over neck, upper arms, chest, abdomen (late sign)
   4. Monitor for complications of compartment syndrome (irreversible if compromise persists beyond 4 to 6 hr).
      a. Pain unrelieved by positioning or medication
      b. Cyanosis
      c. Tingling
      d. Paralysis
   5. Maintain correct body alignment.
   6. Provide nursing care specific to therapeutic measures of fracture reduction.

C. **Therapeutic Measures**

1. Cast: application of plaster or fiberglass to immobilize and maintain alignment of the bone

   a. Collaborative Care

      1) Assess neurovascular status.

      2) Allow plaster cast to air-dry. Handle cast with palms while drying.

      3) Elevate affected extremity.

      4) Monitor for complications.

      5) Client may "petal" plaster cast if irritation around edges develops.

      6) To help reduce risk of infection, remind client to not place objects down cast.

2. Traction

   a. Skin traction: provides a mechanical pulling force to overcome muscle spasms, to immobilize or relieve pain

      1) Buck's

      2) Bryant's

      3) Cervical halter

      4) Pelvic

   b. Skeletal traction: applied directly to a bone to reduce a fracture or maintain surgically manipulated bone alignment

      1) Pins or wires inserted through skin and soft tissue into the bone

      2) Balanced suspension using splints, slings, weights

D. **External fixation device:** rigid metal frames with attached percutaneous pins or wires used to align and immobilize

   1. Collaborative Care

      a. Assess pulses and vascular status.

      b. Maintain proper body alignment.

      c. Verify weights are free-hanging.

      d. Monitor skin for pressure points or breakdown.

      e. Promote strengthening exercises for uninjured areas.

      f. Consult with physical therapy team.

      g. Pin site care per agency protocol.

      h. Administer medications (e.g., opioids, NSAIDs, muscle relaxants).

EXTERNAL FIXATION DEVICES

Cervical Traction

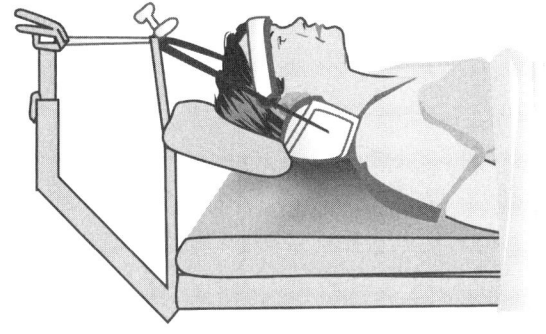

Buck's Traction

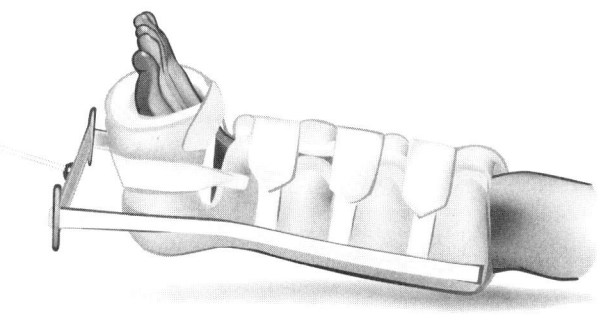

Balanced Suspension Skeletal Traction

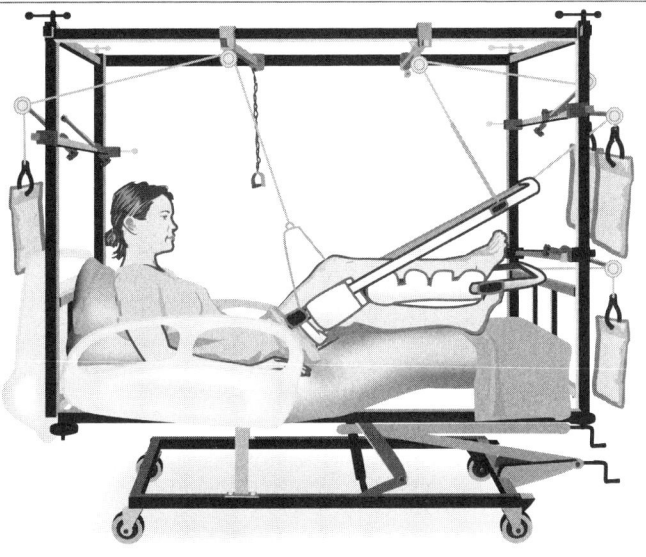

Halo Traction

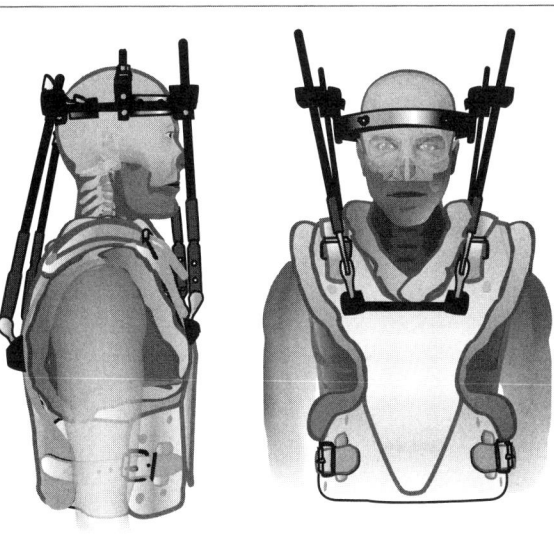

IV Osteoporosis

Chronic disease in which bone loss causes decreased density and possible fracture. Osteopenia is the precursor of osteoporosis.

A. **Contributing Factors**

1. Primary Osteoporosis
   a. Women age 65 and older
   b. Men age 75 and older
   c. Asian and Caucasian ethnicity
   d. Family history
   e. Estrogen or androgen deficiency
   f. Protein deficiency
   g. Sedentary lifestyle
   h. Smoking and alcohol intake

2. Secondary Osteoporosis
   a. Bone cancer
   b. Cushing's syndrome
   c. Diabetes mellitus
   d. Medications: corticosteroids, phenytoin, cytotoxic agents, immunosuppressants, loop diuretics
   e. Paget's disease
   f. Prolonged immobilization
   g. Rheumatoid arthritis

B. **Manifestations**

1. Shortened height
2. History of fractures
3. Thoracic kyphosis
4. Decreased bone mass

C. **Collaborative Care**

1. **Nursing Interventions**
   a. Encourage safe weight-bearing exercises.
   b. Teach strengthening exercises; encourage walking.
   c. Instruct client to increase foods rich in calcium and vitamin D.
   d. Refer to smoking cessation program.
   e. Implement fall precautions.

2. Medications
   a. Biophosphonates
   b. Calcium supplements
   c. Vitamin D supplements
   d. Estrogen agonists/antagonists
   e. Calcitonin
   f. Parathyroid hormone (prepared as teriparatide [Forteo]): Teach to administer subcutaneously each day.

3. Client Education
   a. Instruct client to continue health screenings and diagnostic evaluations.
   b. Instruct client to avoid activities with increased risk of falls (e.g., ice, slippery surfaces).
   c. Instruct client to take medications as prescribed.

V Osteomyelitis

An acute or chronic bone infection

A. **Contributing Factors**

1. Diabetes
2. Hemodialysis
3. Injection drug use
4. Poor blood supply
5. Recent trauma

B. **Manifestations**

1. Bone pain
2. Fever
3. General discomfort, uneasiness, or ill feeling (i.e., malaise)
4. Local swelling, redness, and warmth
5. Other Possible Manifestations
   a. Chills
   b. Excessive sweating
   c. Low back pain
   d. Swelling of the ankles, feet, and legs

C. **Diagnostic Procedures**

1. Bone biopsy (which is then cultured)
2. Bone scan
3. Bone x-ray
4. Complete blood count (CBC)
5. CRP
6. ESR
7. MRI of the bone
8. Needle aspiration of the area around affected bones

D. **Collaborative Care**

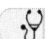

1. **Nursing Interventions**
   a. Initiate IV antibiotic therapy as soon as possible.
   b. In the presence of wound drainage, implement contact precautions.
   c. Teach that the full course of antibiotics must be completed, even if manifestations disappear.
   d. Implement wound irrigation.
   e. Refer to wound care nurse as needed.

2. Medications
   a. Antibiotics
   b. Analgesics

3. Therapeutic Measures
   a. Surgical excision of dead and infected bone may be needed.
   b. Bone grafting may be performed in large impacted areas.

VI Total Joint Arthroplasty (Replacement)

Surgical procedure performed to replace a joint with a prosthetic system. Arthroplasty may be performed for ankle, finger, elbow, shoulder, toe, and wrist. The hip and knee arthroplasties are the most commonly performed procedures.

KNEE REPLACEMENT

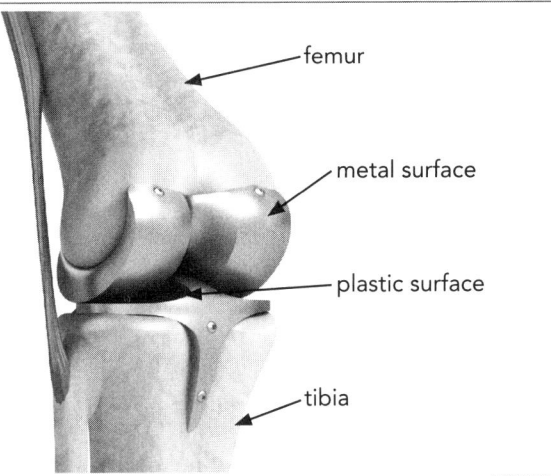

femur

metal surface

plastic surface

tibia

ALEXANDR MITIUC
GETTY IMAGES/ISTOCKPHOTO

A. **Contributing Factors**

1. Impaired mobility and uncontrolled pain related to osteoarthritis
2. Congenital anomalies
3. Trauma
4. Osteonecrosis

B. **Collaborative Care**

1. **Nursing Interventions**

   a. Position client correctly, maintaining alignment.
      1) Hip arthroplasty: keep abductor pillow in place while in bed, do not flex hip more than 90° (do not position on operative site).
      2) Knee arthroplasty: maintain continuous passive motion (CPM) machine to promote joint mobility.
   b. Assess for pain, rotation, and extremity shortening.
   c. Assess neurovascular status.
   d. Use aseptic technique for wound care and emptying of drains.
   e. Monitor for indications of infection.
   f. Ambulate the day of surgery and after stabilization and discharge from PACU.
   g. Use toilet seat extender.
   h. Teach exercises to reduce risk of DVT: ankle dorsiflexion, circles with the feet, push feet into bed while tightening quads, and straight leg raises.

2. Medications
   a. Anticoagulants
   b. NSAIDs
   c. Opioid narcotics; extended-release epidural morphine or PCA
   d. Antibiotics

3. Client Education
   a. Instruct client to participate in exercise regimen.
   b. Instruct client in use of ambulatory devices.

C. **Referral and Follow-up**

1. Physical therapy for ambulation, transfer, and joint movement
2. Occupational therapy to meet goals of independence and self-care

VII Amputations

Removal of a part of the body; may be elective or traumatic

A. **Types of Amputations**

1. Above-the-knee
2. Below-the-knee
3. Mid-foot
4. Toe

B. **Contributing Factors**

1. Peripheral vascular disease
2. Severe crushing of tissues or significant vessels
3. Malignant tumors
4. Osteomyelitis
5. Thermal injuries

C. **Collaborative Care**

1. **Nursing Interventions**

   a. Assess neurovascular status.
   b. Assess psychosocial status.
   c. Assess client's willingness and motivation to withstand prolonged rehabilitation.
   d. Manage phantom limb and residual limb pain.
   e. Monitor for signs of wound healing.
   f. Monitor for complications:
      1) Hemorrhage
      2) Infection
      3) Phantom limb pain
      4) Flexion contractures
   g. Promote mobility and range of motion.
   h. Promote independence.
   i. Maintain aseptic technique with dressing changes.
   j. Wrap residual limb with figure-8 elastic bandage after surgical dressing is removed.

FIGURE-8 BANDAGE

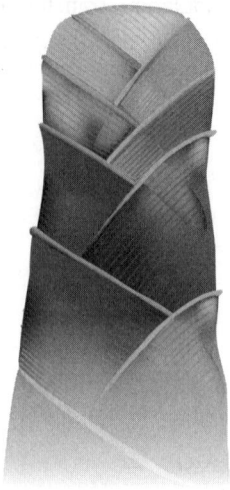

ALLEN CROSWHITE
ASSESSMENT TECHNOLOGIES INSTITUTE

2. Medications

   a. Opioids for residual limb pain

   b. Calcitonin to reduce phantom pain

   c. Antispasmodics for muscle spasms

   d. Beta blockers for constant, dull, burning pain

   e. Antiepileptic drugs for knifelike or sharp burning pain

3. Client Education

   a. Types of pain and management regimen

   b. Measures to prevent contractures

   c. Use of ambulatory devices or prosthetics

D. **Referral and Follow-up**

1. Rehabilitation therapy

2. Support group

SECTION 6

Endocrine System Functions and Disorders

Overview of the endocrine system: The endocrine system is made up of glands, organs, and hormones. The endocrine system works with the nervous system to regulate body function and maintain homeostasis through feedback loops. Endocrine glands include the hypothalamus, pituitary gland, adrenal glands, thyroid gland, parathyroid glands, islet cells of the pancreas, and gonads.

I Pituitary Gland

A. **Anterior pituitary gland:** secretion of these hormones is controlled by the hypothalamus.

1. Adrenocorticotropic hormone (ACTH)

2. Follicle-stimulating hormone (FSH)

3. Luteinizing hormone (LH)

4. Gonadotropic hormones

5. Prolactin

6. Growth hormone (GH)

7. Thyroid-stimulating hormone (TSH)

B. **Posterior pituitary gland**

1. Vasopressin (antidiuretic hormone [ADH])

2. Oxytocin

II Disorders of the Anterior Pituitary Gland

A. **Acromegaly:** hypersecretion of growth hormone (GH) that occurs after puberty

1. Manifestations

   a. Enlargement of skeletal extremities; increase in adult height; change in ring and/or shoe size

   b. Protrusion of the jaw and orbital ridges

   c. Headache, visual problems, and blindness

   d. Muscle weakness

   e. Organ enlargement

   f. Decalcification of the skeleton

   g. Endocrine disturbances similar to hyperthyroidism

2. Diagnostic Procedures

   a. Serum studies, showing elevated GH levels

   b. CT and MRI of pituitary may show pituitary tumor.

   c. X-rays show abnormal bone growth.

3. Collaborative Care

   a. **Nursing Interventions**

     1) Provide emotional support.

     2) Provide symptomatic care.

     3) Prepare client for surgery or radiation if indicated for tumor treatment.

   b. Medications

     1) Octreotide—synthetic GH analogue

     2) Bromocriptine mesylate or pergolide—dopamine agonists

   c. Therapeutic Measures

     1) Surgical removal of pituitary gland (i.e., transsphenoidal hypophysectomy); surgery is generally the first treatment option.

     2) Replacement therapy will be needed following surgical removal of the pituitary gland and may be needed following radiation therapy.

       a) Corticosteroids

       b) Thyroid hormones

     3) Radiation therapy

4. Client Education and Referral

   a. Medication adherence

   b. Continued compliance with follow-up appointments with all providers

B. **Gigantism:** hypersecretion of GH that occurs in childhood prior to closure of the growth plates

1. Manifestations

   a. Proportional overgrowth in all body tissue

2. Diagnostic Procedures/Collaborative Care: same as acromegaly

C. **Dwarfism:** hyposecretion of GH during fetal development or childhood that results in limited growth congenital or result from damage to the pituitary gland

1. Manifestations
   a. Head and extremities are disproportionate to torso.
      1) Face may appear younger than peers'.
   b. Short stature; slow or flat growth rate
   c. Progressive bowed legs and lordosis
   d. Delayed adolescence or puberty
2. Diagnostic Procedures
   a. Comparison of height/weight against growth charts; slowed growth rate will be noted.
   b. Serum growth hormone level; most providers will also evaluate other hormonal levels to ensure that no secondary deficiencies exist.
   c. MRI of the head (to assess pituitary gland)
3. Collaborative Care
   a. **Nursing Interventions**
      1) Teach child and family adaptive measures available for ADLs.
      2) Teach child and family how to administer supplemental GH.
         a) The earlier the therapy is initiated, the better the prognosis.
         b) GH therapy does not work in all children.
      3) Provide positive feedback to child to promote positive self-esteem.
   b. Medications
      1) Human growth hormone injections

III Disorders of the Posterior Pituitary Gland

A. **Diabetes insipidus (DI):** a deficiency of antidiuretic hormone (ADH or vasopressin) due to a disorder of the posterior pituitary gland that results in the inability of the kidneys to conserve water appropriately. DI is caused by head trauma, tumor, surgery, radiation, CNS infections, malignant tumors, or failure of renal tubules. The underlying cause of DI should be identified and treated.

1. Manifestations
   a. Urine Chemistry (dilute)
      1) Decreased urine specific gravity
      2) Decreased urine osmolality
   b. Serum Chemistry (concentrated)
      1) Hypernatremia
      2) Increased serum osmolality
   c. Polyuria and Polydipsia
      1) Increased urinary output
      2) Clients may crave ice water in excessive amounts.
   d. Dehydration, weight loss, muscle weakness, and dry skin
   e. Hemoconcentration

2. Diagnostic Procedures
   a. Water (fluid) Deprivation Test
      1) Monitor body weight, vital signs, hourly urine output
      2) Assess serum and urine osmolality
   b. Vasopressin Test
      1) Performed only if fluid deprivation test is inconclusive.
      2) IV vasopressin is administered.
      3) Client urine and serum chemistries will improve.
   c. MRI of hypothalamus and pituitary
   d. 24-hr urine
3. Collaborative Care
   a. **Nursing Interventions**
      1) Weigh client daily.
      2) Monitor urine output and urine specific gravity.
      3) Assess the client's blood pressure and heart rate.
      4) Maintain fluid and electrolyte balance.
   b. Medications
      1) Desmopressin acetate
      2) Vasopressin
      3) If DI is nephrogenic in origin, thiazide diuretics will be prescribed.
   c. Client Education and Referral
      1) Lifetime vasopressin replacement therapy
      2) Report weight gain or loss, polyuria, or polydipsia to the provider.
      3) Monitor fluid intake and urine output.
      4) Avoid foods with diuretic action.

B. **Syndrome of inappropriate secretion of antidiuretic hormone (SIADH):** the excessive release of ADH resulting in the inability to excrete an appropriate amount of urine, thus developing fluid retention and dilutional hyponatremia. Caused by neoplastic tumors, head injury, meningitis, respiratory disorders, and some medications (e.g., vincristine, phenothiazines, tricyclic antidepressants, thiazide diuretics) and nicotine.

1. Manifestations
   a. Urine Chemistry (concentrated)
      1) Increased urine specific gravity and osmolality
   b. Serum Chemistry (dilute)
      1) Hyponatremia
      2) Decreased serum osmolality
   c. Mental confusion, irritability, lethargy, and seizures (due to hyponatremia)
   d. Weakness, anorexia, nausea, and vomiting (due to hyponatremia)
   e. Increased ADH (vasopressin) levels
   f. Weight gain

2. Collaborative Care
   a. **Nursing Interventions**
      1) Restrict oral fluids to 500 to 1,000 mL/day.
      2) Monitor I&O.
      3) Weigh client daily.
      4) Monitor for increased BP, tachycardia, hypothermia.
      5) Monitor mental status frequently; initiate seizure precautions.
   b. Medications
      1) Hypertonic saline infusion (3% to 5% sodium chloride)
      2) Loop diuretics; used to treat hypervolemic hyponatremia
      3) Demeclocycline
      4) Vasopressin receptor antagonists
         a) Conivaptan
   c. Therapeutic Measures
      1) Treat the underlying cause with surgery, chemotherapy, and/or radiation.

IV Adrenal Gland

The adrenal cortex produces glucocorticoids (cortisol), mineralocorticoids (aldosterone), and sex hormones. The adrenal medulla produces the catecholamines epinephrine and norepinephrine.

V Disorders of the Adrenal Cortex

A. **Addison's disease (adrenal insufficiency):** the hyposecretion of adrenal cortex hormones, caused by autoimmune disease, TB, histoplasmosis, adrenalectomy, tumors, HIV; can be induced by abrupt cessation of steroid medications

> **MEMORY HINT:** With Addison's, you need to **add** cortisol.

1. Manifestations
   a. Weakness and fatigue
   b. Nausea and vomiting
   c. Hyperpigmentation
   d. Hypotension; increased heart rate
   e. Hypoglycemia, hyponatremia, hyperkalemia, hypercalcemia
   f. Craving salty foods
   g. Emotional lability and depression
   h. Diminished libido
2. Diagnostic Procedures
   a. Serum adrenocortical hormone levels
   b. ACTH stimulation test
   c. Electrolyte panels
   d. Abdominal/renal CT scan

3. Collaborative Care
   a. **Nursing Interventions**
      1) Assess blood pressure and heart rhythm.
      2) Monitor fluid and electrolyte balance.
      3) Monitor and treat hypoglycemia.
      4) Monitor for Addisonian crisis (also known as adrenal crisis): characterized by signs of shock (hypotension, tachycardia, tachypnea, pallor). It occurs secondary to stressors such as infection, trauma, surgery, pregnancy, or emotional stress. The client will require IV fluid replacement and IV steroids and may require respiratory support.
      5) Monitor for adverse effects of hormone replacement therapy, which are the same manifestations as hypersecretion of the adrenal cortex.
   b. Medications—adrenocorticoid replacement
      1) Hydrocortisone
      2) Prednisone
      3) Cortisone
   c. Client Education and Referral
      1) Provide emotional support to the client and provide instruction on lifelong disease management (e.g., medications, prompt treatment of infection and illness, and stress management).
      2) Educate about lifelong medication replacement, including the potential need for increased steroid therapy during times of stress or illness.
         a) Teach manifestations of excessive or insufficient hormone replacement
         b) Instruct client to promptly notify the provider in cases of infection, injury, and stress. Doses of hormones will need to be individually adjusted during these times.
      3) Teach the client indications of Addisonian crisis.
      4) Teach the client to avoid using caffeine and alcohol.
      5) Teach the client to have appropriate medical identification at all times in case of emergency.
      6) Advise the client to eat a high-protein and high-carbohydrate diet.

B. **Cushing's disease and Cushing's syndrome:** the hypersecretion of the glucocorticoids caused by hyperplasia of the adrenal cortex or pituitary gland tumor. Cushing's syndrome is caused by exogenous use of steroid medications.

1. Manifestations
   a. Upper body obesity and thin extremities; moon face, buffalo hump, and neck fat
   b. Skin fragility with purple striae
   c. Osteoporosis
   d. Hyperglycemia, hypernatremia, hypokalemia, and hypocalcemia
   e. Hirsutism
   f. Amenorrhea
   g. Elevated triglycerides and hypertension

h. Sexual dysfunction; decreased libido, erectile dysfunction in men

i. Immunosuppression

j. Peptic ulcer disease

k. In children: slower growth rate

l. Backache, bone pain, or tenderness

m. Increased thirst and urination

2. Diagnostic Procedures

a. Dexamethasone suppression test (dexamethasone administered at 2300; plasma cortisol levels obtained at 0800). Suppression of cortisol indicates the hypothalamic–pituitary–adrenal axis is functioning properly.

b. Nighttime salivary cortisol levels

3. Collaborative Care

a. **Nursing Interventions**

1) Monitor the client for infection.

2) Protect the client from accidents and falls.

3) Monitor and treat hyperglycemia.

4) Assess blood pressure and heart rhythm.

b. Medications

1) Adrenal enzyme inhibitors (e.g., metyrapone, aminoglutethimide, mitotane, and ketoconazole)

c. Therapeutic Measures

1) For a pituitary adenoma, the client may need a transsphenoidal adenomectomy.

2) For an adrenal carcinoma, the client may need a unilateral or bilateral adrenalectomy.

3) Monitor for adrenal insufficiency following postsurgery.

4) Slowly taper corticosteroid therapy.

d. Client Education and Referral

1) For clients prescribed exogenous steroid therapy, educate concerning long–term self-administration of hormone suppression therapy in Cushing's disease and the need for tapering steroid doses in Cushing's syndrome.

2) Advise the client to eat foods high in protein and calcium, low in carbohydrates and sodium, with potassium supplementation.

3) Teach client infection prevention, fall precautions, and skin care.

4 S's OF CUSHING'S AND ADDISON'S DISEASE

	cuShingS diSeaSe (Big S's) ↑	ADDIsONs DIsEAsE (Small S's) ↓
Steroid	↑	↓ (Need to "add")
Sugar	↑	↓
Sodium	↑	↓
Skin	Thin, fragile, striae	Hyperpigmented

C. **Hyperaldosteronism (Conn's syndrome):** the hypersecretion of aldosterone from the adrenal cortex (usually due to a tumor), clinical manifestations of Cushing's syndrome.

1. Manifestations

a. Hypokalemia and hypernatremia

b. Hypertension

c. Muscle weakness, numbness, and cardiac problems

d. Fatigue

e. Headache

f. Polyuria and polydipsia

g. Alkalosis

2. Diagnostic Procedures

a. Abdominal CT, MRI

b. ECG

c. Serum aldosterone/renin and potassium

d. Urine aldosterone

3. Collaborative Care

a. **Nursing Interventions**

1) Provide the client with a quiet environment.

2) Assess the client's blood pressure and cardiac activity.

3) Monitor the client's potassium level and be prepared to replace potassium.

4) Closely monitor I&O.

b. Medications

1) Antihypertensive medications: spironolactone

2) Eplerenone: blocks action of aldosterone

c. Therapeutic Measures

1) Surgical removal of tumor/adrenal gland if primary cause

VI Disorders of the Adrenal Medulla

A. **Pheochromocytoma:** a usually benign tumor of the adrenal medulla that causes hypersecretion of epinephrine and norepinephrine

1. Manifestations

a. Most common signs are the 5 H's

1) Hypertension

2) Headache

3) Hyperhidrosis (excessive sweating)

4) Hypermetabolism

5) Hyperglycemia

2. Diagnostic Procedures

a. Plasma levels of catecholamines and metanephrine (catecholamine metabolite)

b. 24–hr urine level of catecholamines and their metabolites

c. CT, MRI, or PET scan

d. Adrenal biopsy

e. Clonidine suppression test (in clients who have pheochromocytoma, catecholamines are not suppressed)

3. Collaborative Care

   a. **Nursing Interventions**
      1) Assess vital signs.
      2) Provide a high-calorie, nutritious diet, and avoid caffeine.
      3) Encourage frequent rest periods.
      4) Provide a quiet environment.
      5) Prevent stroke secondary to hypertensive crisis.
      6) Do not palpate or assess for CVA tenderness, as this can cause rupture of the tumor.
   b. Medications
      1) Alpha (phentolamine) and beta blocker (propranolol) to diminish the effect of norepinephrine prior to surgery
      2) Sodium nitroprusside
      3) Calcium channel blockers (nifedipine)
   c. Therapeutic Measures
      1) Surgical removal of tumor

VII Thyroid Gland

The thyroid gland has a rich blood supply and produces thyroxine (T_4), triiodothyronine (T_3), and calcitonin. T_4 and T_3 regulate metabolism, and calcitonin inhibits mobilization of calcium from bone and reduces blood calcium levels.

VIII Disorders of the Thyroid Gland

A. **Hypothyroidism:** suboptimal levels of thyroid hormone resulting in decreased metabolism. Occurs most frequently in women ages 30 to 60.

   1. Manifestations
      a. Fatigue and weakness
      b. Increased sensitivity to cold
      c. Constipation
      d. Dry skin, brittle hair and nails
      e. Weight gain
      f. Deepened, hoarse voice
      g. Joint pain
      h. Hyperlipidemia and anemia
      i. Depression
      j. Menstrual disturbances
   2. Diagnostic Procedures/Findings
      a. Low serum T_4 and T_3
      b. Elevated TSH (seen in primary hypothyroidism)
   3. Myxedema coma is a rare, life-threatening condition seen in untreated or uncontrolled hypothyroidism. The client is hypothermic, with changes in mental functioning ranging from depression to unconsciousness. The severely decreased metabolism causes respiratory depression and cardiovascular collapse. Management is to provide intensive supportive measures, along with hemodynamic therapy. High mortality rate.

4. Collaborative Care

   a. **Nursing Interventions**
      1) Provide a warm environment.
      2) Provide a low-calorie, low-cholesterol, and low-fat diet.
      3) Increase roughage and fluids.
      4) Avoid sedatives.
      5) Plan rest periods for the client.
      6) Weigh the client daily.
      7) Observe for manifestations of overdose of thyroid preparations (e.g., palpitations, insomnia, increased appetite, and tremors).
   b. Medications
      1) Levothyroxine
   c. Client Education and Referral
      1) Educate the client regarding lifelong medication therapy.
      2) Continue follow-up with provider.
      3) Take medication on an empty stomach each morning.
      4) Know manifestations of medication toxicity.
      5) Eat a diet high in fiber.
      6) Monitor need for sleep.

B. **Hyperthyroidism:** the excessive secretion of thyroid hormones. Graves' disease is the most common type of hyperthyroid disease and causes overstimulation of the thyroid by circulating immunoglobulins.

   1. Manifestations
      a. Anxiety and irritability
      b. Insomnia and fatigue
      c. Tachycardia
      d. Tremors
      e. Diaphoresis
      f. Intolerance of heat
      g. Weight loss (despite food intake)
      h. Exophthalmos
      i. Diarrhea
      j. Light or absent menstrual cycle
   2. Diagnostic Procedures/Findings
      a. Elevated T_4 and T_3
      b. Decreased TSH
   3. Thyroid storm is a life-threatening condition seen in untreated or uncontrolled hyperthyroidisms. Manifestations include hyperpyrexia, tachycardia, hypertension, and other exaggerated symptoms of hyperthyroidism.
   4. Collaborative Care

      a. **Nursing Interventions**
         1) Assess vital signs. Report temperature increase of 1 degree or greater to provider immediately.
         2) Promote comfort.
         3) Encourage the client to get adequate rest in a cool, quiet environment.
         4) Provide a high-caloric diet without extra stimulants.

5) Weigh the client daily.

6) Provide the client emotional support.

7) Provide eye protection for the client who has exophthalmos by giving ophthalmic medicine, taping the client's eyes at night, and decreasing sodium and water.

8) Elevate head of the bed.

b. Medications

1) Beta blocker medications to manage tachycardia, anxiety, and tremors.

2) Propylthiouracil (Propyl-Thyracil or PTU): blocks thyroid hormone production.

3) Methimazole: short-term use to block production of thyroxine; usually used no more than 8 weeks. Monitor CBC frequently for occurrence of agranulocytosis.

4) Iodides decrease vascularity and inhibit the release of thyroid hormones. Give through a straw to prevent staining of teeth.

a) Lugol's solution

b) Saturated solution of potassium iodide (SSKI); used prior to thyroidectomy

5) A radioactive iodine treatment shrinks the thyroid gland; may be used alone or prior to surgery. Teach client appropriate radiation precautions.

c. Therapeutic Measures

1) Thyroidectomy: the removal of all or part of the thyroid gland. Requires a lifelong intake of levothyroxine and possible calcium supplementation.

a) Preoperative goal: Decrease thyroid function toward normal range (euthyroid) using saturated solution of potassium iodide (SSKI) and antithyroid medication.

b) Postoperative Interventions

(1) Place the client in the semi-Fowler's position.

(2) Assess the client's dressing, especially the back of the neck.

(3) Observe for respiratory distress. Keep a tracheostomy tray, oxygen, and suction apparatus at the client's bedside.

(4) Assess for signs of hemorrhage.

(5) Note any hoarseness, which is indicative of laryngeal nerve injury; limit talking.

(6) Observe for signs of tetany (Chvostek's and Trousseau's sign), which may indicate damage or accidental removal of parathyroid glands and subsequent hypocalcemia.

(7) Keep calcium gluconate IV at the client's bedside.

(8) Observe for thyroid storm caused by an increased release of the thyroid hormone due to manipulation of the thyroid gland.

(9) Gradually increase the range of motion to the neck and support the client when sitting up.

IX Parathyroid Gland

Parathormone (parathyroid hormone) maintains calcium and phosphate balance.

X Disorders of the Parathyroid Gland

A. **Hypoparathyroidism:** the hyposecretion of parathyroid hormone (PTH), resulting in hypocalcemia and hyperphosphatemia and usually caused by surgical removal of parathyroid gland tissue during parathyroidectomy, thyroidectomy, or radical neck dissection

1. Manifestations—from hypocalcemia

a. Paresthesia

b. Muscle cramps and tetany

c. Chvostek's sign: Tapping the side of the cheek causes muscle spasms and twitching around the mouth, throat, and cheeks.

d. Trousseau's sign: Pressure from the blood pressure cuff induces muscle spasms in the distal extremity.

e. Circumoral paresthesia with numbness and tingling of the fingers.

f. Severe tetany may lead to bronchospasm, laryngeal spasm, carpopedal spasm, dysphagia, cardiac dysrhythmias, and seizures.

2. Collaborative Care

a. **Nursing Interventions**

1) Monitor ECG.

2) Assess the client for signs of neuromuscular irritability.

3) Provide a high-calcium, low-phosphorous diet.

4) Institute seizure precautions.

b. Medications

1) Acute: IV calcium gluconate

2) Chronic

a) Oral calcium salts (generally calcium carbonate) and phosphate binders

b) Vitamin D

B. **Hyperparathyroidism:** a hypersecretion of PTH (caused by tumor or renal disease) that leads to the loss of calcium from the bones into the serum, resulting in hypercalcemia and hypophosphatemia

1. Manifestations—may not have symptoms

a. Kidney stones (containing calcium)

b. Osteoporosis

c. Hypercalcemia and hypophosphatemia

d. Abdominal pain, constipation, nausea, and vomiting

e. Muscle weakness and fatigue; skeletal and joint pain

f. Polyuria and polydipsia

g. Hypertension

h. Cardiac dysrhythmias

2. Collaborative Care

  a. **Nursing Interventions**

    1) Encourage a minimum of 2,000 mL of fluids daily.

    2) Provide the client a low-calcium, low-vitamin D diet.

    3) Prevent constipation and fecal impaction.

    4) Strain all of the client's urine.

    5) Instruct the client about safety measures to prevent fractures.

    6) Encourage cranberry juice to lower the urinary pH.

    7) Monitor for hypercalcemic crisis, which is life-threatening. It usually occurs with serum calcium levels greater than 15 mg/dL.

      a) IV rehydration

      b) Phosphate therapy

      c) Calcitonin

      d) Dialysis

  b. Medications

    1) Calcimimetics such as cinacalcet mimic calcium in the blood and may cause the parathyroid to decrease the release of parathormone.

    2) Calcitonin decreases the release of skeletal calcium and increases the kidney excretion of calcium; enhanced if given along with glucocorticoids.

    3) Hydration and diuretics: Furosemide (Lasix) promotes excretion of excess calcium (avoid thiazide diuretics).

    4) Biphospates

  c. Therapeutic Measures

    1) Surgical removal of the parathyroid gland

XI Pancreas

The pancreas has exocrine (secretion of the pancreatic enzymes amylase, trypsin, and lipase, which aid in digestion) and endocrine (secretion of insulin, glucagon, and somatostatin) functions. Insulin lowers blood glucose by facilitating glucose entry into the cell. Somatostatin also lowers blood glucose levels. Glucagon raises blood glucose by converting glycogen to glucose in the liver.

XII Disorders of the Pancreas

A. **Diabetes mellitus:** a group of metabolic disorders characterized by hyperglycemia caused by altered insulin production, action, or a combination of both

  1. **Type 1:** usually characterized by an acute onset before 30 years of age. In Type 1 diabetes, the pancreatic beta cells are destroyed by either genetic predisposition (not inherited), immunologic, environmental, or a combination of these factors.

  2. **Type 2:** usually occurs after 30 years of age and is comprised of inadequate insulin production and insulin resistance

    a. Contributing Factors

      1) Family history of diabetes

      2) Obesity

      3) More prevalent in African American, Native American, and Hispanic populations

      4) Hypertension

      5) History of gestational diabetes

      6) Sedentary lifestyle

  3. **Metabolic Syndrome**

    a. Insulin resistance leads to increased insulin production in attempt to maintain glucose at a normal level.

    b. Characterized by hypertension, hypercholesterolemia, and abdominal obesity.

    c. If the beta cells cannot produce enough insulin to meet the demands, type 2 diabetes will develop.

  4. Diagnostic Criteria

    a. Symptoms of diabetes, plus casual plasma glucose of 200 mg/dL or greater, or

    b. Fasting plasma glucose of 126 mg/dL or greater, or

    c. 2-hr postload glucose of 200 mg/dL or greater during an oral glucose tolerance test

  5. Glycemic Control

    a. Glucose control is monitored on a day-to-day basis by capillary blood glucose levels.

      1) Normal preprandial (fasting) blood glucose is 70 to 105 mg/dL.

      2) Normal postprandial blood glucose is less than 180 mg/dL.

    b. Glucose control is monitored on a long-term basis by HbA1c (glycosylated hemoglobin).

6. Manifestations
    a. "3 Polys"
        1) Polyuria
        2) Polydipsia
        3) Polyphagia
    b. Fatigue and weakness
    c. Sudden vision changes
    d. Recurrent infections
    e. Slow wound healing
    f. Type 1 Diabetes
        1) Sudden weight loss
        2) Nausea, vomiting, or abdominal pain
7. Long-Term Complications
    a. Neuropathy
    b. Nephropathy
    c. Retinopathy
    d. Cardiovascular disease
    e. Infection and slow wound healing
8. Collaborative Care
    a. **Nursing Interventions**
        1) Monitor blood glucose.
        2) Administer medication as prescribed.
        3) Provide education. (See Client Education.)
        4) Monitor vital signs and I&O.
        5) Refer to a diabetic educator.
        6) Monitor for complications.
    b. Possible Complications
        1) Hypoglycemia occurs when the blood glucose level falls below 60 mg/dL.
            a) Causes: decreased dietary intake, excess insulin, and increased exercise
            b) Manifestations
                (1) Tachycardia
                (2) Diaphoresis
                (3) Weakness, fatigue
                (4) Irritability, anxiety
                (5) Confusion
                (6) Headache, blurred vision
        2) **Transient hyperglycemia:** an elevated blood glucose; generally treated with sliding scale insulin to return serum blood glucose to normal range
            a) Prompt treatment is necessary to avoid hyperglycemic emergencies.
                (1) Treat with regular insulin.
                (2) Do not hold insulin when blood glucose is in the normal range.
                (3) Provide education on importance and strategies to maintain blood glucose in the normal range.

    b) **Nursing Interventions for Hypoglycemia**
        (1) Give the client 15 g of fast-acting simple carbohydrates.
            (a) 3 or 4 glucose tablets for the equivalent to 15 g of carbohydrates
            (b) 4 oz of fruit juice or regular soda
            (c) 6 to 10 hard candies
            (d) 2 to 3 teaspoons of sugar or honey
        (2) If the client is unconscious or unable to swallow, administer glucagon IM or subcutaneous. Repeat in 10 min if client is still unconscious and notify provider.
        (3) Follow the 15/15/15 rule.
            (a) Administer 15 g of fast-acting carbohydrates.
            (b) Wait 15 min and recheck blood glucose.
            (c) Administer 15 more grams of carbohydrates if blood glucose remains less than 70 mg/dL.
            (d) Give 7 g of protein when blood glucose is within normal limits
                v) 2 tablespoons of peanut butter
                vi) 1 oz of cheese
                vii) 8 oz of milk
    c. Medications (see Unit Four: Pharmacology in Nursing)
        1) Insulin pump: an external device that provides a basal dose of rapid-acting or regular insulin with a bolus dose for meals, which is calculated by the client using a predetermined insulin-to-carbohydrate ratio; does not read blood glucose
            a) Needles are inserted into subcutaneous abdominal tissue (change site at least every 3 days).
            b) Complications are secondary to continuous administration of insulin or from disruption of insulin infusion.
            c) Allows for flexibility of diet.
    d. Client Education
        1) Nutritional therapy as prescribed (e.g., exchange, carbohydrate counting, calories, healthy food choices)
        2) Importance of consistent exercise
        3) Self-glucose monitoring and interpretation of results
        4) Medication Administration
            a) Medication importance and schedule
            b) Medication route (e.g., PO, subcutaneous, insulin pump)
            c) Rotation of injection within an anatomic area
        5) Manifestations and management of hypo and hyperglycemia
        6) Wear medic alert bracelet.

7) Foot Care

   a) Cleanse feet daily in warm, soapy water; rinse and dry carefully.

   b) Trim nails straight across.

   c) Wear supportive, protective shoes.

   d) Do not go barefoot and inspect feet daily, including between the toes.

8) Guidelines During Illness ("Sick Day Rules")

   a) Take usual doses of insulin or antidiabetic agents.

   b) Test blood glucose and urine for ketones every 3 to 4 hr.

   c) Report elevated blood glucose or urine ketones to provider.

   d) Encourage to consume 4 oz of sugar-free, non-caffeinated fluids every 30 min to prevent dehydration.

   e) Eat small, frequent meals of soft foods or liquids to meet carbohydrate needs.

B. **Diabetic ketoacidosis:** an acute, life-threatening complication of diabetes mellitus due to insufficient insulin. Main clinical manifestations are hyperglycemia (i.e., blood glucose levels vary between 300 to 800 mg/dL), acidosis, dehydration, and fluid loss; most common in type 1 diabetes mellitus.

   1. Contributing Factors

      a. Decreased or missed dose of insulin

      b. Illness or infection

      c. Undiagnosed or untreated diabetes

   2. Manifestations

      a. Exacerbated polyuria, polydipsia, polyphagia

      b. Anorexia, nausea, vomiting, abdominal pain

      c. Metabolic acidosis with ketonuria

      d. Kussmaul's respirations

      e. Acetone breath (fruity odor)

      f. Altered mental status, blurred vision, headache

      g. Weak, rapid pulse

      h. Orthostatic hypotension

3. Collaborative Care

   a. **Nursing Interventions**

      1) Monitor blood glucose, LOC, vital signs, and strict I&O.

      2) Administer prescribed IV fluids to promote perfusion.

         a) Normal saline infusion to maintain perfusion.

         b) Follow with 45% saline infusion to replace total body fluid losses.

         c) Add fluids containing dextrose when blood glucose is approximately 250 mg/dL.

      3) Administer insulin.

         a) Insulin infusion usually at 0.1 mg/kg/hr. Regular insulin is the only insulin that may be given IV.

         b) Usually blood glucose checks hourly while on an insulin infusion.

         c) Resume subcutaneous when possible.

      4) Monitor potassium levels and replace as prescribed.

      5) Monitor acid–base balance.

      6) Teach strategies to prevent DKA and hyperglycemic hyperosmolar state (HHS).

C. **Hyperglycemic hyperosmolar state (HHS):** an acute, life-threatening complication of diabetes (more commonly in type 2). It is characterized by elevated blood glucose levels of greater than 600 mg/dL, a hyperosmolar state, which leads to fluid and electrolyte losses.

   1. Contributing Factors

      a. Acute illness (e.g., surgery, infection, CVA)

      b. Medications that exacerbate hyperglycemia (such as thiazides)

      c. Treatments (such as dialysis)

   2. Manifestations

      a. Clinical Signs of Dehydration

         1) Hypotension and tachycardia

         2) Elevated BUN

      b. Generally not seen with ketosis

      c. Altered mental status

   3. Collaborative Care

      a. **Nursing Interventions**

         1) Replace fluids as prescribed (monitor for fluid overload).

         2) Administer insulin and electrolytes as prescribed.

         3) Monitor blood glucose, LOC, vital signs, electrolyte levels, and acid–base balance.

         4) Teach strategies to prevent HHS.

ENDOCRINE END-OF-SECTION REVIEW

1. The client who is diagnosed with syndrome of inappropriate antidiuretic hormone (SIADH) would have _____ serum and concentrated _____. The opposite would be true for diabetes insipidus (DI).

2. A medication that is beneficial in the treatment of diabetes insipidus (DI) is _____.

3. The client who is receiving long-term _____ therapy may have symptoms similar to those of the client with Cushing's disease. This client is at risk to develop Addisonian crisis, which may cause dehydration and cardiovascular collapse, if this medication therapy is _____ stopped.

4. The client diagnosed with pheochromocytoma is at risk for cerebral vascular accident (CVA) secondary to _____ crisis.

5. The client diagnosed with _____ would be expected to have the following laboratory findings: thyroid stimulating hormone (TSH) level would be increased and thyroxine (T_4) and triiodothyronine (T_3) decreased. The medication usually given for this disorder is _____. A potentially life-threatening condition that may be caused when this disorder is untreated and that may lead to decreased cardiac output and organ failure due to severely decreased metabolism is called _____.

6. The client may develop hypoparathyroidism following surgical removal of the thyroid gland. The client may experience clinical manifestations related to alteration in _____ levels. Potentially life-threatening manifestations that the nurse needs to monitor for in the client with alteration in this electrolyte are _____, _____, and _____.

7. It is important to teach appropriate foot care to the client who has diabetes mellitus. This would include teaching the client to always wear socks and protective _____ and inspect, wash, and thoroughly _____ the feet daily.

8. The client needs to be taught to _____ injection sites within the same anatomical location when giving insulin injections.

9. The diabetic client is found to have a blood glucose level less than 70 mg/dL. The appropriate intervention would be to give the client 15 grams of carbohydrates, which may include _____. The blood glucose is rechecked in 15 min and is now 90 mg/dL. The appropriate interventions would be to give the client 7 grams of protein, which may include _____.

10. The priority interventions during the management of diabetic ketoacidosis (DKA) and hyperglycemic hyperosmolar state (HHS) focus on restoration of _____, _____ (particularly potassium), and acid-base balance and reduction of _____ levels.

WORD BANK

4 oz of fruit juice

1 oz of cheese

Addison's disease

Blood glucose

Calcium

Corticosteroid

Desmopressin acetate (DDAVP)

Dilute

Dry

Dysrhythmias

Electrolyte

Fluid

Hypertensive

Hypothyroidism

Laryngospasms

Myxedema coma

Rotate

Seizures

Shoes

Suddenly

Levothyroxine (Synthroid)

Urine

Answer Key: 1. Dilute, urine; 2. Desmopressin acetate (DDAVP); 3. Corticosteroid, suddenly; 4. Hypertensive; 5. Hypothyroidism, levothyroxine (Synthroid), myxedema coma; 6. Calcium, dysrhythmia, laryngospasms, seizures; 7. Shoes, dry; 8. Rotate; 9. 4 oz of fruit juice, 1 oz of cheese; 10. Fluid, electrolyte, blood glucose

---

SECTION 7

Hematologic Disorders

A. **Anemia:** a deficiency of RBCs characterized by a decreased functional RBC count, Hgb/Hct, or both. Anemia is a clinical condition that results in decreased oxygen delivery to the cells.

1. Contributing Factors
   a. Acute or chronic blood loss (gastrointestinal bleeding)
   b. Greater than normal destruction of RBCs (spleen diseases)
   c. Abnormal bone marrow function (chemotherapy)
   d. Decreased erythropoietin (renal failure)
   e. Inadequate maturation of RBCs (cancer)
   f. Nutritional deficiencies (iron, B_{12}, folic acid, intrinsic factor)

2. Manifestations
   a. Fatigue and weakness
   b. Dizziness and headaches
   c. Pallor: first seen in conjunctiva (light-skinned clients) and mucosal membranes (dark-skinned clients), as well as the nail beds, the palmar creases, and around the mouth
   d. Tachycardia, murmurs and gallops, and orthostatic hypotension
   e. Decreased activity tolerance
   f. Decreased Hgb, Hct, and RBC levels
   g. Shortness of breath and dyspnea; decreased oxygen saturation levels

3. Collaborative Care

   a. **Nursing Interventions**
      1) Monitor labs (RBC, Hgb, and Hct).
      2) Encourage activity as tolerated by the client with frequent rest periods.
      3) Monitor skin integrity and implement measures to prevent breakdown.
      4) Provide oxygen therapy to the client as needed.
      5) Administer blood products and medications as prescribed. (See individual anemias.)
      6) Encourage foods high in iron (e.g., meats, poultry, fish).

B. **Types of Anemia**

1. **Anemia secondary to renal disease:** anemia due to lack of erythropoietin

    a. Medications

        1) Erythropoietin

2. **Iron deficiency anemia:** anemia resulting from low iron levels; the iron stores are depleted first, followed by hemoglobin stores

    a. Contributing Factors

        1) Chronic blood loss (bleeding ulcer)
        2) Nutritional deficiency
        3) Common in infants, older adults, and young adult women (due to pregnancy or menses)

    b. Manifestations

        1) Microcytic red blood cells
        2) Weakness and pallor
        3) Low serum ferritin levels

    c. Collaborative Care

        1) **Nursing Interventions**
            a) Monitor for symptoms of bleeding.
            b) Monitor labs.
        2) Medications
            a) Administer iron preparations.
        3) Therapeutic Measures
            a) Follow provider prescriptions for ulcer treatment.

3. **Aplastic anemia:** bone marrow suppression of new stem cell production resulting in a deficiency of circulating WBCs, platelets, and/or RBCs. Can be due to medications, viruses, toxins, and/or radiation exposure.

    a. Manifestations

        1) Hypoxia, fatigue, and pallor (related to anemia)
        2) Increased susceptibility to infection (related to leukopenia)
        3) Hemorrhage, ecchymosis/petechiae (related to thrombocytopenia)
        4) Pancytopenia (decrease in RBCs, WBCs, and platelets)

    b. Collaborative Care

        1) **Nursing Interventions**
            a) Monitor labs.
            b) Provide protective isolation.
            c) Monitor for manifestations of infection.
            d) Provide emotional and psychological support to the client.
            e) Implement protective barrier precautions.
            f) Prepare client for bone marrow aspiration/biopsy.
        2) Medications
            a) Immunosuppressive therapy (prednisone, cyclosporine)
            b) Chemotherapy medications
        3) Therapeutic Measures
            a) Hematopoietic stem cell transplantation
            b) Splenectomy
            c) Cautious use of blood transfusions

4. **B₁₂ deficiency anemias (macrocytic):** anemia due to a lack of dietary intake or absorption of vitamin B_{12}

    a. Contributing Factors

        1) Atrophy of the gastric mucosa/hypochlorhydria (underproduction of hydrochloric acid by the stomach)
        2) Total gastrectomy (lack of intrinsic factor decreases intestinal vitamin B_{12} absorption)
        3) Malnutrition

    b. Manifestations

        1) Numbness and tingling of extremities (paresthesia)
        2) Hypoxemia
        3) Pallor
        4) Jaundice
        5) Glossitis
        6) Poor balance

    c. Diagnostic Procedures

        1) Shilling test is used to differentiate malabsorption versus pernicious anemia by measuring absorption of B_{12} with and without intrinsic factor after the client is given an oral dose of radioactive vitamin B_{12}.
        2) CBC: megaloblastic RBCs (macrocytic)

    d. Collaborative Care

        1) **Nursing Interventions**
            a) Monitor labs.
            b) Promote rest and encourage a balanced dietary intake.
        2) Medications
            a) Cyanocobalamin (vitamin B_{12}): standard dose is 1,000 mcg IM daily for 2 weeks, then weekly until Hct level is therapeutic, then monthly for life. Cyanocobalamin intranasally maintains vitamin B_{12} levels.

5. **Folic acid deficiency anemia:** anemia due to folic acid deficiency. Symptoms similar to vitamin B_{12} deficiency, but nervous system functions remain normal.

    a. Contributing Factors

        1) Poor nutrition
        2) Malabsorption (secondary to Crohn's disease)
        3) Drugs (e.g., chronic alcohol abuse, anticonvulsants, and oral contraceptives)

    b. Collaborative Care

        1) **Nursing Interventions**
            a) Identify high-risk clients: alcoholics, elderly, debilitated clients
        2) Medications
            a) Folic acid replacement

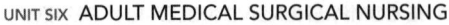

6. **Hemolytic and aplastic anemia:** a group of anemias that occur when the bone marrow is unable to increase production to make up for the premature destruction of red blood cells. Sickle cell and thalassemia are hemolytic anemias. Aplastic anemia often occurs with leukopenia, thrombocytopenia, and pancytopenia.

   a. Contributing Factors
      1) Trauma; crushing injuries
      2) Lead poisoning
      3) Tuberculosis
      4) Infections
      5) Transfusion reactions
      6) Toxic agents
      7) Radiation exposure

   b. Manifestations
      1) Chills
      2) Dark urine
      3) Enlarged spleen
      4) Pallor
      5) Rapid heart rate
      6) Shortness of breath
      7) Jaundice

   c. Collaborative Care

      1) **Nursing Interventions**
         a) Treat the underlying cause.
         b) Hydrate the client.
         c) Blood transfusion when kidney function is normal.
      2) Medications
         a) In severe immune-related hemolytic anemia, steroid therapy is sometimes necessary.
         b) Hematopoietic stem cell transplantation for aplastic anemia if other treatments fail.

7. **Sickle cell anemia:** a genetic defect found in clients of African American or Mediterranean origin, in which the Hgb molecule assumes a sickle shape and delivers less oxygen to tissues. The sickle cells become lodged in the blood vessels, especially the brain and the kidneys.

   a. Contributing Factors (precipitate crisis by enhancing sickling)
      1) Stress
      2) Dehydration
      3) Hypoxia
      4) High altitudes
      5) Infections

   b. Manifestations
      1) Severe pain and swelling
      2) Fever
      3) Jaundice
      4) Susceptibility to infection
      5) Hypoxic damage to organs: spleen, liver, heart, kidney, brain

   c. Diagnostic Procedures
      1) Percentage of hemoglobin S (Hgb S) seen on electrophoresis. Sickle cell trait has less than 40% Hgb S and sickle cell disease may have 80% to 100% Hgb S.

   d. Collaborative Care
      1) **Nursing Interventions**
         a) Maintain adequate hydration.
         b) Provide oxygen therapy to the client.
         c) Encourage the client to rest, and avoid high altitudes, alcohol, and temperature extremes.
         d) Teach the client to identify triggers, get immunizations in a timely manner, and refer for genetic counseling.
      2) Medications
         a) Morphine sulfate or hydromorphone to manage the client's pain
         b) Hydroxyurea to reduce the amount of sickling and number of painful episodes

8. **Thalassemia:** inherited blood disorder in which the body makes an abnormal form of hemoglobin, resulting in excessive destruction of red blood cells, which leads to anemia

   a. Contributing Factors
      1) Must inherit the defective gene from both parents to develop thalassemia major
      2) Asian, Mediterranean, or African ethnicity
      3) Family history of the disorder

   b. Manifestations
      1) Develops during the first year of life
      2) Bone deformities in the face
      3) Fatigue
      4) Growth failure
      5) Shortness of breath
      6) Yellow skin (jaundice)

   c. Diagnostic Procedures
      1) Red blood cells appear small and abnormally shaped.
      2) Complete blood count (CBC) reveals anemia.
      3) Hemoglobin electrophoresis shows the presence of an abnormal form of hemoglobin.
      4) Mutational analysis detects alpha thalassemia that cannot be seen with hemoglobin electrophoresis.

d. Collaborative Care

　1) **Nursing Interventions**

　　a) Encourage increase of folate in the diet by including dark green leafy vegetables, dried beans and peas (legumes), and citrus fruits and juices.

　　b) Administer blood transfusions.

　　c) Encourage rest.

　　d) Provide genetic counseling.

　2) Therapeutic Measures

　　a) Treatment often involves regular blood transfusions.

　　b) Clients receiving blood transfusions should not take iron supplements as this can cause high iron levels in the blood.

　　c) Chelation therapy may be necessary to remove excess iron from the body.

　　d) Bone marrow transplant may help treat the disease in some clients, especially children.

　3) Medications

　　a) Folic acid

Cardiovascular System Disorders

ᵢ Cardiovascular Overview

A. Efficiently pumps blood to all parts of the body, indicating healthy working cardiac muscles and system.

B. Circulates adequate blood volume to meet the body's needs.

C. Adequate blood pressure is maintained by peripheral vasculature.

D. Normal heart rate is 60 to 100/min.

ᵢᵢ Diagnostic Procedures

A. **Laboratory tests**

1. Serum electrolytes

2. Erythrocyte sedimentation rate (ESR)

3. C-reactive protein

4. Blood coagulation tests

　a. PTT: most significant if the client is on heparin therapy

　b. PT: most significant if the client is on warfarin (Coumadin) therapy

　c. INR

5. BUN and creatinine: reflect renal function and perfusion; levels may increase in MI, CHF, and cardiomyopathy.

6. Total serum cholesterol desirable

　a. Low-density lipids (LDL)

　b. High-density lipids (HDL)

　c. Triglycerides

7. B-type natriuretic peptide (BNP): indicator for diagnosing heart failure

　a. Critical value greater than 100 pg/mL

8. Enzymes: test indicates death of myocardial muscles; heart attack

　a. Creatinine phosphokinase MB (CK–MB) isoenzyme increases within 4 to 6 hr following MI and remains elevated from 24 to 72 hr.

　b. Troponin is a protein that is considered the gold standard in diagnosing MI. It remains elevated for 2 to 3 weeks following an event. Normal level is less than 0.2 ng/dL.

　c. Myoglobin rises early in response to tissue injury within the first 2 hours, but also declines quickly after 7 hours of injury. It is less useful than CK–MB and troponin since myoglobin is present in skeletal as well as cardiac muscle.

DIAGNOSTIC TESTING: CARDIAC ENZYMES

Important Lab Findings

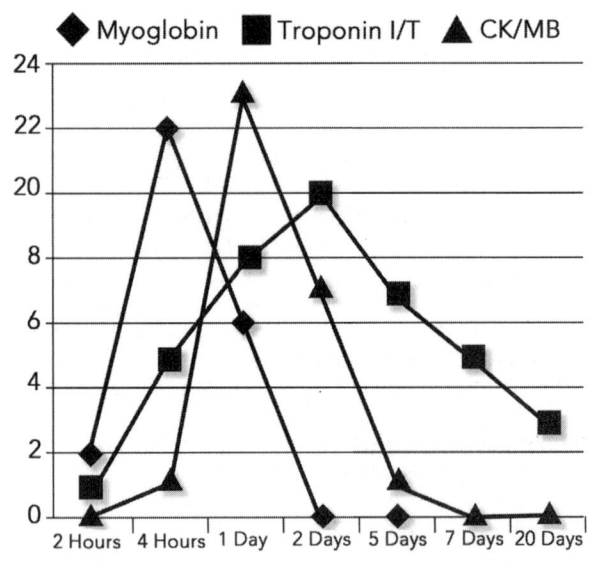

B. **Electrocardiogram (ECG):** a recording of the electrical activity occurring in the heart. A 12-lead ECG should be obtained within 10 min of onset of chest pain to identify any areas of myocardial damage.

1. T-wave inversion—ischemia
2. ST-segment elevation—injury
3. Q-wave enlargement—infarction

ECG WAVE ELEMENTS

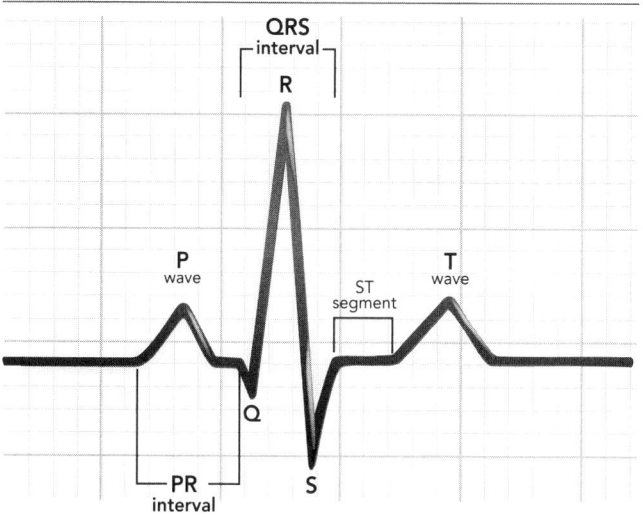

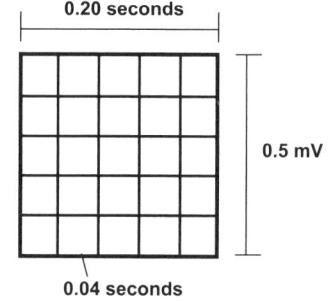

P wave represents atrial depolarization (contraction).

QRS complex (interval) represents ventricular depolarization (contraction) and should be less than 0.12 seconds.

T wave represents ventricular repolarization (relaxation). T wave depression (inversion) indicates myocardial ischemia.

PR interval represents time between SA node and AV node. Should be between 0.12 and 0.20 seconds.

ST segments represents elevation. Indicates myocardial injury.

C. **Cardiac catheterization:** a procedure involving the advancement of a catheter, usually through the femoral artery, into the coronary arteries. Dye may be injected to visualize blockages, which can then be treated with percutaneous coronary intervention (PCI). The femoral vein can also be accessed to perform other assessments of cardiac function.

1. Types of PCI
   a. **Coronary angioplasty:** A balloon-tipped catheter is used to press the coronary blockage open to improve blood flow.
   b. **Coronary stent:** a procedure performed during angioplasty that leaves a metal mesh in place as a structural support to prevent the blockage from recurring

2. Purpose
   a. Perform angiography.
   b. Perform PCI.
   c. Obtain information about cardiac structure and blood flow.
   d. Obtain blood samples.
   e. Determine cardiac output.

3. **Nursing Interventions**
   a. Prior to Catheterization
      1) Verify that procedural consent has been obtained.
      2) Know approach for shave prep—right (venous) side or left (arterial) side.
      3) NPO for 6 hr prior to the procedure.
      4) Mark distal (baseline) pulses.
      5) Explain to the client that the procedure may leave a metallic taste, and the client may feel flushed when the dye is injected.
      6) Verify that the client does not have any history of allergy to dye or shellfish.

D. **After Catheterization**
   1. Monitor the client's blood pressure and apical pulse every 15 min for 2 to 4 hr.
   2. Perform a neurovascular assessment on the client every 15 min for the first 2 hr, then every 30 min until the client is able to sit up.
   3. Monitor for bleeding and/or hematoma at catheter insertion site.
   4. Apply pressure for a minimum of 15 min to prevent bleeding or hematoma formation.
   5. Monitor for vasospasm, dysrhythmia, or rupture of the coronary vessel.
   6. Assess the client for chest pain.
   7. Keep the extremity extended for 4 to 6 hr.
   8. Maintain bed rest; no hip flexion and no sitting up in bed.
   9. Increase fluid intake to enhance flushing of dye.

E. **Transesophageal echocardiogram (TEE):** diagnostic tool to visualize structures (including valves) and function of the heart. Used for diagnosis of heart failure and murmurs.
   1. Preprocedure:
      a. NPO for 6 to 8 hr prior to the procedure.
      b. Clarify medications to be administered with the provider.
   2. Postprocedure:
      a. Assess for adequate gag reflex.
      b. Monitor respiratory effort as client recovers from sedation.
      c. Observe oral secretions (blood-tinged oral secretions common in early recovery).

III Cardiovascular Disorders

A. **Angina:** a manifestation of myocardial ischemia caused by arterial stenosis or blockage, uncontrolled blood pressure, or cardiomyopathy

1. **Chronic stable angina (CSA)** is characterized by the chest discomfort described by the client as typical and usually is relieved with rest or a single nitroglycerin. CSA is attributable most often to fixed or stable atherosclerotic plaque.

2. **Acute coronary syndrome (ACS)** describes clients experiencing unstable angina or an acute myocardial infarction (AMI). Unstable angina is characterized by the chest discomfort described by the client as occurring at rest or with activity and may last longer than 15 minutes unrelieved by nitroglycerin.

3. Types of Angina

   a. **Stable (exertional) angina.** Occurs with exercise or emotional stress and is relieved by rest or nitroglycerin.

   b. **Unstable (preinfarction) angina.** Occurs with exercise or at rest, but increases in occurrence, severity, and duration over time.

   c. **Variant (Prinzmetal's) angina.** Due to a coronary artery spasm, often occurring during periods of rest.

B. **Contributing Factors**

1. Coronary Artery Disease (CAD)

   a. Family history
   b. Advanced age
   c. Hyperlipidemia
   d. Tobacco use
   e. Hypertension
   f. Diabetes mellitus
   g. Obesity
   h. Physical inactivity

C. **Manifestations**

1. Chest pain or discomfort
2. Pain in arms, neck, jaw, shoulder, or back
3. Nausea
4. Fatigue
5. Shortness of breath
6. Anxiety
7. Diaphoresis
8. Dizziness

D. **Diagnostic Procedures**

1. 12-lead ECG
2. Stress test
3. Cardiac catheterization
4. Echocardiogram
5. Cardiac enzymes and biomarkers

E. **Collaborative Care**

1. **Nursing Interventions**

   a. Assess the client's pain.

      1) Location: jaw and/or arm, as well as chest
      2) Character
      3) Duration: relieved with rest and/or nitroglycerin
      4) Precipitating factors (once identified, eliminate or minimize to avoid attacks)

   b. Administer oxygen as needed.

   c. Provide environment conducive to rest; avoid activities.

   d. Administer medications.

      1) Aspirin
      2) Nitrates
      3) Beta blockers
      4) Statins
      5) Calcium channel blockers
      6) Angiotensin-converting enzyme (ACE)

   e. Client Education

      1) Lifestyle changes

         a) Avoid constipation.
         b) Avoid excessive activity in cold weather.
         c) Decrease stress.
         d) Exercise.
         e) Consume low-sodium, low-fat diet.
         f) Maintain healthy weight.
         g) Rest after meals.
         h) Promote tobacco cessation.

      2) Provide teaching on the correct use of nitroglycerin.

         a) Take as needed at onset of chest pain or tightness or in preparation of exertional activity.

         b) Take nitroglycerin as prescribed, at onset of attack, and every 5 min up to three doses. If pain is not relieved after first sublingual tablet, call 911.

         c) Store nitroglycerin in a dark, dry spot, and replace every 6 months.

         d) Side effects of taking nitroglycerin include headache and hypotension.

         e) Types of nitroglycerin are tablets, ointment, patch, or spray.

         f) If the client is given nitroglycerin for prevention, the client must be nitroglycerin-free daily for 12 hr to prevent developing a tolerance.

         g) If the client uses a nitro patch, instruct to apply it in the morning and remove it at bedtime.

         h) Instruct the client to take nitroglycerin while sitting down and stopping all activity.

         i) Erectile dysfunction medication is contraindicated with the use of nitrates.

F. **Myocardial infarction (MI):** the process by which myocardial tissue is destroyed due to reduced coronary blood flow and lack of oxygen; actual necrosis of the heart muscle (i.e., myocardium) occurs

1. Contributing Factors
   a. Atherosclerotic heart disease
   b. Coronary artery embolism
2. Manifestations
   a. Severe chest pain, unrelieved with nitroglycerin or rest
   b. Crushing quality, radiates to jawline, left arm, neck, and/or back
   c. Women, older adults, and clients who have diabetes mellitus often report no pain.
   d. Diaphoresis, nausea, vomiting, anxiety, fear
   e. Vital sign changes: tachycardia, hypotension, dyspnea, dysrhythmias
3. Diagnostic Procedures
   a. Laboratory results: elevated troponin and CK-MB enzymes, elevated myoglobin
   b. 12-lead ECG: Should be obtained ASAP to identify ST changes. May be an ST elevation MI (STEMI) or non–ST elevation MI (NSTEMI).
4. Collaborative Care

   a. **Nursing Interventions** (aimed at resting the myocardium and preserving the heart muscle)
      1) Early
         a) Administer oxygen.
         b) Administer medications.
            (1) Aspirin
            (2) Antidysrhythmics: amiodarone, lidocaine
            (3) Analgesics: morphine sulfate
            (4) Anticoagulants: heparin IV
            (5) Thrombolytics within 6 hr of a cardiac event: streptokinase, alteplase recombinant
            (6) Vasodilators: nitroglycerine
            (7) Beta blockers: metoprolol
            (8) Calcium channel blockers: verapamil, nifedipine
         c) Frequently monitor vital signs, O₂ saturation, and ECG.
         d) Provide emotional support to the client.
      2) Later
         a) Administer stool softeners to prevent straining with bowel movements and/or Valsalva maneuver.
         b) Provide a soft, low-fat, low-cholesterol, low-sodium diet.
         c) Use a bedside commode, which requires less energy than using a bedpan.
         d) Promote self-care, but instruct the client to stop at the onset of pain.
         e) Plan for cardiac rehabilitation.
         f) Initiate an exercise program, but stop if fatigue or chest pain occurs.
         g) Teach and encourage the use of stress management techniques.

      h) Teach the client to modify any risk factors.
         (1) Obesity
         (2) Stress
         (3) Diet
         (4) Hypertension
         (5) Tobacco use
         (6) Physical inactivity
      i) Recognize risk factors that cannot be modified.
         (1) Heredity
         (2) Race
         (3) Age
         (4) Gender
      j) Ensure bleeding precautions with anticoagulant and antiplatelet therapy.
      k) Initiate long-term medication therapy.
         (1) Anticoagulants/antiplatelets: heparin, aspirin, warfarin, enoxaparin, clopidogrel
         (2) Antihypertensives
            (a) Beta-blockers: metoprolol
            (b) Calcium channel blockers: diltiazem
         (3) Vasodilators: nitroglycerin
         (4) Antilipidemics: simvastatin, atorvastatin

G. **Heart failure:** the inability of the heart to meet the tissue requirements for oxygen. Characterized by manifestations of fluid overload or inadequate tissue perfusion. Has been called congestive heart failure due to the frequent occurrence of pulmonary and peripheral congestion. Most often a chronic condition with a goal of preventing acute exacerbations.

1. Left-sided heart failure: Manifestation primarily related to pulmonary congestion.
   a. Dyspnea
   b. Cough
   c. Crackles
   d. Orthopnea
   e. Paroxysmal nocturnal dyspnea
   f. Low oxygen saturation levels
   g. Elevated PAWP
2. Right-sided heart failure: Manifestations primarily related to systemic congestion.
   a. Dependent edema
   b. Hepatomegaly
   c. Ascites
   d. Anorexia and vomiting
   e. Weakness
   f. Weight gain
   g. Jugular vein distention
   h. Elevated CVP

HEMODYNAMIC MONITORING

	EXPECTED REFERENCE RANGE	CAUSES OF ABNORMAL RANGE
Central venous pressure (CVP)	1 to 8 mm Hg	Increased: hypervolemia, right-sided heart failure
		Decreased: hypovolemia
Pulmonary artery wedge pressure (PAWP)	4 to 12 mm Hg	Increased: hypervolemia, left-sided heart failure
		Decreased: hypovolemia

3. Collaborative Care

a. **Nursing Interventions**

1) Respiratory Status

a) Auscultate lung sounds to detect crackles and/or wheezes.

b) Oxygen therapy as needed

c) Fowler's position to help work of breathing

2) Fluid Volume

a) Fluid restriction depending on severity

b) Low-sodium diet 2,000 to 3,000 mg day

c) Report 2 to 3 lb weight increase in 1 day

3) Pharmacological Therapy

a) ACE inhibitors

b) ARBs

c) Hydralazine and nitrates

d) Beta blockers

e) Calcium channel blockers

f) Diuretics

g) Digitalis

h) IV nesiritide

i) IV milrinone

j) IV dobutamine

H. **Valvular disorders:** result in narrowing of valve that prevents or impedes blood flow (stenosis) or impaired closure that allows backward leakage of blood (regurgitation); may affect mitral, aortic, or tricuspid valve

1. Contributing Factors

a. History of endocarditis and rheumatic fever is frequently the cause.

2. Manifestations

a. Right-sided heart failure (mitral stenosis, mitral regurgitation, tricuspid stenosis)

b. Left-sided heart failure (aortic stenosis, aortic regurgitation)

c. Murmurs

d. Decreased cardiac output

3. Collaborative Care

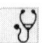

a. **Nursing Interventions**

1) Management: similar as for heart failure.

2) Valvuloplasty: Postprocedure care is similar to that of PCI. Watch for signs of systemic emboli, which may have dislodged from the valve.

3) Valve Replacement

a) Mechanical: will require lifelong anticoagulants using warfarin. Maintain INR 2.0 to 3.0.

b) Biologic: will only require prophylactic anticoagulants for 3 months

c) All clients who have undergone valve surgery will require prophylactic antibiotics prior to any future invasive procedures or tests, including dental procedures to prevent infective endocarditis.

I. **Aortic aneurysm:** local distention of the aortic artery wall, usually thoracic or abdominal. Monitored until above 5 cm, when the rate of rupture increases and surgery is usually required.

1. Contributing Factors

a. Atherosclerosis (most common cause)

b. Infections/inflammatory disorders

c. Connective tissue disorders

2. Manifestations (frequently asymptomatic)

a. Thoracic: pain, dyspnea, hoarseness, cough, dysphagia

b. Abdominal: abdominal pain; persistent or intermittent low back or flank pain; pulsating abdominal mass

3. Diagnostic Procedures

a. CT scan, MRI

b. X-ray, ultrasound

4. Collaborative Care

a. **Nursing Interventions**

1) Treatment often includes surgery.

a) Preoperative: Maintain systolic pressure at 100 to 120 mm Hg with beta blockers and/ or antihypertensives such as hydralazine. Continuous IV nipride may be required. Monitor closely for manifestations of rupture (e.g., intense pain, decreasing blood pressure).

b) Postoperative: careful monitoring of peripheral circulation below the level of the aneurysm. Continue close monitoring of BP. Low BP may indicate hemorrhage. High BP places stress on the arterial suture line.

c) Postoperative Complications

(1) Arterial occlusion

(2) Hemorrhage

(3) Infection

(4) Renal failure

J. **Hypertension:** persistent blood pressure above 140/90 mm Hg; often called the "silent killer"

1. Primary Hypertension

a. Most common type (90% of cases)

b. Hereditary disease; cause unknown

c. More common among African Americans

d. Late manifestations: headaches, fatigue, dyspnea, edema, nocturia, blackouts

e. Usually no manifestations until end-organ involvement occurs

2. Secondary Hypertension

a. Due to identifiable cause

b. Pheochromocytoma

c. Renal pathology

3. Collaborative Care
   a. **Nursing Interventions**
      1) Teach weight control methods.
      2) Encourage tobacco cessation.
      3) Decrease alcohol and caffeine intake.
      4) Promote a program of regular physical exercise.
      5) Promote a lifestyle with reduced stress.
      6) Encourage a sodium-restricted diet.
      7) Encourage the DASH diet—increased fruits, vegetables, low-fat dairy, limited saturated fats.
   b. Medications: Initial medications include diuretics and beta blockers.
      1) Loop diuretic: furosemide, bumetanide
      2) Thiazide-hydrochlorothiazide (HCTZ), chlorothiazide
         a) Interventions for Loop and HCTZ Diuretics
            (1) Administer potassium supplements as prescribed.
            (2) Teach dietary sources of potassium.
            (3) Hypokalemia increases the risk of digitalis toxicity.
      3) Potassium-Sparing Diuretics
         a) Spironolactone
         b) Triamterene
         c) Monitor for increased potassium level.
      4) Beta Blockers
         a) Propranolol HCl
         b) Atenolol
         c) Metoprolol
         d) **Nursing Interventions** for Beta Blockers
            (1) Monitor for major side effects of bradycardia.
            (2) Monitor pulse daily.
            (3) Monitor for manifestations of heart failure.
            (4) Non-cardioselective beta blockers may be contraindicated in clients who have asthma.
            (5) Monitor for hypoglycemia in clients who have diabetes mellitus; may mask manifestations.
      5) Central-Acting Alpha Blockers (sympatholytics)
         a) Clonidine HCl
         b) Guanfacine HCl
         c) Methyldopa
      6) Angiotensin-Converting Enzyme (ACE) Inhibitors
         a) Captopril
         b) Enalapril
         c) Lisinopril
      7) Calcium Channel blockers
         a) Nifedipine
         b) Verapamil, diltiazem

GERONTOLOGIC CONSIDERATIONS

1. Medications start at half the dose used in younger clients.
2. Monotherapy desirable due to simplicity and decreased expense.
3. At increased risk for postural hypotension secondary to medications.

K. **Peripheral vascular disease:** includes peripheral arterial disease and peripheral venous disorders
   1. **Peripheral arterial disease:** impairs blood flow in the arteries that carry blood away from the heart. Most common in arteries of the legs.
      a. Manifestations
         1) Intermittent claudication: pain/cramping when walking; resolves with rest
         2) Calf muscle atrophy
         3) Skin appears shiny, with hair loss and thickened toenails.
         4) Poor neurovascular integrity
         5) Necrotic ulcers (looks punched-out; no edema present)
         6) Tingling and numbness of the toes
         7) Cool extremities with poor pulses
      b. Collaborative Care
         1) **Nursing Interventions**
            a) Exercise therapy: walk to the point of pain three times per week.
            b) Encourage tobacco cessation.
            c) Promote weight reduction.
            d) Dependent position relieves pain.
         2) Administer Medications
            a) Administer pentoxifylline and cilostazol
         3) Therapeutic Measures
            a) Surgical Treatment
               (1) Femoral popliteal bypass surgery
               (2) Angioplasty or stenting
   2. **Peripheral venous disease:** disorder that interferes with adequate return of blood flow from legs. Includes venous insufficiency, venous thromboembolism (VTE), and varicose veins.
      a. Contributing Factors
         1) Prolonged sitting or standing
         2) Obesity
         3) Pregnancy
         4) Thrombophlebitis
      b. Manifestations
         1) Stasis dermatitis (brown discoloration)
         2) Edema
         3) Stasis ulcers (typically found around ankles)
      c. Collaborative Care
         1) **Nursing Interventions**
            a) Elevate legs four to five times throughout the day.
            b) Avoid the following: crossing legs, constrictive clothing, or tight socks.
            c) Apply compression stockings.

L. **Venous thromboembolism (VTE):** the collective condition of deep-vein thrombosis (DVT) and pulmonary embolism (PE)

1. Contributing Factors
    a. Immobility
    b. Surgery
    c. Trauma
    d. Obesity
    e. Age greater than 65
    f. Spinal cord injury
    g. Disorders of coagulation
    h. Pregnancy
    i. Oral contraceptives
2. Manifestations of DVT
    a. Edema of affected limb
    b. Local swelling, bumpy, knotty
    c. Red, tender, local induration
    d. Venous ulcers usually around the ankle; reddened and bluish; edema often present
3. Diagnostic Procedures
    a. MRI, CT scan, ultrasound
4. Collaborative Care
    a. **Nursing Interventions**
        1) Heparin: Monitor PTT.
        2) Warfarin: Monitor INR.
        3) Thrombolytic therapy: alteplase
        4) Assess for bleeding and thrombocytopenia.
        5) Elevate affected extremity and apply warm, moist compresses.
        6) Monitor for manifestations of PE: dyspnea, chest pain, tachycardia, anxiety.

KEY NURSING INTERVENTIONS: Prevention of VTE: early mobilization, leg exercises, compression stockings or intermittent pneumatic compression devices, prophylactic subcutaneous heparin.

M. **Varicose veins:** enlarged, twisted, and superficial veins; most common in the lower extremities and the esophagus

1. Contributing Factors
    a. Prolonged standing
    b. Pregnancy
    c. Obesity
    d. Heredity
2. Manifestations
    a. Enlarged, tortuous veins in lower extremities, visible just below skin
    b. Muscle cramping, pain after sitting
    c. Edema (after standing)

3. Collaborative Care
    a. **Nursing Interventions**
        1) Avoid prolonged sitting or standing.
        2) Instruct the client to wear supportive anti-embolism stockings, especially during air flights and pregnancy.
        3) Avoid crossing legs. Engage in daily exercise. Maintain an ideal body weight.
        4) Elevate lower extremities to reduce edema and promote venous return.
        5) Promote circulation with thigh-high anti-embolism stockings, ambulation, and elevation.
4. Medical Management
    a. **Sclerotherapy:** chemical injection
    b. **Ligation and stripping:** surgery
    c. **Thermal ablation:** nonsurgical use of energy or lasers

N. **Buerger's disease (thromboangiitis obliterans):** recurring inflammation of the arteries and veins of the lower and upper extremities, resulting in thrombus with occlusion (cause unknown).

1. Contributing Factors
    a. Thought to have a genetic predisposition
    b. Cigarette smoking and chewing tobacco use
    c. Occurs most often in men ages 20 to 35.
2. Manifestations
    a. Intermittent pain in the legs, feet, arms, and hands. Pain eases when activity is stopped (claudication).
    b. Inflammation along a vein below the skin's surface (due to a blood clot in the vein)
    c. Cold sensitivity of the Raynaud type frequently occurs in the hands.
    d. Painful open sores on fingers and toes
    e. Ulcerations and gangrene with amputation are common.
3. Collaborative Care
    a. Interventions
        1) Promote smoking cessation.
        2) Avoid cold or constrictive clothing.

O. **Raynaud's syndrome:** vasospastic or obstructive condition of the arteries/arterioles of upper and lower extremities resulting from exposure to cold/stress; more common in women

1. Contributing Factors
    a. Factors that cause Raynaud's attacks are not clearly understood.
    b. Blood vessels in hands and feet appear to overreact to cold or stress.
2. Manifestations
    a. Coldness, pallor, and pain in extremities secondary to vasospasm
    b. Occasional ulceration of the fingertips
    c. Color changes from white to blue to red (can be bilateral or symmetrical)

3. Diagnostic Procedures
   a. Cold-stimulation test: placing the hands in cool water or exposing to cold air to trigger an episode of Raynaud's
4. Collaborative Care

   a. **Nursing Interventions**
      1) Teach the client to avoid the cold and keep extremities warm; wear warm, but nonconstrictive gloves.
      2) Encourage the client to stop smoking and to limit caffeine intake.
   b. Medications
      1) Administer nifedipine.

IV Cardiac Surgery

A. **Coronary artery bypass graft (CABG):** a surgical procedure to bypass occluded coronary arteries and re-establish perfusion to the heart muscle.
   1. Most procedures require an open chest/heart approach with a bypass machine; however, the latest techniques may not use bypass, resulting in fewer complications and a shorter recovery period for some clients.
   2. Collaborative Care
      a. Preoperative/General Care
         1) Obtain baseline vital signs, physical assessment, and history.
         2) Provide psychological support and administer anxiolytic agents as needed (diazepam and lorazepam).
         3) Inform client and family what to anticipate postoperatively: intubation, IV lines, urinary catheter, arterial line, chest tubes.
         4) Shower with an antiseptic solution.
      b. Postoperative care
         1) Assess hourly for first 8 hr.
            a) Neurologic: responsiveness, pupils, reflexes
            b) Cardiac: BP, CVP, PAWP, heart rate, and rhythm and cardiac sounds
            c) Respiratory: chest movement, breath sounds, ventilator settings, chest tube drainage, ABGs
            d) Peripheral vascular status: pulses, edema, skin color and temperature
            e) Renal: urinary output, urine specific gravity
            f) F&E: I&O, electrolytes
            g) Pain: type, location, intensity
         2) Monitor for complications.
            a) Decreased cardiac output
            b) Fluid volume and electrolyte imbalance
            c) Impaired gas exchange
            d) Impaired cerebral circulation

V Shock

Inadequate delivery of oxygen and nutrients to support vital organs and cellular function. Results in impaired tissue perfusion.

A. **Types**
   1. Cardiogenic: failure of the heart to pump adequately
   2. Hypovolemic: decreased circulating blood volume
   3. Distributive (circulatory): vasodilation that causes blood to pool in the peripheral vessels
      a. Neurogenic: caused by spinal cord injury, certain medications, or hypoglycemia. Characterized by warm, dry skin and bradycardia.
      b. Anaphylactic: hypersensitivity reaction that causes a sudden onset of hypotension and is life-threatening. May also experience respiratory distress and cardiac arrest.
      c. Septic: most common type of circulatory shock. It results from a systemic infection and is characterized by warm, dry skin, bounding pulses, and tachypnea.

B. **Manifestations (related to decreased tissue perfusion)**
   1. Tachycardia with hypotension
   2. Tachypnea
   3. Oliguria
   4. Cold, moist skin (except neuro and septic)
   5. Color ashen, pallor
   6. Metabolic acidosis
   7. Decreased level of consciousness

C. **Collaborative Care**
   1. **Nursing Interventions**
      a. Position the client in modified Trendelenburg.
      b. Secure a large-bore IV line (16- or 18-gauge).
      c. Administer oxygen.
      d. Record vital signs every 5 min.
      e. Promote rest and decrease movement.
      f. Monitor urine output.
   2. Treatment
      a. Hypovolemic: volume replacement
      b. Cardiogenic: increase contractility and reduce afterload (BP).
      c. Septic: IV fluids, vasopressors, and antibiotics
      d. Anaphylactic: epinephrine and diphenhydramine
      e. Neurogenic: treat cause (e.g., stabilize spinal cord).

VI Cardiopulmonary Resuscitation (CPR)

A. **Indications**

  1. Absence of palpable carotid pulse

  2. Absence of breath sounds

B. **Purpose**

  1. Establish effective circulation and respiration.

  2. Prevent irreversible cerebral anoxic damage.

C. **Procedure**

  1. Follow the American Heart Association's current recommendations.

    a. Call 911.

    b. Send someone for the automated external defibrillator (AED).

    c. Immediately begin CPR if an adult victim is unresponsive and not breathing normally.

    d. Early, uninterrupted chest compressions are important. Follow the acronym CAB (compressions, airway, breathing).

    e. Untrained rescuers should perform hands-only compressions. Push hard and fast on the center of the victim's chest or follow the directions of EMS dispatchers.

    f. Trained rescuers should provide 30 compressions and two rescue breaths to improve outcomes.

    g. Depth: Compress the chest at least 2 inches (5 cm) in adults and the depth of chest in children and infants.

    h. Rate: Provide compressions 100/min, to the beat of the Bee Gees song "Stayin' Alive."

    i. Recoil: Allow the chest to recoil fully between compressions.

    j. Minimize interruptions: Do not delay or interrupt chest compressions to check pulse or rhythm.

    k. When necessary to check for a pulse, do not exceed 10 seconds.

  2. Complications

    a. Fractured ribs

    b. Punctured lungs

    c. Lacerated liver

    d. Abdominal distension

  3. Stop CPR when

    a. A provider pronounces the client dead.

    b. The rescuer is exhausted.

    c. Help arrives.

    d. The client's heartbeat returns.

  4. Automated external defibrillator: a computerized defibrillator that analyzes cardiac rhythm once pads are placed on the client's chest

    a. Do not stop compressions while defibrillator is being applied and set up.

    b. Stop compressions and rescue breaths while rhythm is being analyzed.

    c. A mechanical voice tells the rescuer if/when to deliver shock to the client.

    d. AED is frequently found in public locations because it is easy for nontrained individuals to use.

  5. Obstructed airway

    a. Conscious

      1) Establish that the client is choking.

      2) Perform the Heimlich maneuver until it is successful or the client becomes unconscious.

    b. Unconscious

      1) If a conscious choking adult becomes unresponsive, look for the foreign object in the pharynx. If object is seen, perform a finger sweep.

      2) If not breathing, begin CPR. Every time you open the airway to give breaths, look for the object.

      3) Continue CPR.

HEART

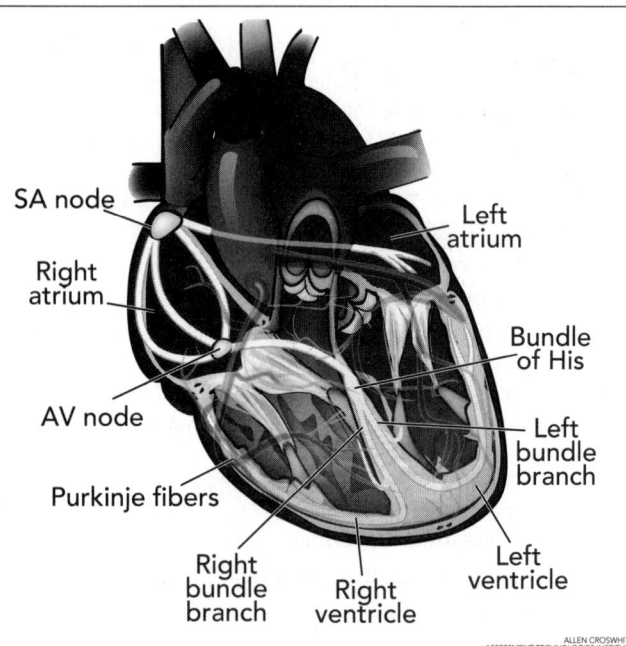

ALLEN CROSWHITE
ASSESSMENT TECHNOLOGIES INSTITUTE

VII Adjunctive Management

If medications are ineffective in eliminating dysrhythmias, electrical cardioversion and defibrillation may be used for tachydysrhythmias and pacemaker therapy for bradycardias.

A. **Cardioversion:** treats tachydysrhythmias by delivering an electrical current to the heart in an effort to convert the client to a normal rhythm

  1. Synchronized (timed to coincide with the client's own electrical cardiac cycle).

  2. Used when the client has a pulse.

  3. May be scheduled.

  4. TEE may be performed to rule out right atrial or ventricular clot formation prior to cardioversion.

  5. Sedation is commonly used.

B. **Defibrillation:** also delivers an electrical current to the heart, but used only for life-threatening dysrhythmias in an effort to convert the client to a more stable rhythm

1. Used for VF or pulseless VT.
2. Unsynchronized (not timed as with cardioversion).
3. Delivery is required immediately (not scheduled).
4. Used ONLY when client is pulseless.
5. Not effective for treatment of asystole.

C. **Pacemaker therapy:** an electronic device that provides repetitive electrical stimuli to the heart muscle in order to control the heart rate

1. Types
   a. Permanent Pacemakers
      1) Surgically placed in the subcutaneous tissue of the chest.
      2) Instruct client to avoid raising arm above head until wound heals.
      3) Observe for hiccups (sign of accidental dislodgement).
      4) Client Education
         a) Avoid large magnets (MRIs).
         b) Carry wallet notification or health ID, especially for airport travel.
         c) Know set rate and check pulse daily.
         d) Recognize and report signs of battery failure.
         e) Wear loose-fitting clothing.
         f) Avoid contact sports.
   b. Temporary Pacemakers (transvenous)
      1) Monitor ECG.
      2) Check heart rate.
      3) Assess site for hematoma and infection.
      4) Administer analgesics as needed.
      5) Maintain electrically safe environment.
   c. Transcutaneous (skin)
      1) Externally placed for use in emergency situations only
      2) Causes significant discomfort.
      3) Prepare for alternate interventions (temporary pacemaker).
      4) Remove transdermal patches from chest area. Arching can cause burns.
      5) Clip chest hair as needed to improve pad adherence and reduce burns.

2. Settings
   a. Ventricular demand: fires at a preset rate when heart rate drops below a predetermined/ preprogrammed rate
   b. Ventricular fixed: fires constantly at a preset/ preprogrammed rate, regardless of the client's heart rate
   c. Dual chamber: stimulates both the atria and the ventricles
   d. Atrial demand: fires as needed when the atria do not originate a rhythm
   e. Variable rate: senses oxygen demands and increases the firing rate to meet the client's needs

Genitourinary System Disorders

A. **Assessment of the Kidney and Urinary System**
   1. Functions of the Kidney
      a. Regulates acid–base balance
      b. Regulates fluid and electrolyte balance
      c. Excretes metabolic wastes (creatinine, urea)
      d. Regulates blood pressure: renin (stimulated by decreased blood pressure or blood volume) stimulates the production of angiotensin I, which is converted to angiotensin II in the lungs. Angiotensin II is a strong vasoconstrictor and stimulates aldosterone secretion; vasoconstriction and sodium reabsorption result in increased blood volume and increased blood pressure.
      e. Secretes erythropoietin
      f. Converts vitamin D to its active form for absorption of calcium
      g. Excretes water-soluble medications and medication metabolites
      h. Minimum urine output 0.5 ml/kg/hr
   2. Contributing Factors
      a. History of genitourinary disorder
      b. History of hypertension
      c. History of diabetes
      d. Family history of renal disease, such as PKD
      e. Incontinence, BPH, cancer, or kidney stones
      f. Nephrotoxic medications
   3. Manifestations
      a. Flank pain radiating to upper thigh, testis, or labium
      b. Changes in voiding: hematuria, proteinuria, dysuria, frequency, urgency, burning, nocturia, incontinence, polyuria, oliguria, anuria
      c. Thirst, fatigue, generalized edema

B. **Diagnostic Tests**
   1. **Urinalysis**
      a. Specific gravity
      b. Color: yellow, amber, or clear
      c. Negative glucose, protein, nitrites, RBCs, and WBCs
      d. pH
      e. First voided morning sample preferred: 15 mL
      f. Sent to laboratory immediately or refrigerated
      g. If clean catch, get urine for culture prior to starting antibiotics.
         1) Cleanse labia, glans penis.
         2) Obtain midstream sample.

IDENTIFY THE FOLLOWING ECG RHYTHMS

Calculating heart rate: To estimate heart rate, count the number of R waves in 6 seconds and multiply by 10. For example, if there are seven R waves in a 6-second strip, the estimated heart rate is 70/min (7 × 10 = 70).

1. Name the Rhythm:

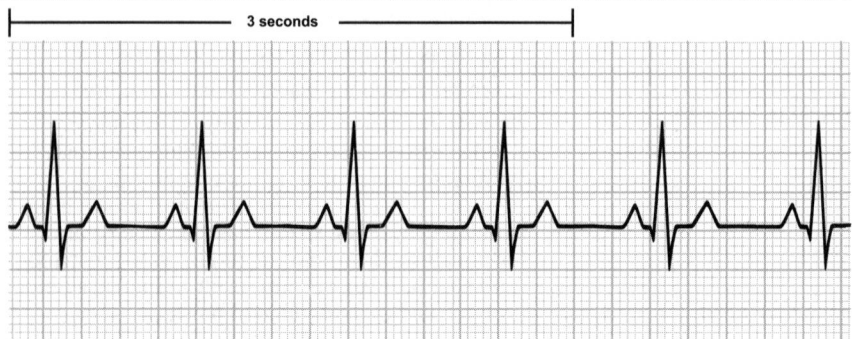

3 seconds

Characteristics

- › Rate: Atrial (P wave) and ventricular (QRS complex) rates are 60 to 100/min.
- › Rhythm: Atrial (P wave) and ventricular (QRS complex) rhythms are regular.
- › P waves: consistent and one before each QRS complex
- › PR interval: 0.12 to 0.20 seconds and consistent
- › QRS complex: less than 0.12 seconds and consistent

2. Name the Rhythm:

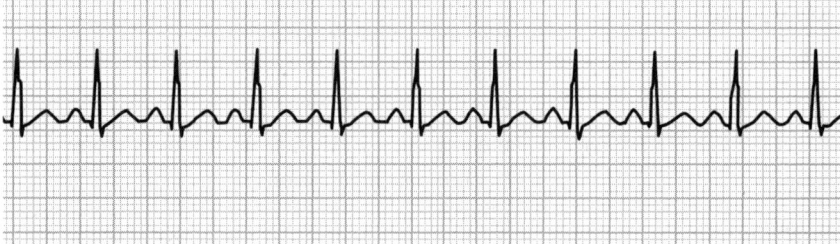

Characteristics

- › Rate: atrial (P wave) and ventricular (QRS complex) rates greater than 100/min
- › Rhythm: Atrial (P wave) and ventricular (QRS complex) rhythms are regular.
- › P waves: consistent and one before each QRS complex
- › PR interval: 0.12 to 0.20 seconds and consistent
- › QRS complex: less than 0.12 seconds and consistent

Causes: shock, fever, stress, exercise, anxiety, pain, stimulants

Treatment: usually none other than treating the cause

3. Name the Rhythm:

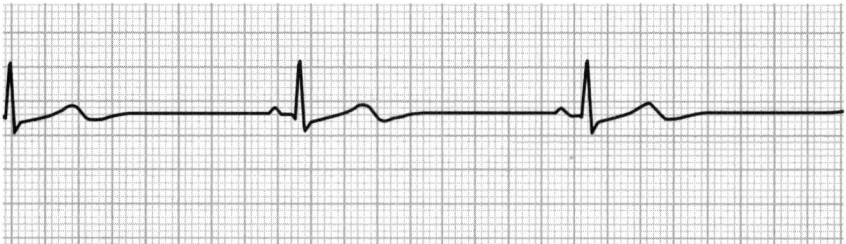

Characteristics

- › Rate: atrial (P wave) and ventricular (QRS complex) rates less than 60/min
- › Rhythm: Atrial (P wave) and ventricular (QRS complex) rhythms are regular.
- › P waves: consistent and one before each QRS complex
- › PR interval: 0.12 to 0.20 seconds and consistent
- › QRS complex: less than 0.12 seconds and consistent

Causes: Lower metabolic needs (e.g., sleep, hypothyroidism, athletic individuals), vagal stimulation (e.g., vomiting, straining during a bowel movement), medications (e.g., beta blockers, calcium channel blockers)

Treatment: directed at the cause if possible (e.g., discontinuing medication, preventing vagal stimulation) or signs of hemodynamic instability (e.g., hypotensive, dyspneic, altered mental status, angina). If the client is unstable, IV atropine 0.5 mg is the medication of choice, given 3 to 5 min apart to a maximum total of 3 mg.

4. Name the Rhythm:

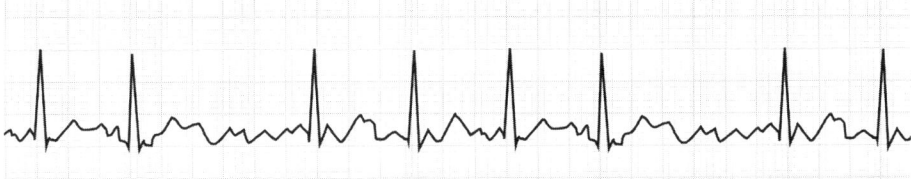

Characteristics

› Rate
› Atrial: Multiple rapid impulses from many areas of the atria result in a fibrillatory line.
› Ventricular: usually responds at a rate of 120 to 200/min
› Rhythm: Ventricular rhythm is irregular.
› P waves: no clear P wave
› PR interval: no clear P wave, so unable to determine
› QRS complex: less than 0.12 seconds and consistent

Causes: usually occurs in people of advanced age who have heart disease

Treatment: depends on the cause and the duration of the dysrhythmia. Many clients convert to an NSR spontaneously within 24 hr. If a client is unstable (e.g., hypotensive, dyspneic, altered mental status, angina), electrical cardioversion may be indicated. If a client has been in this rhythm for more than 48 hr, treatment with anticoagulants should occur first with warfarin for 3 to 4 weeks to avoid the formation of emboli, which can cause a cerebrovascular accident (CVA). Heart failure may occur due to loss of atrial kick. Medications may also be effective in converting the client back to an NSR. If atrial fibrillation is chronic, treatment with daily anticoagulant is common to prevent CVA.

5. Name the Rhythm:

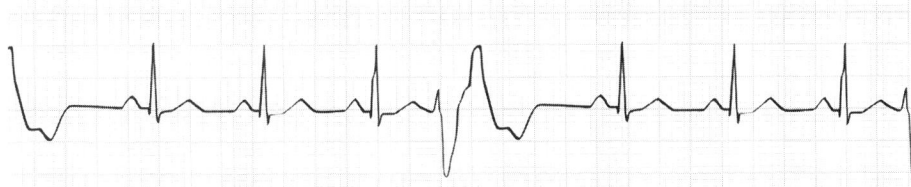

Characteristics: not a rhythm, but isolated abnormal beats that arise from an irritable area within a ventricle that causes the ventricle to contract prematurely. May cause palpitations.

Causes: may occur in healthy individuals. Often associated with nicotine, caffeine, and alcohol intake. May be caused by myocardial ischemia or infarction, heart failure, acidosis, hypoxia, and electrolyte imbalances, especially hypokalemia.

Treatment: If they occur in the absence of heart disease and are not causing a problem for the client, there may not be any treatment indicated. Treating the cause if possible and administering amiodarone or sotalol may be indicated depending on the severity and symptoms of the client. Manifestations may include slowing of the heart rate, decreased BP, and signs of impaired tissue perfusion.

6. Name the Rhythm:

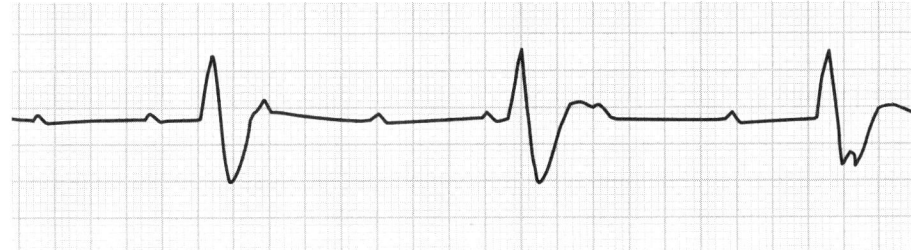

Characteristics

› Rate: Atrial rate is faster than the ventricular rate.
› Rhythm: Atrial and ventricular rhythms are usually regular.
› P waves: consistently present, but not consistently followed by a QRS complex
› PR interval: inconsistent and no identifiable relationship between the P wave and QRS complex
› QRS complex: usually consistent and may be wider than normal (greater than 0.12 seconds)

› Atrioventricular (AV) heart block: Cardiac electrical conduction transmission is blocked, not allowing any impulses to be conducted through the AV node. The atria and ventricles are beating independently from each other. Ventricular pacing is slow and unreliable.

Causes: can be caused by medication (e.g., digitalis, beta blockers, calcium channel blockers), myocardial ischemia and infarction, cardiomyopathy, inflammatory heart disease, or valvular disorders.

Treatment: depends on the cause, but often requires the placement of a pacemaker

7. Name the Rhythm:

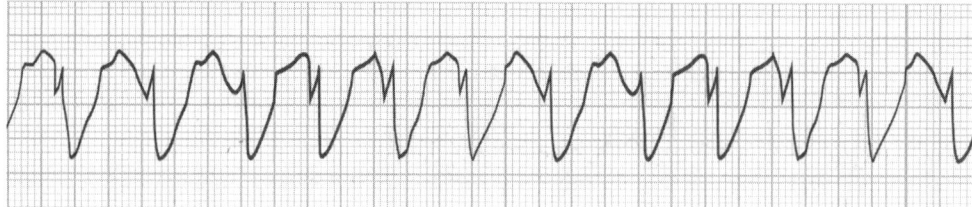

Characteristics

› Rate: ventricular rate usually 140 to 180/min
› Rhythm: irregular.
› P waves: not usually seen
› PR interval: not identifiable
› QRS complex: wide

Causes: similar to those for PVCs and more lethal if associated with myocardial infarction or low ejection fraction (percent of blood ejected from the heart with each contraction)

Treatment: If the client has a pulse, cardioversion is indicated, as well as the administration of antidysrhythmic IV medications (e.g., procainamide, amiodarone). If the client does not have a pulse, the treatment is immediate defibrillation.

8. Name the Rhythm:

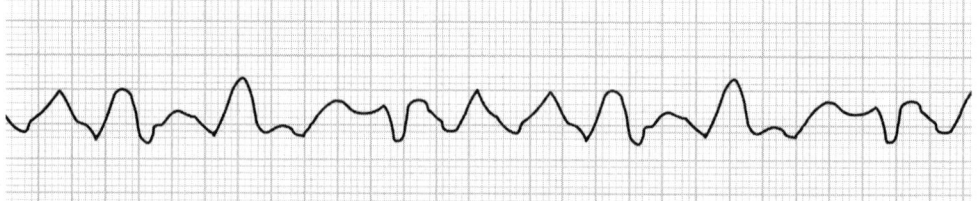

Characteristics: The electrical chaos in the heart causes the ventricles to fibrillate, resulting in a fibrillatory wave pattern. There are no recognizable waves or patterns. They do not contract and there is no pulse. There is no cerebral or systemic perfusion occurring. This rhythm is usually fatal if not reversed in 3 to 5 min.

Causes: most commonly caused by myocardial infarction and is the most common dysrhythmia resulting in cardiac arrest

Treatment: There is never a pulse with this rhythm. In addition to CPR, immediate defibrillation is critical to survival. The chance for survival decreases by 7% to 10% for every 1 min delay in defibrillation.

9. Name the Rhythm:

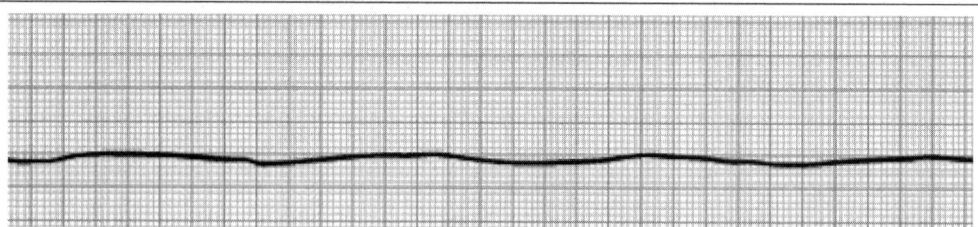

Characteristics: There is no electrical activity in the heart. This results in a flat line with no identifiable waves or pattern. Because there is no electrical activity, there is no contraction, pulse, or perfusion occurring. The prognosis for these clients is usually poor.

Causes: hypoxia, acidosis, severe electrolyte imbalances, drug overdose, hypovolemia, cardiac tamponade, tension pneumothorax, myocardial infarction, hypothermia, or trauma

Treatment: high-quality CPR. Identify and treat cause. Medications such as epinephrine and vasopressin can be beneficial. If this does not correct the rhythm, resuscitation efforts are usually ceased.

Answer Key: 1. Normal sinus rhythm; 2. Sinus tachycardia; 3. Sinus bradycardia; 4. Atrial fibrillation; 5. Premature ventricular contractions; 6. Third-degree heart block; 7. Ventricular tachycardia; 8. Ventricular fibrillation; 9. Asystole

2. **Renal Function Tests** (several tests over a period of time are necessary)
   a. BUN
   b. An increased BUN may indicate
      1) Hepatic or renal disease.
      2) Dehydration or decreased kidney perfusion.
      3) A high-protein diet.
      4) Infection
      5) Stress
      6) Steroid use
      7) GI bleeding
   c. Creatinine
      1) Creatinine is the best measure of renal function.
   d. 24-hr creatinine clearance: 75 to 120 mL/min
      1) Have the client void and discard the first specimen.
      2) Obtain serum creatinine.
      3) Collect all urine from the client for the next 24 hr (refrigerate or keep container on ice).
      4) At the completion of the 24 hr, the test is stopped following the client's last void.
   e. Uric acid (serum)
   f. Prostate-specific antigen: greater than 10 indicates risk of prostate cancer

3. **Radiologic Tests**
   a. Kidneys, ureters, bladder (x-ray): shows the size, shape, and position of kidneys, ureters, and bladder; no preparation necessary (verify that the client is not pregnant)
   b. IV pyelography (contrast dye): to help in visualization of the urinary tract
      1) Collaborative Care
         a) **Nursing Interventions**
            (1) Verify that informed consent has been signed.
            (2) Verify the client's last creatinine level.
            (3) The client should remain NPO for 8 hr; fluids may be permitted.
            (4) Administer laxatives as prescribed.
            (5) Administer an enema or suppository on the morning of the test (as necessary).
            (6) Assess for allergies to iodine or shellfish.
            (7) Inform the client of potential sensations during the exam (e.g., flushing, warmth, nausea, a metallic or salty taste, or incontinence).
            (8) Emergency equipment should be readily available during the test.
            (9) Encourage fluids to help flush out the dye.

4. **Renal angiography:** visualization of renal arterial supply; contrast material injected through a catheter
   a. **Nursing Interventions** (preprocedure)
      1) Approach is through the femoral or brachial artery.
      2) Locate and mark peripheral pulses.
      3) Have the client void before the procedure.
      4) Explain that the procedure may create the feeling of warmth along the vessel.
   b. **Nursing Interventions** (postprocedure)
      1) Maintain bed rest for 6 to 8 hr.
      2) Monitor the client's vital signs until stable.
      3) Observe the client for swelling and hematoma.
      4) Palpate peripheral pulses/vascular checks.
      5) Monitor the client's I&O, including urinary status.

5. **Cystoscopy:** an invasive procedure in which a scope is passed to view the interior of the bladder, urethra, or the position of urethral orifices to remove calculi from the urethra, bladder, and ureter; to treat lesions of the bladder, urethra, and prostate
   a. **Nursing Interventions** (preoperative)
      1) Maintain NPO if the client is given general anesthesia.
      2) Administer preoperative cathartics/enemas as ordered.
      3) Teach the client deep breathing exercises to relieve bladder spasms.
      4) Monitor for postural hypotension.
      5) Inform the client that pink-tinged or tea-colored urine is common following the procedure, but bright, red urine or clots should be reported.
      6) Provide nonpharmacological pain management techniques following the procedure.
   b. **Nursing Interventions** (postoperative)
      1) Assess for leg cramps due to lithotomy position.
      2) Assess for back pain or abdominal pain.
      3) Offer warm sitz baths for comfort.
      4) Push fluids and provide analgesics.
      5) Monitor the client's I&O.

6. **Renal biopsy**
   a. **Nursing Interventions** (preprocedure)
      1) Obtain bleeding, clotting, and prothrombin times.
      2) Obtain results of prebiopsy x-rays of kidney.
      3) Administer IV fluids.
      4) Maintain NPO status for 6 to 8 hr.
      5) Position the client with a pillow under the abdomen and shoulders on the bed.
      6) Verify that the informed consent is signed.
      7) Instruct client to remain still during the procedure.

 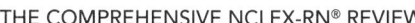

b. **Nursing Interventions** (postprocedure)

1) Maintain the client in the supine position. The client should remain in bed for 24 hr.

2) Monitor the client's vital signs every 5 to 15 min for 4 hr.

3) Maintain pressure to the puncture site for 20 min.

4) Observe the client for any pain, nausea, vomiting, and blood pressure changes.

5) Encourage fluid intake.

6) Assess Hct and Hgb 8 hr after procedure.

7) Monitor the client's urine output.

8) Make sure the client avoids strenuous activity, sports, and heavy lifting for at least 2 weeks.

7. **Indwelling urinary catheterization:** a sterile procedure to empty the contents of the bladder, obtain a sterile specimen, determine residual urine, initiate irrigation of the bladder, or bypass an obstruction.

a. Collaborative Care

1) **Nursing Interventions**

a) Maintain a closed system.

b) Measure the client's output every shift.

c) Provide meticulous perineal care.

d) Keep a drainage bag below the level of the client's bladder.

e) Increase daily fluid intake.

f) Prevent dependent loops in the catheter tubing.

g) Discontinue as soon as possible due to increased risk for urinary tract infection.

C. **Specific Disorders**

1. **Cystitis:** inflammation of the urinary bladder

a. Contributing Factors

1) Wiping back to front after toileting, secondary to ascending infection from *Escherichia coli*

2) Prolonged baths with excessive soap (common in females)

3) Benign prostatic hyperplasia (males)

4) Indwelling urinary catheter

b. Manifestations

1) Frequency and urgency, and only voiding small amounts of urine each time

2) Dysuria with hematuria

3) Suprapubic tenderness; pain in the bladder region or flank pain

4) Fever, malaise, chills

5) Cloudy, foul-smelling urine

6) Urinalysis: increased protein and WBC, presence of leukoesterase, casts, and bacteria

c. Collaborative Care

1) **Nursing Interventions**

a) Obtain the client's clean catch urine sample for culture and sensitivity before initiating antibiotic therapy.

b) Maintain acidic urine pH.

c) Push fluids (greater than 3,000 mL/day).

d) Encourage the client to drink cranberry juice.

e) Apply heat to the perineum for comfort.

2) Medications

a) Antimicrobial medications: Sulfonamides are the medications of choice unless the client is allergic (sulfamethoxazole-trimethoprim and nitrofurantoin macrocrystal).

b) Urinary analgesics (phenazopyridine): Inform the client that the medication will temporarily turn urine orange.

c) Antispasmodics: hyoscyamine

3) Client Education and Referral

a) Follow appropriate perineal care (such as wiping front to back).

b) Wear cotton underwear.

c) Avoid bubble baths (they can irritate urethra).

d) Maintain an increased fluid intake.

e) Void after sexual intercourse.

f) Drink cranberry juice daily.

2. **Acute glomerulonephritis:** an acute renal disease involving the renal glomeruli of both kidneys. Thought to be an antigen-antibody reaction that damages the glomeruli of the kidney. May be a secondary response to infection in other areas of the body that usually occurs in children. The prognosis is good if treatment is implemented.

a. Contributing Factors

1) Beta-hemolytic streptococcal

2) Can follow tonsillitis or pharyngitis

b. Manifestations

1) Hematuria (cola or tea-colored urine), with proteinuria

2) Edema (especially facial and periorbital; ascites)

3) Oliguria or anuria

4) Hypertension with headache

5) Azotemia

6) Flank or abdominal pain

7) Anemia

c. Collaborative Care

1) **Nursing Interventions**

a) Maintain bed rest to protect the kidney.

b) Restrict fluids.

c) Increase calories and reduce protein and sodium in the diet.

d) Monitor daily weight.

2) Medications

    a) Penicillin for streptococcal infection (substitute other antibiotics for clients allergic to penicillin)

    b) Corticosteroids for inflammatory disease

    c) Antihypertensives for increased blood pressure

3. **Nephrosis:** a clinical disorder associated with protein wasting; secondary to diffuse glomerular damage

  a. Contributing Factors

    1) May be autoimmune; the glomerular membrane is more permeable, especially to proteins.

  b. Manifestations

    1) Insidious onset of pitting edema (generalized edema is anasarca)

    2) Proteinuria

    3) Anemia

    4) Hypoalbuminemia

    5) Anorexia, malaise, and nausea

    6) Oliguria

    7) Ascites

  c. Collaborative Care

    1) **Nursing Interventions**

      a) Maintain bed rest (during severe edema only) to preserve renal function.

      b) Maintain a low-sodium, low-potassium, moderate-protein, high-calorie diet.

      c) Protect the client from infection.

      d) Monitor I&O.

      e) Weigh the client and measure abdominal girth daily.

    2) Medication Therapy

      a) Loop diuretics: furosemide

      b) Steroids: prednisone

      c) Immunosuppressive agents: cyclophosphamide

4. **Urolithiasis (urinary calculi):** stones in the urinary system

  a. Contributing Factors

    1) Obstruction and urinary stasis

    2) Uric acid stones (excessive purine intake)

    3) Immobilization

    4) More common in males ages 20 to 40 and tends to reoccur

  b. Manifestations (based on location and size of the stone)

    1) Pain: severe renal colic (ureter); dull, aching (kidney); radiates to the groin

    2) Nausea, vomiting, diarrhea, or constipation

    3) Hematuria

    4) Manifestations of a urinary tract infection

  c. Collaborative Care (goals: to eradicate the stone and prevent nephron destruction)

    1) **Nursing Interventions**

      a) Force fluids—at least 3,000 mL/day (IV or by mouth).

      b) Strain all urine.

      c) Provide pain control.

      d) Maintain proper urine pH (depends on type of stone).

    2) Medications

      a) Opioids (morphine IV for rapid pain relief). NSAID ketorolac in acute phase.

      b) Administer allopurinol for uric acid stones.

    3) Therapeutic Measures

      a) Lithotripsy to crush the stone through sound waves

    4) Client Education

      a) Avoid foods high in oxalates if it is a calcium oxalate stone (e.g., spinach, black tea, rhubarb, chocolate).

      b) Maintain fluid intake to maintain hydration.

5. **Acute kidney injury:** an abrupt decrease in renal function; may be the result of trauma, allergic reactions, drug overdose, kidney stones, or shock

  a. Contributing Factors

    1) Prerenal: disrupted blood flow to the kidneys; hypovolemic shock, dehydration, heart failure, burn injury, and anaphylaxis

    2) Renal: renal tissue damage; trauma, hypokalemia, acute glomerulonephritis, hemolytic uremic syndrome (infection caused by *Escherichia coli*; common in children), substance abuse

    3) Postrenal: urine flow from the kidney is compromised; kidney stones, prostate hyperplasia, tumors, and strictures

  b. Manifestations (four phases)

    1) Onset: begins with the onset of the event and lasts for hours to days

    2) Oliguric (1 to 3 weeks): sudden onset, less than 400 mL in 24 hr, edema, elevated BUN, creatinine and potassium; increased specific gravity; acidosis; heart failure; dysrhythmias

    3) Diuretic: Urine output increases, followed by diuresis of up to 4,000 to 5,000 mL/day, indicating recovery of damaged nephrons; decreased specific gravity; hypotension and fluid and electrolyte imbalances are a concern.

    4) Recovery: may take up to 1 year until renal function returns to normal (baseline); older adults are at increased risk for residual impairment

c. Collaborative Care

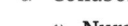

  1) **Nursing Interventions**

    a) Eliminate or prevent cause.

    b) Correct metabolic acidosis, hyperkalemia, hyperphosphatemia, and hypocalcemia.

      (1) Kayexalate (an ion exchange resin given orally or by enema to treat hyperkalemia)

      (2) IV glucose and insulin (causes potassium to enter cells)

      (3) Calcium IV or sodium bicarbonate to stabilize cell membrane

    c) Implement dietary modifications.

      (1) For oliguric phase, low-protein, high-carbohydrate diet and restricted potassium intake

      (2) For diuresis phase, low-protein, high-calorie diet and restricted fluids as indicated

        (a) Encourage bed rest in the oliguric phase.

        (b) Monitor daily weights.

        (c) Monitor I&O.

        (d) Implement dialysis (as ordered) until renal function returns.

        (e) Assess for pericarditis (friction rubs).

  2) Medications

    a) Phosphate binders to lower phosphorus while replacing calcium (e.g., calcium acetate)

    b) Epoetin alfa to treat anemia

6. **Chronic kidney disease:** progressive failure of kidney function that results in death unless hemodialysis or transplant is performed; is irreversible

  a. Stages of Chronic Kidney Disease

    1) Stage 1: glomerular filtration rate (GFR) greater than 90 mL/min

    2) Stage 2: GFR 60 to 89 mL/min

    3) Stage 3: 30 to 59 mL/min

    4) Stage 4: 15 to 29 mL/min

    5) Stage 5: less than 15 mL/min (end-stage renal disease [ESRD])

  b. Contributing Factors

    1) Diabetes mellitus (leading cause)

    2) Uncontrolled hypertension (second cause)

    3) Chronic glomerulonephritis

    4) Pyelonephritis

    5) Congenital kidney disease, such as PKD

    6) Ethnicity—African American, Native American, and Asian

  c. Manifestations (progressively worsen)

    1) Fatigue secondary to anemia

    2) Headache and hypertension

    3) Nausea, vomiting, diarrhea

    4) Irritability

    5) Edema

    6) Hypocalcemia, hyperkalemia

    7) Pruritus, uremic frost

    8) Pallid, gray-yellow complexion

    9) Metabolic acidosis; elevated BUN and creatinine; decreased glomerular filtration rate

    10) Convulsions, coma

  d. Collaborative Care

    1) **Nursing Interventions**

      a) Maintain bed rest.

      b) Implement a renal diet for the client—low-protein, low-potassium, high-carbohydrate, vitamins and calcium supplements, low-sodium, and low-phosphate.

      c) Monitor for and treat hypertension as prescribed.

      d) Strict I&O; fluid replacement—500 to 600 mL more than previous 24-hr urine output.

      e) Monitor electrolytes.

      f) Do not administer antacids with magnesium or enemas with phosphorous.

      g) Maintain dialysis.

      h) Administer diuretics in early stages.

      i) Provide meticulous skin care.

      j) Provide emotional support to the client and the client's family.

      k) Assess for bleeding tendencies.

    2) Medications

      a) Phosphate binders (aluminum hydroxide gel, calcium acetate, sevelamer hydrochloride)

      b) Epoetin alfa/erythropoietin (for anemia to stimulate RBC formation and transfuse as necessary

7. **Dialysis**

  a. Goals

    1) Remove end products of metabolism (i.e., urea and creatinine) from the client's blood.

    2) Maintain safe concentration of serum electrolytes.

    3) Correct acidosis.

    4) Remove excess fluid from the client's blood.

  b. **Hemodialysis:** the process of cleansing the blood of accumulated waste products and fluids; used for ESRD or clients who are acutely ill and require short-term treatment

    1) Collaborative Care

      a) **Nursing Interventions**

        (1) Weigh the client before and after the procedure.

        (2) Monitor the client's blood pressure continuously during the procedure.

        (3) Provide care to the access site to prevent clotting and infection.

        (4) Assess for presence of thrill and bruit.

        (5) Provide adequate nutrition as prescribed.

(6) Post a sign above the client's bed that warns of no blood pressure readings or blood work on the side of the fistula.

(7) Maintain fluid restrictions.

(8) Withhold regular morning medications prior to dialysis.

(9) Instruct the client to notify the nurse of muscle cramps, headache, nausea, or dizziness that occurs during the procedure.

(10) Provide emotional support. Offer activities, such as books, magazines, music, cards, or television, to occupy the client.

c. **Peritoneal dialysis:** an alternative method using the peritoneum to remove fluids, electrolytes, and waste products from the blood. Dialysis is accomplished via a catheter surgically placed into the peritoneal cavity.

1) Collaborative Care

a) **Nursing Interventions**

(1) Assist the client to void prior to the procedure.

(2) Weigh the client daily.

(3) Monitor the client's vital signs and baseline electrolytes.

(4) Maintain asepsis.

(5) Sterile dressing changes per facility policy.

(6) Keep an accurate record of the client's fluid balance.

(7) Procedure

(a) Warm dialysate (1 to 2 L of 1.5%, 2.5%, or 4.25% glucose solution).

(b) Allow to flow in by gravity.

(c) 5 to 10 min inflow time; close clamp immediately.

(d) 30 min of equilibration (dwell time).

(e) 10 to 30 min of drainage (should be clear and pale yellow).

(f) Monitor for complications (e.g., peritonitis, bleeding, respiratory difficulty, abdominal pain, and bowel or bladder perforation).

d. **Continuous ambulatory peritoneal dialysis (CAPD):** peritoneal dialysis performed by the client without the use of a machine (cycler)

1) Procedure (differs from acute peritoneal dialysis)

a) Permanent indwelling catheter inserted into peritoneum

b) Fluid infused by gravity (1.5 to 3 L)

c) Dwell time: 4 to 8 hr

d) Dialysate drains by gravity: 20 to 40 min

e) Four to five exchanges daily, 7 days/week (some clients may elect to do at night with automatic cycling machines; 10 to 14 hr, 3 times/week); continuous cycling peritoneal dialysis (CCPD)

2) Collaborative Care

a) **Nursing Interventions**

(1) Monitor the client for complications.

(2) Monitor the client for peritonitis (rebound tenderness, fever, cloudy outflow).

(3) Monitor for bladder perforation (yellow outflow).

(4) Monitor for hypotension.

(5) Monitor for bowel perforation (brown outflow).

b) Advantages to CAPD

(1) More independence

(2) Clients may continue normal activities during CAPD.

(3) Free dietary intake and better nutrition

(4) Satisfactory control of uremia

(5) Least expensive dialysis

(6) Decreased likelihood of future transplant rejection

(7) More closely approximates normal renal function

8. **Renal and Urinary Tract Surgery**

a. Kidney Transplantation

1) For individuals with ESRD

2) Requires a well-matched donor

a) Living donors (most desirable)

b) Cadaver donors

3) Preoperative Management

a) Interventions are prescribed to correct the client's metabolic status.

b) Administer immunosuppressive therapy.

c) Schedule hemodialysis within 24 hr if client currently requires dialysis.

d) Provide the client with emotional support.

4) **Nursing Interventions** (postoperative management)

a) Monitor labs (CBC, electrolytes, BUN/creatinine).

b) Administer immunosuppressive medications to the client, such as azathioprine, cyclosporine, or steroids.

c) Monitor the client for rejection. This could include oliguria, edema, fever, tenderness over graft site, fluid and electrolyte imbalance, hypertension, elevated BUN, creatinine, and elevated WBCs.

d) Monitor the client for infection and maintain protective isolation.

e) Provide emotional support and monitor for depression.

9. **Urinary diversion:** removal of the bladder and surrounding structures to reroute urinary flow through a pouch and abdominal stoma

a. Collaborative Care

  1) **Nursing Interventions**

    a) Monitor the client's vital signs. (Hemorrhage and shock are frequent complications.)

    b) Monitor stoma.

    c) Provide the client with pain control.

    d) Observe for manifestations of paralytic ileus, which are very common.

    e) Provide adequate fluid replacement.

    f) Weigh the client daily.

    g) Maintain function and patency of the drainage tubes.

      (1) Indwelling urinary catheter (dependent position, tape tubing to the thigh)

      (2) Nephrostomy Tube

        (a) Never clamp.

        (b) Irrigate only with prescription for 10 mL of 0.9% sodium chloride.

        (c) Assess for leakage of urine.

      (3) Ureteral Catheters

        (a) Each catheter drains half of the urinary system.

        (b) Bloody drainage is expected after surgery, but should clear within 24 to 48 hr.

        (c) Never irrigate the surgical implant.

        (d) Aseptic technique is required.

10. **Benign prostatic hyperplasia:** enlargement of the prostate that may accompany the aging process in males; exact cause is unknown

a. Manifestations

  1) Difficulty starting stream/dribbling

  2) Decrease in force of the urinary stream

  3) Frequent urinary tract infections

  4) Nocturia

  5) Hematuria

b. Diagnosis

  1) Digital rectal exam or cystoscopy

  2) Prostate-specific antigen (PSA) for diagnosis

c. Treatments

  1) Urinary antibiotics

  2) Alpha blocker medications to promote urinary flow: terazosin, tamsulosin, alfuzosin, silodosin, and doxazosin

  3) Enzyme inhibitors to decrease the size of the prostate gland: dutasteride and finasteride

4) **Transurethral resection of prostate (TURP):** Enlarged portion of the prostate is removed through an endoscopic instrument.

  a) **Nursing Interventions** (preoperative)

    (1) Insert indwelling urinary catheter.

    (2) Administer antibiotics as prescribed.

  b) **Nursing Interventions** (postoperative)

    (1) Monitor the client for shock and hemorrhage.

    (2) Teach the client to avoid heavy lifting, prolonged sitting, constipation, or straining (which could cause a rebleed).

    (3) Monitor for continuous bladder irrigation (expect bloody drainage; monitor I&O carefully).

    (4) Encourage fluid intake (at least 3,000 mL/day).

    (5) Assess for TURP syndrome: a cluster of manifestations resulting from absorption of irrigating fluids through prostate tissue (e.g., hyponatremia, confusion, bradycardia, hypo/hypertension, nausea, vomiting, and visual changes).

    (6) Medicate for pain control: the client may need medication and narcotics to decrease bladder spasm.

    (7) Keep the catheter taped tightly to the client's leg (for hemostasis at the surgical site by catheter balloon).

    (8) Teach the client Kegel exercises (there may be temporary or permanent loss of sexual function or urinary control).

11. **Prostate cancer:** a slow-growing cancer of the prostate gland

a. Contributing Factors

  1) Men age 50 and older

  2) African American

  3) Family history

  4) Elevated testosterone levels

  5) High-fat diet

b. Manifestations

  1) Asymptomatic in early stages

  2) Hematuria

  3) Prostate-specific antigen (PSA) greater than 10

  4) Rectal exam: hard, pea-sized nodule

  5) Frequent UTIs

c. Treatment

  1) Radical prostatectomy

  2) External radiation therapy

  3) Internal radioactive seeds

  4) Hormone therapy

12. **Testicular cancer:** rare cancer affecting one or both testes. Testicular self-examination (TSE) should begin during adolescence.
    a. Contributing Factors
        1) Men 20 to 54 years of age
        2) Higher risk in males who have an undescended testis
        3) Family history
    b. Manifestations
        1) Swelling or painless lump in one or both testes
        2) Possible heaviness or aching in lower abdomen or scrotum
    c. Treatment
        1) Offer sperm banking prior to surgery.
        2) Orchiectomy to remove affected testicle.
        3) Chemotherapy
        4) Emotional support
13. **Incontinence**
    a. Types
        1) Urge: cannot hold urine when stimulus to void occurs
        2) Functional: cannot physically get to the bathroom or is not aware of the stimulus to void
        3) Stress: Pressure such as coughing, straining, lifting, bearing down, or laughing causes incontinence; very common in middle-age women.
    b. Collaborative Care

        1) **Nursing Interventions**
            a) Use adult incontinence devices.
            b) Decrease the client's fluid intake after 6 p.m.
            c) Maintain a regular toilet schedule.
            d) Perform the Credé maneuver as needed.
            e) Monitor the client for signs of cystitis.
            f) Teach the client Kegel exercises to strengthen the sphincter.
            g) Ensure that the physical environment enhances the ability to get to the bathroom.
        2) Medications
            a) Urge Incontinence
                (1) Anticholinergics: tolterodine and oxybutynin
            b) Stress Incontinence
                (1) Tricyclic antidepressant: imipramine
14. **Urine retention:** caused by a physical obstruction of the urethra from acute or chronic causes (e.g., edema, BPH, tumor, inflammation, or inability of the bladder to work; postanesthesia, stroke); at risk for hydronephrosis
    a. Collaborative Care
        1) **Nursing Interventions**
            a) Stimulate relaxation of the urethral sphincter by providing the client privacy, placing the client's hands in warm water (or just turning on the water), and encouraging guided imagery.
            b) Administer bethanechol chloride.
            c) Position the client upright.
            d) Ensure adequate fluid intake.

Neurosensory Disorders

A. **Neurological Assessment**
    1. History of present illness
    2. Mental Status
        a. Level of consciousness (e.g., alert, lethargic, obtunded, stuporous, comatose)
        b. Orientation (e.g., person, place, time)
        c. Affect
        d. Mood
        e. Speech (e.g., clarity, consistency, word-finding ability)
        f. Cognition (e.g., judgment and abstraction ability)
    3. Cranial Nerves (I through XII)
        a. CN I, olfactory: sensory, smell
        b. CN II, optic: sensory, vision
        c. CN III, oculomotor: motor, eye
        d. CN IV, trochlear: motor, eye
        e. CN V, trigeminal: sensory, face; motor, chewing
        f. CN VI, abducens: motor, eye
        g. CN VII, facial: sensory, face and hands
        h. CN VIII, acoustic: sensory, hearing and balance
        i. CN IX, glossopharyngeal: sensory, posterior taste
        j. CN X, vagus: sensory, throat; motor, swallow, speech; cardiac innervation (slows down)
        k. CN XI, accessory: motor, throat, neck muscles, upper back
        l. CN XII, hypoglossal: motor, tongue
    4. Motor Function
        a. Muscles
            1) Size
            2) Symmetry
            3) Tone
            4) Strength
        b. Coordination
        c. Movement
            1) Voluntary control/involuntary movements
            2) Tremors
            3) Twitches
            4) Balance and gait

d. Posturing

   1) Flexion (decorticate): an abnormal posturing indicated by rigidity, flexion of the arms to the chest, clenched fists, and extended legs. Indicative of damage to the corticospinal tract (the pathway between the brain and the spinal cord).

DECORTICATE POSTURING

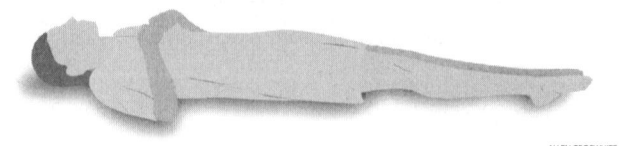

ALLEN CROSWHITE
ASSESSMENT TECHNOLOGIES INSTITUTE

   2) Extension (decerebrate): an abnormal body posturing indicated by rigid extension of the arms and legs, downward pointing of the toes, and backward arching of the head. Indicative of deterioration of structures of the nervous system, particularly the upper brain stem.

DECEREBRATE POSTURING

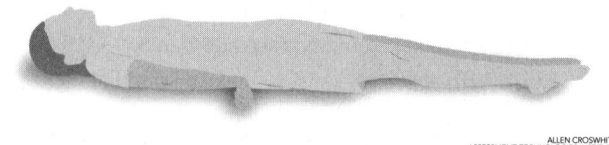

ALLEN CROSWHITE
ASSESSMENT TECHNOLOGIES INSTITUTE

5. Reflexes
   a. Deep Tendon Reflexes (DTRs)
      1) Biceps, triceps, brachioradial, quadriceps
   b. Superficial Reflex
      1) Plantar, abdominal, Babinski
   c. Reflex Activity
      1) Absent, no response = 0
      2) Weaker than normal = 1+
      3) Normal = 2+
      4) Stronger/more brisk = 3+
      5) Hyperactive = 4+
6. Glasgow Coma Scale: neurologic assessment tool
   a. Rating: 3 (least responsive) to 15 (most responsive)

GLASGOW COMA SCALE

EYE OPENING RESPONSE (E)	VERBAL RESPONSE (V)	MOTOR RESPONSE (M)
4 = Spontaneous	5 = Normal conversation	6 = Normal
3 = To voice		5 = Localizes to pain
2 = To pain	4 = Disoriented conversation	4 = Withdraws to pain
1 = None	3 = Words, but not coherent	3 = Decorticate posture
	2 = No words, only sounds	2 = Decerebrate
	1 = None	1 = None
E Score	V Score	M Score

E + V + M = Total score

7. Pupil Check: PERRLA
   a. **P**upils **e**qual in size, **r**ound and regular in shape, **r**eactive to **l**ight and **a**ccommodation
8. Vital Signs
   a. Blood pressure or pulse changes may indicate increased intracranial pressure.

B. **Diagnostic Procedures**

1. **Lumbar puncture:** procedure that inserts a needle into the subarachnoid space to measure pressure, obtain CSF for analysis, and inject contrast, anesthetics, and certain medications
   a. **Nursing Interventions**
      1) Verify that informed consent has been signed.
      2) Have the client empty his bladder and bowel.
      3) Position the client on his side with knees pulled toward his chest and chin tucked downward.
      4) Assist providers with measuring pressure and collecting fluid.
      5) Postprocedure
         a) Encourage fluid intake.
         b) Check puncture site for redness, swelling, and clear drainage.
         c) Assess movement of extremities.
         d) Monitor for complications.

2. **Computed Tomography (CT) Scan**
   a. **Nursing Interventions**
      1) Preprocedure
         a) Verify that informed consent has been signed.
         b) Check for any allergies to iodine, contrast dyes, or shellfish.
         c) Assess BUN and creatinine.
         d) Instruct the client to lie still and flat.
      2) Postprocedure
         a) Increase fluids to clear dye from the client's system.
         b) Assess dye injection site.
         c) Assess for allergic reaction to dye.

3. **Cerebral arteriography:** injection of dye, usually via the femoral artery to allow visualization of the cerebral arteries
   a. **Nursing Interventions**
      1) Preprocedure
         a) Verify that informed consent has been signed.
         b) Check for allergies to iodine, contrast dyes, or shellfish.
         c) Assess BUN and creatinine.
         d) Keep client NPO 4 to 6 hr before the procedure.
         e) Mark distal peripheral pulses.
         f) Instruct the client that her face may feel warm during the procedure.

2) Postprocedure

   a) Monitor for an altered level of consciousness and sensory or motor deficits.

   b) Check for bleeding or hematoma at the insertion site. Movement is restricted for 8 to 12 hr.

   c) Check peripheral pulses, color, and temperature of extremities.

4. **Electroencephalogram (EEG):** noninvasive assessment of the electrical activity of the brain. Electrodes are placed over multiple areas of the scalp to detect and record patterns of electrical activity, and they also check for abnormalities such as seizure disorders, evaluation of head injuries, tumors, infections, degenerative diseases, metabolic disturbances, or to confirm brain death.

  a. **Nursing Interventions**

   1) Verify which medications should be administered before the EEG. Depressive, stimulant, and antiseizure medications are usually not given.

   2) Instruct the client to avoid caffeine 8 hr before the test.

   3) Advise the client to wash hair before the test because it must be free of oils, sprays, and conditioners.

   4) Verify if the test is to be done awake, asleep, or sleep-deprived.

5. **Magnetic resonance imaging (MRI):** a noninvasive procedure that uses a magnetic field to construct clear, detailed, cross-sectional images of the body

  a. **Nursing Interventions**

   1) Verify that informed consent has been signed.

   2) Assess the client for claustrophobia.

   3) Remove all metal objects such as body piercings, jewelry, credit cards, and watches.

   4) No special test, diet, or medications are required.

C. **Disorders**

1. **Head injury:** any trauma that leads to injury of the scalp, skull, or brain, ranging from concussion to skull fracture; classified as either closed or open (scalp, skull, and dura open)

  a. **Closed-Head Injury**

   1) Head sustains blunt force trauma

   2) Concussion (temporary loss of neurological function with no apparent structural damage)

   3) Contusion (brain is damaged; characterized by loss of consciousness and confusion)

   4) Diffuse axonal injury (shearing and rotational forces produce brain damage)

  b. **Basilar Skull Fracture**

   1) Manifestations

    a) Bleeding from the nose and ears

    b) Otorrhea, rhinorrhea: CSF from the ears or nose; differentiate between CSF and mucus by assessing glucose content of the drainage

    c) Raccoon eyes (periorbital edema and ecchymosis)

    d) Battle's sign (postauricular ecchymosis) noted on mastoid bone

c. **Hematomas**

1) Epidural hematoma: bleeding into the space between the skull and the dura

  a) Commonly involves the middle meningeal artery

  b) Typical presentation: client sustains the injury, followed by a brief loss of consciousness; this is followed by a lucid interval, then rapid deterioration

  c) Emergency management: burr holes and placement of drain to relieve increasing intracranial pressure

2) Subdural hematoma: bleeding below the dura

  a) Usually venous

  b) May be acute, subacute, or chronic

  c) Manifestations

   (1) Acute: symptoms develop over 24 to 48 hr and include change in LOC, pupillary changes, and hemiparesis

   (2) Subacute: symptoms develop from 48 hr to 2 weeks after injury

   (3) Chronic: seen frequently in the elderly; symptoms may mimic CVA

   (4) Management: surgical evacuation of hematoma and/or burr holes and drain placement

3) **Nursing Interventions**

  a) Assess the client frequently for signs of increased intracranial pressure (ICP).

  b) Prevent or minimize increased ICP.

2. **Increased ICP:** a rise in pressure within the skull that can result from or cause a brain injury

  a. Contributing Factors

   1) Head injury with subdural or epidural hematoma

   2) Cerebrovascular accident or cerebral edema

   3) Brain tumor

   4) Hydrocephalus

   5) Ruptured aneurysm and subarachnoid hemorrhage

   6) Meningitis, encephalitis

  b. Manifestations (vary depending on cause and location; will affect level of consciousness)

   1) Earliest sign: changes in LOC such as restlessness, confusion, drowsiness, lethargy, or stupor; motor and sensory changes

   2) Headache, diplopia, irritability

   3) Nausea and vomiting, often projectile

   4) Pupil changes: dilated, unequal, nonreactive

   5) Changes in Vital Signs

    a) Cushing's triad: hypertension with widening pulse pressure, bradycardia, and irregular breathing (Cheyne-Stokes respirations)

    b) Ineffective thermoregulation

c. Collaborative Care

   1) **Nursing Interventions**

     a) Monitor vital signs and neurological function.

     b) Keep head of bed elevated 30° to 45°.

     c) Keep the client's head in a neutral position to enhance drainage.

     d) Avoid coughing, sneezing, straining, and suctioning.

     e) Maintain maximum respiratory exchange. (Hypercapnia causes vasodilation, thus increasing ICP.)

     f) Administer oxygen to increase the supply to the brain.

     g) Monitor fluid I&O. May restrict fluids to prevent increased cerebral edema.

     h) Administer medications as prescribed.

     i) Use hypothermia as prescribed to decrease ICP.

     j) Decrease environmental stimuli.

     k) Intensive care is required when monitoring ICP (ventriculostomy).

   2) Medications

     a) Avoid opiates and sedatives unless ventilated. Will restrict neurological assessment.

     b) Barbiturates to place the client into a therapeutic coma with ventilator support and close monitoring of cardiac status.

     c) Acetaminophen may be used for fever.

     d) Osmotic diuretics (such as mannitol) and steroids (such as dexamethasone) may be used to decrease cerebral edema.

3. **Hyperthermia**: Elevated temperature may be caused by infection or damage to the hypothalamic temperature-regulating center. This increases cerebral oxygen demand.

  a. Contributing Factors

   1) Infections

   2) Cerebral edema

   3) Environmental heat

  b. Manifestations

   1) Temperature elevation, shivering

   2) Hypoxia

  c. Collaborative Care

   1) **Nursing Interventions**

     a) Assess neurologic status and vital signs.

     b) Use a hypothermia blanket or cool sponge bath.

     c) Monitor the ECG for tachycardia and dysrhythmias.

     d) Monitor for manifestations of dehydration by checking I&O and weighing the client daily.

     e) Initiate seizure precautions. May be prescribed benzodiazepines to suppress seizure activity.

     f) Prevent shivering, which may occur if temperature is reduced quickly, to decrease risk of increased ICP and oxygen consumption

       (1) Chlorpromazine

       (2) Benzodiazepines: diazepam

4. **Seizure disorders**: abnormal, sudden, uncontrolled, excessive discharge of electrical activity within the brain

  a. Contributing Factors

   1) Drug or alcohol withdrawal

   2) Trauma

   3) Brain tumors

   4) Toxicity or infection

   5) Fever

  b. Classifications

   1) Generalized Seizures

     a) Tonic-clonic (formerly grand mal)

     b) Absence (formerly petit mal)

     c) Myoclonic

     d) Atonic or akinetic (drop attacks)

   2) Partial Seizures

     a) Complex (usually with impairment of consciousness)

     b) Simple (usually without alteration of consciousness)

  c. Collaborative Care

   1) **Nursing Interventions**

     a) Maintain patent airway (position side-lying).

     b) Monitor respiratory status and loosen constrictive clothing.

     c) Protect the client from injury.

     d) Do not restrain the client.

     e) Do not put anything in the client's mouth.

     f) Turn client's head to the side to prevent aspiration.

     g) Document observations before, during, and after seizure.

     h) Observe for prodromal signs of an aura (a sensory warning that the seizure is about to occur).

     i) Document how long the client remains unconscious.

     j) Determine if there is any incontinence.

     k) Identify precipitating factors.

     l) Monitor and document behavior during the postictal phase (period following seizure).

     m) Initiate seizure precautions.

       (1) Bed rest should include padded side rails.

       (2) Ensure that immediate access is available for oxygen administration and suction.

   2) Medications

     a) Phenytoin

     b) Carbamazepine

     c) Valproic acid

     d) Phenobarbital

     e) Levetiracetam

     f) Topiramate

3) Client Education

  a) Take medications consistently. Never stop abruptly.

  b) Teach manifestations of medication toxicity.

  c) Get adequate rest to minimize fatigue.

  d) Avoid alcohol.

  e) Wear medical alert bracelet.

  f) Follow state laws regarding operating vehicles and machinery.

  g) Keep all follow-up appointments.

  h) Identify seizure triggers.

5. **Status epilepticus**: a life-threatening condition characterized by a series of generalized seizures without full recovery of consciousness between; may be caused by a sudden withdrawal of anticonvulsant medications; can lead to brain damage or death

  a. Collaborative Care

    1) **Nursing Interventions**

      a) Initiate seizure precautions.

    2) Medications

      a) Lorazepam is the medication of choice.

      b) Diazepam

      c) Phenytoin: Administer IV slowly, giving no more than 50 mg/min.

        (1) Do not mix with glucose. Administer in 0.9% sodium chloride.

        (2) Monitor for bradycardia and heart block.

      d) Fosphenytoin

6. **Transient ischemic attack (TIA)**: sudden temporary episode of neurological dysfunction lasting usually less than 1 hr secondary to decreased blood flow to the brain; may be a warning sign of an impending stroke

  a. Contributing Factors

    1) Non-modifiable

      a) Advanced age

      b) Gender (male)

      c) Genetics

    2) Modifiable

      a) Hypertension

      b) Hyperlipidemia

      c) Diabetes mellitus

      d) Smoking

      e) Atrial fibrillation

  b. Manifestations

    1) Sudden change in visual function

    2) Sudden loss of sensory or motor functions

  c. Diagnostic Procedures

    1) Carotid ultrasound

    2) CT scan and/or MRI

    3) Arteriography

    4) 12-lead ECG

  d. Collaborative Care

    1) **Nursing Interventions**

      a) Encourage the client to stop smoking and limit alcohol intake.

      b) DASH diet (high in fruits and vegetables, moderate in low-fat dairy products, and low in animal protein)

      c) Stress the importance of maintaining ideal body weight with regular exercise.

    2) Medications

      a) Antiplatelet Medications

        (1) Clopidogrel

        (2) Dipyridamole, plus aspirin

        (3) Ticlopidine

      b) Anticoagulant Medications

        (1) Warfarin

      c) Lipid-lowering agents

    3) Therapeutic Measures

      a) Angioplasty

      b) Carotid endarterectomy (removal of plaque from one or both carotid arteries)

7. **Cerebrovascular accident (CVA)**: commonly referred to as a stroke or "brain attack"; the sudden loss of brain function resulting from a disruption of blood supply to the involved part of the brain; causes temporary or permanent neurological deficits

  a. Contributing Factors

    1) Hypertension and obesity

    2) Smoking or cocaine use

    3) Hyperlipidemia

    4) Diabetes mellitus

    5) Peripheral vascular disease

    6) Aneurysm or cranial hemorrhage

  b. Manifestations: the severity of the neurological deficit is determined by location and the extent of tissue ischemia; physical manifestations occur on the side opposite of damage to the brain

    1) Change in mental status

    2) Slurred speech, aphasia, and dysphagia

    3) Numbness or weakness of the face or extremities, especially on one side of the body

    4) Visual disturbance

    5) Cranial nerve disturbance

    6) Loss of balance or coordination

    7) Sudden severe headache

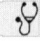

c. Collaborative Care

  1) **Nursing Interventions**

    a) Maintain airway.

    b) Monitor neurological function and vital signs.

    c) Establish baseline level of function and Glasgow coma scale.

    d) Maintain fluid and electrolyte balance.

    e) Monitor for aspiration due to risk of dysphagia. Feed the client slowly, placing food in the back of the mouth and to the unaffected side.

    f) Provide psychological support to the client and family.

    g) Establish means of communication with a client who is experiencing aphasia (expressive, receptive, global).

    h) Encourage slow, deliberate speech.

    i) Range of motion: To prevent flexion contractures, keep extremities in a position of extension or neutrality.

    j) Maintain skin integrity.

    k) Hemiparesis, hemiplegia: Will cause safety issues in the client.

    l) Help the client to achieve bowel and bladder control.

    m) Hemianopsia: Place articles within client's visual range.

  2) Therapeutic Measures

    a) Thrombolytic therapy (ischemic CVA); contraindicated if longer than 4.5 hr

    b) Surgical management (usually hemorrhagic CVA)

    c) Endovascular interventions (embolectomy and carotid artery angioplasty/stent)

  3) Client Education and Referral

    a) Occupational and physical therapy

    b) Speech therapy

8. **Spinal cord injury**: partial or complete disruption of nerve tracts and neurons; resulting in paralysis, sensory loss, altered activity, and autonomic nervous system dysfunction

  a. Contributing Factors

    1) Male age 16 to 30 years

    2) Motor vehicle crashes

    3) Falls

    4) Violence

    5) Sporting activities

  b. Types

    1) Contusion

    2) Laceration

    3) Compression of the cord

    4) Complete transection (paralyzed below the level of injury)

c. Manifestations (determined by the level of injury)

  1) Cervical: partial or complete quadriplegia/ tetraplegia

    a) Respiratory dysfunction (the client may be ventilator-dependent)

    b) Partial or complete paralysis of all four extremities

    c) Loss of bladder and bowel control, alteration in sexual function

  2) Thoracic injury: partial or complete paraplegia

    a) Loss of bladder and bowel control, alteration in sexual function

    b) Partial or complete paralysis of lower extremities and major control of body trunk

    c) Potential complication of autonomic dysreflexia—injury above T6

    d) Respiratory complications

  3) Lumbar

    a) Partial or complete paralysis of lower extremities

    b) Loss of bladder and bowel control, alteration in sexual function

d. Collaborative Care

  1) **Nursing Interventions**

    a) Immobilize the client.

      (1) Spinal board

      (2) Halo traction

      (3) Gardner-Wells traction or Crutchfield tongs

      (4) Cervical collar

    b) Maintain and monitor respiratory function.

    c) Monitor for spinal shock (loss of sensation, flaccid paralysis, and reflexes below the level of injury).

    d) Monitor for neurogenic shock (decreased blood pressure, heart rate, and cardiac output, as well as venous pooling).

    e) Monitor for autonomic dysreflexia, a life-threatening syndrome with sudden, severe hypertension triggered by noxious stimuli below damage of cord. May be caused by impaction, bladder distension, pressure points or ulcers, or pain.

      (1) Manifestations

        (a) Hypertension with bradycardia

        (b) Headache, flushing

        (c) Piloerection ("goose bumps"), sweating

        (d) Nasal congestion

      (2) **Nursing Interventions**

        (a) Place the client in the high-Fowler's position to help decrease blood pressure.

        (b) Determine and remove causative stimuli.

        (c) Teach the client bowel and bladder management.

        (d) Administer medications as prescribed.

(3) Therapeutic Measures

    (a) Surgical management

(4) Client Education and Referral

    (a) Occupational and physical therapy

9. **Multiple sclerosis (MS)**: chronic, progressive, immune-mediated disease of the CNS, characterized by patches of demyelination in the brain and spinal cord in which symptoms occur in relapse and remission-type pattern (exact cause unknown)

  a. Contributing Factors

    1) Age: young adults 20 to 40 years

    2) Gender: women

    3) Geographic: Europe, New Zealand, southern Australia, northern U.S., southern Canada

    4) Genetic predisposition

  b. Manifestations vary in relation to location of lesion (plague).

    1) MRI shows sclerotic patches through the brain and spinal cord.

    2) Fatigue

    3) Visual disturbances: nystagmus, blurred vision, diplopia

    4) Slurred speech

    5) Spasticity and/or weakness of extremities, paresthesia, numbness, and pain

    6) Emotional lability, depression

    7) Intention tremors

    8) Spastic bladder

  c. Management

    1) Currently there is no cure. Treatment is aimed at relieving symptoms and decreasing the frequency and severity of relapses.

    2) During exacerbation, administer corticosteroids as prescribed.

    3) Stress management techniques may be helpful to prevent exacerbations.

  d. Collaborative Care

    1) **Nursing Interventions**

      a) Promote independence and maintaining an active, normal lifestyle as possible.

      b) Teach self-catheterization techniques, if needed.

      c) Promote daily exercise with fall precautions.

      d) Instruct the client to avoid stressors that exacerbate the condition (infections).

      e) Teach the self-injection technique.

      f) Prevent injury.

    2) Medications

      a) Immunosuppressants to reduce the frequency and duration of relapses: interferon beta-1a (IM weekly), interferon beta-1b (subcutaneously), glatiramer acetate (subcutaneously daily)

      b) Muscle spasticity and tremors: baclofen, gabapentin, clonazepam

      c) Urinary problems and constipation: oxybutynin, tolterodine, propantheline, psyllium

      d) Depression: amitriptyline, sertraline, fluoxetine

      e) Sexual difficulties: sildenafil

      f) Fatigue: amantadine, modafinil

    3) Client Education and Referrals

      a) Referrals to occupational, physical, and speech therapy

      b) Proper medication administration to include self-injection

      c) Prevention of relapse

      d) Self-catheterization if needed

10. **Parkinson's disease**: chronic, progressive neurological disorder caused by loss of pigmented cells of substantia nigra and depletion of dopamine

  a. Manifestations

    1) Bradykinesia with rigidity

    2) Resting tremor

    3) Postural and gait disturbances

    4) Expressionless, fixed gaze; masklike

    5) Depression

    6) Drooling and slurred speech

  b. Collaborative Care

    1) **Nursing Interventions**

      a) Teach fall precautions.

      b) Encourage clothing that fosters independence (no snaps, buttons, or zippers).

      c) Encourage a high-fiber diet.

    2) Medications

      a) Antiparkinsonian agent: levodopa

      b) Dopamine agonist: bromocriptine mesylate

      c) Anticholinergic: benztropine

      d) Antiviral: amantadine hydrochloride; side effects include tremor, rigidity, and bradykinesia

      e) Antihistamine: diphenhydramine

    3) Therapeutic Measures

      a) Thalamotomy and pallidotomy

      b) Neural transplantation

      c) Deep brain stimulation

    4) Client Education and Referral

      a) Injury prevention

      b) Medication regimen

      c) Promotion of adequate nutrition (may need supplementation)

      d) Strategies to improve bowel and bladder function

      e) Use of assistive devices

      f) Referral to occupational, physical, and speech therapy

11. **Amyotrophic lateral sclerosis (ALS)**: progressive, invariably fatal neurological disease that attacks nerve cells (neurons) that control voluntary muscles; also known as Lou Gehrig's disease

    a. Manifestations

        1) Fasciculations (i.e., twitching), cramping, and muscle weakness

        2) Fatigue

        3) Slurred or nasal speech with difficulty forming words (i.e., dysarthria)

        4) Difficulty chewing and swallowing (i.e., dysphagia)

        5) Overactive deep tendon reflex

        6) Some may experience cognitive impairment.

        7) Eventual respiratory compromise. Death usually occurs from respiratory failure, infection, or aspiration.

    b. Etiology unknown; no known cure; treatment is symptomatic

    c. Collaborative care

        1) **Nursing Interventions**

            a) Provide education.

            b) Provide information and support. Assess home support systems.

            c) Implement aspiration precautions and alternate methods of communication if needed.

            d) Support respiratory function (mechanical ventilation or noninvasive positive-pressure ventilation).

            e) Administer medications to provide relief from excessive salivation, pain, muscle cramps, constipation, and depression.

            f) Provide supportive services to the client and family with anticipatory grieving.

        2) Medications

            a) Glutamate antagonist: Riluzole may have a neuroprotective effect in early stages.

            b) Manage spasticity: baclofen, dantrolene sodium, diazepam

            c) Client Education and Referral

                (1) Disease progression and prognosis

                (2) Complete advance directive

                (3) Interventions to maximize respiratory function and prevent infection

                (4) Strategies to prevent aspiration

                (5) Alternate communication methods

                (6) Referral to occupational, physical, speech therapy, home care, and hospice when needed

12. **Myasthenia gravis**: autoimmune disorder in which antibodies are produced, it is thought, by the thymus gland, which damages the acetylcholine receptor sites leading to impaired transmission at the myoneural junction. This results in voluntary muscle weakness that increases with activity, improves with rest, and is characterized by periods of exacerbation and remission.

    a. Manifestations

        1) Muscular weakness that increases with activity and improves with rest

        2) Early manifestations involve the ocular muscles leading to an increased risk of aspiration. Symptoms include: diplopia, ptosis, dysphagia, and dysphonia.

        3) Progressive deterioration, particularly the respiratory system, and muscle wasting

    b. Diagnostic Procedures

        1) Edrophonium chloride: an acetylcholinesterase inhibitor is injected IV; immediate improvement of symptoms that lasts approximately 5 min is considered a positive test and diagnostic of myasthenia gravis. May be used to differentiate between cholinergic and myasthenic crisis. The antidote atropine should be available to counteract possible adverse effects (e.g., bradycardia, sweating, and cramping).

        2) Serum acetylcholine receptor antibodies

        3) MRI of thymus gland

        4) EMG

    c. Types of Crisis

        1) Cholinergic: usually from overmedication; muscle fasciculations, which may lead to respiratory distress, increased GI motility, hypersecretion, hypotension. No improvement or worsening of symptoms with Tensilon test.

        2) Myasthenic: may be caused by an exacerbation trigger or inadequate medication. It is characterized by varying degrees of respiratory distress, dysphagia, dysarthria, ptosis, diplopia, hypertension, and increased muscle weakness. Symptoms improve during Tensilon test.

    d. Factors Contributing to Exacerbations

        1) Infections

        2) Pregnancy

        3) Stress, emotional distress, fatigue

        4) Increases in body temperature

        5) Inconsistency with medication administration

    e. Collaborative Care

        1) **Nursing Interventions**

            a) Maintain patent airway.

                (1) Prevent aspiration.

                (2) Keep suction and manual ventilation equipment at bedside.

            b) Plan activities for the client early in the day to avoid fatigue.

            c) Provide small, frequent, high-calorie meals during the peak time for medications (within 45 min of administration).

            d) Administer medications on time.

            e) Provide eye care (instilling artificial tears and/or taping the eye shut at intervals as prescribed).

2) Medications

  a) Anticholinesterase medications increase the amount of acetylcholine in the neuromuscular function.

    (1) Pyridostigmine: first-line therapy

    (2) Atropine is the antidote for anticholinesterase medications.

  b) Immunosuppressants

    (1) Steroids: prednisone

    (2) Cytotoxic medications: azathioprine

3) Therapeutic Measures

  a) Thymectomy (excision of the thymus)

  b) Intravenous immunoglobulin (IVIG)

  c) Plasmapheresis

4) Client Education and Referral

  a) Importance of appropriate medication administration

  b) Prevention of aspiration (meals need to be timed with peak action of medication, head flexed forward, foods with thickened consistency, suction available in home)

  c) Energy conservation; promote mobility strategies

  d) Factors that contribute to exacerbations and actions to take if an exacerbation occurs

  e) Referral to speech therapy and Myasthenia Gravis Foundation of America

13. **Guillain–Barré syndrome**: acute, autoimmune attack on the peripheral nerve and some cranial nerve myelin

  a. Manifestations

    1) Usually preceded by an infection (respiratory or gastrointestinal)

    2) Usually presents with ascending weakness, which may progress to paralysis, leading to acute respiratory failure

    3) Hyporeflexia

    4) Recovery takes several months to 2 years

    5) Paresthesia and pain

  b. Collaborative Management

    1) **Nursing Interventions**

      a) Assess respiratory status and provide respiratory support as indicated.

      b) Monitor vital signs and ECG.

      c) Provide nutrition and prevent aspiration, may need parenteral supplementation.

      d) Manage bowel and bladder problems.

      e) Collaborate with physical therapy to maintain the client's muscle strength, flexibility, and contractures.

      f) Prevent complications of immobility: pneumonia, deep-vein thrombosis, urinary tract infection atelectasis, and skin breakdown.

      g) Decrease anxiety by providing information and support.

2) Therapeutic Measures

  a) Respiratory support (may need mechanical ventilation)

  b) Plasmapheresis

  c) Intravenous immunoglobulin (IVIG)

3) Client Education and Referral

  a) Refer to occupational, physical, speech, and respiratory therapy.

  b) Teach strategies to prevent complications of immobility.

  c) Inform that recovery may take up to 2 years.

D. **Common Surgical Procedures**

1. **Laminectomy**: a surgical procedure to remove a portion of vertebrae for the treatment of severe pain and disability resulting from compression of spinal nerves by a ruptured disk or bony compression; also an option to relieve persistent pain or to treat progressive neurological problems due to nerve compression

2. **Discectomy**: surgical procedure to remove a herniated disk

3. **Spinal fusion**: surgical fusion of the vertebral spinous process with a bone graft (either autologous or banked), which provides stabilization of the spine and decreases the risk of recurrence

  a. Collaborative Care (interventions for all procedures)

    1) Monitor vital signs.

    2) Assess for neurological deficits.

    3) Monitor the dressing for spinal fluid, bleeding, or signs of infection.

    4) Log roll the client. Teach client to maintain proper alignment and decrease stress on the spine.

    5) Address sexual concerns.

    6) Manage pain.

    7) Refer for rehabilitation if indicated.

E. **Sensory Assessment**

1. Ocular Assessment

  a. Assessment of visual acuity with the use of the Snellen chart. The client stands 20 feet from the chart and is asked to read the smallest line. Corrective lenses for distance vision should be worn during test.

    1) Manifestation

      a) Myopia (nearsightedness): Distant objects appear blurred.

      b) Hyperopia (farsightedness): Close objects appear blurred.

      c) Presbyopia (farsightedness associated with aging): a progressive condition in which the lens of the eye loses its ability to focus

      d) Macular degeneration: a progressive disorder of the retina causing the loss of central vision

      e) Legal blindness is when the vision in the better eye does not exceed 20/200 or whose widest visual field diameter is 20° or less.

  b. External eye exam

  c. Direct and indirect ophthalmoscopy

  d. Tonometry: measures intraocular pressure

2. Treatment of Visual Acuity Problems
   a. Abnormal refractory findings are typically treated with corrective lenses.
   b. Laser eye surgery (Lasik): This procedure changes the shape of the cornea with the goal of restoring 20/20 vision.
3. Common Optical Problems
   a. **Detached retina:** occurs when the sensory retina separates from the pigment epithelium of the retina; vitreous humor fluid flows between the layers when a tear occurs in the retina; can be related to age and/or trauma
      1) Manifestations
         a) Sudden visual disturbances
         b) Flashes of light
         c) Blurred vision with floaters
         d) Curtain or shadow over visual field across one eye
      2) **Nursing Interventions** (preoperative)
         a) Maintain bed rest with patch to affected eye.
         b) Instruct the client to avoid coughing, sneezing, and straining.
         c) Surgical intervention includes scleral buckling, photocoagulation, cryosurgery, vitrectomy, and pneumatic retinopexy.
      3) **Nursing Interventions** (postoperative)
         a) Maintain bed rest in prescribed position with eye patch and shield in place.
         b) Avoid jarring, bumping head, straining, or coughing.
         c) Administer medications as prescribed (e.g., antiemetic, antibiotic, anti-inflammatory).
         d) Teach regular self-administration of eye drops on schedule.
   b. **Cataract:** slow, progressive clouding of the lens
      1) Manifestations
         a) Painless, diplopia, and/or blurred vision
         b) Decreased visual acuity; frequent change in eyeglasses prescription
         c) May perceive surroundings being dimmer
      2) **Nursing Interventions** (preoperative—dilate the eye)
         a) Administer medications as prescribed.
            (1) Mydriatics
            (2) Antibiotics
            (3) Corticosteroids
      3) **Nursing Interventions** (postoperative)
         a) Keep the operative eye covered.
         b) Elevate head of bed 30° to 45° and do not turn the client onto operative side.
         c) Instruct the client to avoid bending at the waist, lifting, sneezing, and coughing, and to not touch the eye area.
         d) Prevent vomiting or straining.
         e) Report severe pain immediately.
      4) Therapeutic Measures
         a) Surgical treatment: removal of the lens, usually under local anesthesia, with intraocular lens implant

   c. **Glaucoma:** group of ocular conditions characterized by optic nerve damage, which may be caused by increased intraocular pressure (IOP)
      1) Manifestations
         a) Acute (closed-angle) Ocular Emergency
            (1) Results from an obstruction to the outflow of aqueous humor resulting in increased intraocular pressure (IOP)
            (2) Rapidly progressive visual impairment
            (3) Severe pain in and around the eye
            (4) Blurred vision with dilated pupils
            (5) Nausea and vomiting
         b) Open Angle
            (1) Insidious onset with slowly decreasing visual acuity
            (2) Usually bilateral, but one eye may be more affected
            (3) Halos around lights and loss of peripheral vision (late manifestations)
            (4) Fluctuating intraocular pressures
            (5) May have no symptoms
      2) Collaborative Care
         a) **Nursing Interventions**
            (1) Administer medications consistently on time.
            (2) Avoid anticholinergic medications.
         b) Medications to Promote Pupils to Contract
            (1) Cholinergics: miotics (e.g., pilocarpine, carbachol)
            (2) Adrenergic agonists: dipivefrin, epinephrine
            (3) Beta blockers: betaxolol, timolol
            (4) Carbonic anhydrase inhibitors: acetazolamide
            (5) Prostaglandin analogues: latanoprost, bimatoprost
            (6) Alpha adrenergic agonists: apraclonidine, brimonidine
         c) Therapeutic Measures
            (1) Laser trabeculoplasty
            (2) Iridotomy
            (3) Drainage implants or shunts
         d) Client Education
            (1) Teach appropriate administration of medications.
            (2) Discuss importance of avoiding activities that may increase IOP.
            (3) Inform of importance of follow-up appointments.

F. **Auditory Assessment**
   1. Assessment
      a. Inspection of external ear
      b. Otoscopic examination
      c. Evaluation of gross auditory acuity
      d. Audiometry

2. Disorders
   a. **Ménière's disease**: abnormal inner ear fluid balance, which may lead to disabling symptoms
      1) Manifestations
         a) Vertigo
         b) Tinnitus
         c) Pressure in the ear
3. Collaborative Care
   a. **Nursing Interventions**
      1) Provide with small, frequent meals low in sodium.
      2) Initiate and teach fall precautions.
      3) Maintain a quiet environment.
   b. Medications
      1) Antihistamines: meclizine
      2) Tranquilizers to control acute vertigo: diazepam
      3) Antiemetics to control nausea, vomiting, and vertigo: promethazine
      4) Diuretics to reduce pressure from fluid
   c. Client Education
      1) Encourage a low-sodium diet.
      2) Encourage the client to drink plenty of fluids but to avoid caffeine and alcohol.
      3) Avoid monosodium glutamate (MSG), aspirin, and aspirin-containing medications, which may increase symptoms.

NEUROSENSORY END-OF-SECTION REVIEW

1. It is important to assess _____ function and allergies to shellfish prior to a client receiving contrast dye.

2. Preprocedure instructions for a client scheduled for an electroencephalogram (EEG) would include avoiding _____, holding _____ and depressant medications, and _____ hair prior to procedure.

3. One of the earliest indicators of increased intracranial pressure is a change in _____. Cushing's triad is a late sign of increasing intracranial pressure characterized by _____ (with widening pulse pressure), _____, and _____.

4. The best position for a client with intracranial pressure would be with the head of bed _____ 30° to 45°, with the head positioned _____. This client should be suctioned as determined by _____.

5. Seizure precautions would include placing the bed in the _____ position, _____ side rails, and ensuring that _____ and _____ equipment are at bedside. The medication of choice for acute seizures is _____.

6. The client who has experienced a stroke is at risk for _____. Strategies to prevent this include feeding slowly, placing food on the _____ side, with the head slightly flexed _____.

7. The client with a spinal cord injury at T6 or above is at risk for a potentially life-threatening condition called _____, which is caused by noxious _____ below the level of injury. This condition is characterized by severe hypertension. Priority interventions include elevating the _____, identifying and _____ the stimuli, and administering _____ medications as prescribed.

8. It is important to time meals with the administration of medications (usually given within 45 min of meals) for the client who has _____ to prevent aspiration.

9. Acute glaucoma is considered an optical emergency. The client experiencing this disorder may experience _____ and _____ vision. Medication to reduce intraocular pressure may include pilocarpine hydrochloride (_____) and acetazolamide (_____).

10. The client diagnosed with Ménière's disease should be advised to follow a low-_____ diet. Due to the client potentially experiencing vertigo, it is important to teach the client _____ precautions.

WORD BANK

Antihypertensive	Lowest
Aspiration	Midline
Assessment	Myasthenia gravis
Autonomic dysreflexia	Oxygen
Blurred	Padding
Bradycardia	Pain
Bradypnea	Pilocar
Caffeine	Removing
Diamox	Renal
Elevated	Sodium
Fall	Stimulant
Forward	Suction
Head of bed	Stimuli
Hypertension	Unaffected
Level of consciousness	Washing
Lorazepam	

Answer Key: 1. Renal; 2. Caffeine, stimulant, washing; 3. Level of consciousness, hypertension, bradycardia, bradypnea; 4. Elevated, midline, assessment; 5. Lowest, padding, oxygen, suction, lorazepam; 6. Aspiration, unaffected, forward; 7. Autonomic dysreflexia, stimuli, head of bed, removing, antihypertensive; 8. Myasthenia gravis; 9. Pain, blurred, Pilocar, Diamox; 10. Sodium, fall

Oncology Nursing

A. **Overview of Cancer**

1. Healthy cells transform into malignant cells upon exposure to certain etiological agents—viruses, chemicals, and physical agents.

2. Malignant cells metastasize and extend directly into adjacent tissue, moving through the lymph system, entering the blood circulation, and diffusing into body cavities.

B. **Risk Factors**

1. Age

   a. Older adult women most commonly develop colorectal, breast, lung, pancreatic, and ovarian cancers.

   b. Older adult men most commonly develop lung, colorectal, prostate, pancreatic, and gastric cancers.

2. Race

3. Genetic disposition

4. Exposure to chemicals, viruses, tobacco, alcohol

5. Exposure to certain viruses, bacteria

6. Sun exposure

7. Diet high in red meat and fat and low in fiber

C. **General Disease-Related Consequences of Cancer**

1. Decreased Immunity and Blood-Producing Function

   a. Occurs most often with leukemia and lymphoma or any cancer that invades the bone marrow and reduces the production of WBCs, RBCs, and platelets, causing thrombocytopenia

   b. Clients are at increased risk for infection.

   c. Changes are caused by either the cancer or chemotherapy.

   d. Clients may experience weakness, fatigue, and bleeding.

2. Altered GI Structure and Function

   a. Impaired absorption and elimination related to tumor obstruction or compression

   b. Tumors increase the metabolic rate, increasing the need for proteins, fats, and carbohydrates.

   c. Liver tumors reduce function and lead to malnutrition.

3. Motor and Sensory Deficits

   a. Occur when cancers invade the bone or brain or compress nerves.

   b. Bone metastases cause pain, fractures, spinal cord obstruction, and hypercalcemia, which decreases mobility.

   c. Sensory changes occur if the spinal cord is damaged by tumor pressure or compression.

   d. Sensory, motor, and cognitive functions are impaired when cancer is in the brain.

   e. Pain is often significant, especially in the terminal stages of the disease process.

4. Decreased respiratory function

   a. Disrupts respiratory function and gas exchange (i.e., tumors in an airway cause an obstruction).

   b. Lung capacity is decreased; gas exchange is impaired.

   c. Tumors can compress blood and lymph vessels in the chest, blocking blood flow through the chest and lungs, causing pulmonary edema and dyspnea.

D. **Cancers/Tumors**

1. Classified according to type of tissue from which they evolve

2. Carcinomas begin in epithelial tissue (e.g., skin, gastrointestinal tract lining, lung, breast, uterus).

3. Sarcomas begin in nonepithelial tissue (e.g., bone, muscle, fat, lymph system).

4. Adenocarcinomas arise from glandular organs.

5. Leukemias are malignancies of the blood-forming cells.

6. Lymphomas arise from the lymph tissue.

7. Multiple myeloma arises from plasma cells and affects the bone.

E. **Manifestations Suggesting Malignant Disease**

1. American Cancer Society 7 Warning Signs

   a. **C**—Changes in bowel or bladder habits

   b. **A**—A sore that does not heal

   c. **U**—Unusual bleeding or discharge

   d. **T**—Thickening or lumps in breast or elsewhere

   e. **I**—Indigestion or difficulty swallowing

   f. **O**—Obvious change in wart or mole

   g. **N**—Nagging cough or hoarseness

2. Other Manifestations

   a. Weight loss

   b. Fatigue/weakness

   c. Pain (may not occur until late in the disease process)

   d. Nausea/anorexia

F. **Cancer management:** systemic or local medications used to cure and/or increase survival rate by damaging cell DNA and interfering with cell mitosis. Rapid growth tumors are more sensitive to chemotherapy.

1. **Chemotherapy**

   a. Systemic or local cytotoxic medications that damage a cell's DNA or destroy rapidly dividing cells. Combination of medications usually given.

   b. Classification (all cause bone marrow depression)

      1) Alkylating agents: mechlorethamine cyclophosphamide, cisplatin

      2) Antimetabolite: fluorouracil, methotrexate

      3) Antibiotics: doxorubicin hydrochloride, bleomycin, dactinomycin

      4) Antimitotics: vincristine, vinblastine

      5) Hormones: estrogen, progesterone, tamoxifen citrate, peclitaxel

      6) Biological modifiers: epoetin alfa, filgrastim

c. Common Side Effects and Interventions to Counteract

1) Bone marrow suppression: neutropenia and leukopenia (WBC less than 1,000 mm³)

   a) Interventions to enhance the immune system include a balanced diet, rest, and handwashing.

   b) Interventions to avoid infections include

      (1) Limit visitors who might be ill.

      (2) Avoid fresh fruits, vegetables, and live plants.

   c) Monitor temperature. Consider any temperature elevation in a client with neutropenia a possible sign of infection and report to provider.

2) Anemia (Hgb less than 10 g/dL)

   a) Administer oxygen therapy; provide iron-rich foods.

   b) Monitor CBCs and administer blood transfusions as needed.

   c) Administer erythropoietin and epoetin alfa to increase RBCs.

3) Thrombocytopenia

   a) Administer prescribed platelet transfusions; oprelvekin to increase platelets.

   b) Implement bleeding precautions; avoid use of aspirin.

4) Alopecia (hair loss 2 weeks after start of treatment. Regrowth occurs 1 month after last chemotherapy treatment.)

   a) Apply ice to the client's scalp during chemotherapy to slow hair loss. Use gentle shampoo, hats, scarves, and sunscreen.

   b) Refer client to the American Cancer Society, which provides wigs and supportive services.

5) Anorexia, Nausea, Vomiting, and GI Issues

   a) Administer antiemetic prior to therapy; ondansetron, dolasetron.

   b) Administer loperamide to manage diarrhea.

   c) The client should drink cool beverages and eat small, favorite meals high in potassium with high-calorie supplements. Avoid unpleasant odors.

   d) Provide soft, bland, high-protein foods at room temperature for stomatitis, and use a straw for fluids. Rinse mouth with a topical anesthetic. May need topical steroids and zinc supplements.

6) Elevated Uric acid, Crystal, and Urate Stone Formation

   a) Administer allopurinol; increase fluid intake.

7) Mucositis: Often develops in the GI tract, especially in the mouth (stomatitis). Mucous membranes, because they undergo rapid cell division, are killed more rapidly than the cells are replaced.

   a) Provide frequent mouth assessment and oral hygiene, including teeth cleaning and mouth rinsing.

   b) Avoid traumatizing oral mucosa due to risk of bleeding; use soft-bristled toothbrush or swabs.

   c) Use plain water or saline for oral rinses.

8) Specific medications have specific toxic effects.

   a) Doxorubicin hydrochloride: irreversible cardiomyopathy

   b) Anzemet, methotrexate: renal toxicity

   c) Vincristine sulfate: peripheral neuropathy

9) Cognitive Function

   a) Reduced ability to concentrate, recall information, and learn new information during treatment and for months to 3 years following treatment.

   b) Referred to as "Chemo brain"; most common in women treated for breast cancer.

2. **Radiation:** Therapy destroys cancer cells with minimal exposure of normal cells to the damaging actions of radiation. Cells damaged by radiation either die or become unable to divide. Gamma rays are used most commonly because of their ability to penetrate tissues and damage cells.

a. Radiation Delivery

1) Teletherapy: distance treatment; the radiation source is external to the client.

2) Brachytherapy: short or close therapy; radiation comes into direct, continuous contact with the tumor tissues. Provides a high dose of radiation with a limited amount to surrounding tissues. (With brachytherapy, the radiation source is within the client who emits radiation and is a hazard to those around for a period of time.)

b. **Nursing Interventions**

1) Ensure precise client position with each radiation treatment to align with fixing devices and markings.

2) Assess condition of skin, and cleanse the area gently each day with water or mild soap.

3) Wet reaction: skin's response to radiation; skin becomes dry or develops blisters that may break, causing pain and the potential for infection. If dry reaction, keep clean and lubricated. If wet reaction, clean and cover to prevent infection.

4) Instruct client to not remove skin markings; avoid powders, lotions, and creams unless prescribed by provider.

5) Instruct client to wear soft, loose clothing and avoid exposure to the sun.

6) Advise client to avoid prolonged sun exposure during treatment and for 1 year after completing radiation therapy.

7) For clients who have sealed implants of radioactive sources

   a) Assign client to a private room.

   b) Place "Caution: Radioactive Material" sign on the client's door in hospital setting.

   c) Wear a lead apron while providing care; pregnant nurses should not care for these clients.

   d) Limit visitors to ½ hr each day, and instruct to remain at least 6 feet from the source.

   e) Do not touch the radioactive source with bare hands.

   f) Save all radioactive dressings and linens until the radioactive source is removed.

   g) Follow institution guidelines for radiation containment.

8) Managing Cancer Pain

   a) Provide effective pain management and monitor client response. (See Opioid Analgesics in Unit Four: Pharmacology in Nursing.)

   b) Assess body image disturbance, coping mechanisms, and support system, and make appropriate referrals.

SECTION 12

Immunologic Disorders

! Point to Remember

The Centers for Disease Control and Prevention (CDC) is the best source for the most up-to-date information regarding HIV and AIDS.

A. **Acquired Immune Deficiency Syndrome (AIDS)**

1. Human immunodeficiency virus (HIV) can progress to acquired immune deficiency syndrome (AIDS). HIV is a viral infection that is transmitted via blood and other body fluids. It affects the ability of the immune system to fight infection, specifically CD4+T cells (healthy adult has 800–1000 cells per cubic mm of blood).

  a. HIV infection is divided into four stages.

   1) *Stage 1, acute infection*: described as the "worst flu ever"; retroviral syndrome usually occurs 2 to 4 weeks after the infection is acquired. CD4+T cells greater than 500 cells/mm³

   2) *Stage 2, latency*: sometimes called asymptomatic HIV infection or chronic HIV infection. CD4+T cell count between 200 and 499 cells/mm³. This stage can last for 8 years or longer.

   3) *Stage 3, AIDS*: CD4+T cell counts drop below 200 cells/mm³. The body becomes susceptible to opportunistic infections. Survival in this stage is usually 1 to 3 years.

   4) *Stage 4, HIV infection, stage unknown*: No information available on CD4+T-lymphocyte count or percentage and no information available on AIDS-defining conditions.

2. Contributing Factors

  a. Unprotected sexual contact

  b. IV drug use; use of contaminated needles

  c. Multiple sexual partners

  d. Pregnancy and breastfeeding: transmission from mother to baby

  e. Blood transfusion (very small risk: 0.02%)

3. Manifestations

  a. Stages

   1) Stage 1: Acute Infection

    a) Fever

    b) Lymphadenopathy

    c) Pharyngitis

    d) Rash

    e) Arthralgia, myalgia

    f) HIV viral load is high; may or may not test positive for antibodies.

    g) CD4+T cell count is greater than 500 cells/mm³

    h) Virus is transmissible to others

   2) Stage 2: Latency

    a) Lymphadenopathy, but may be asymptomatic

    b) Will test positive for HIV antibodies

    c) CD4+T cell count is between 200 and 499 cells/mm³

   3) Stage 3: AIDS

    a) Opportunistic infections occur.

     (1) Respiratory: pneumocystis carinii pneumonia, tuberculosis; Kaposi's sarcoma

     (2) GI: cryptosporidiosis, candida, cytomegalovirus (CMV), isosporiasis, Kaposi's sarcoma

     (3) Neuro: cytomegalovirus, toxoplasmosis, cryptococcosis, non-Hodgkin's lymphoma, varicella zoster (shingles), herpes simplex

     (4) Skin: shingles, herpes simplex, Kaposi's sarcoma

KAPOSI'S SARCOMA

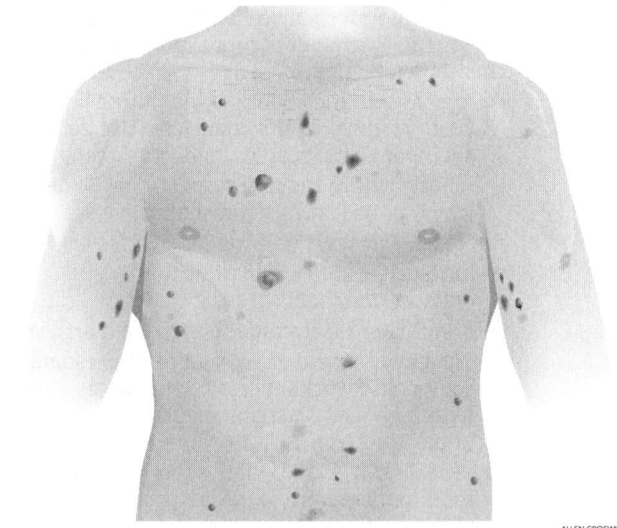

ALLEN CROSWHITE
ASSESSMENT TECHNOLOGIES INSTITUTE

    b) Wasting syndrome

    c) AIDS dementia

    d) Weakness and malaise

    e) Psychosocial: anxiety, depression, poor self-image

    f) CD4+T cell count drops below 200 cells/mm³

4. Diagnostic Procedures
   a. ELISA (antibody assay): positive within 3 weeks to 3 months following infection. Most common and least expensive.
   b. Western Blot blood test used when ELISA is positive to confirm or rule/out infection.
   c. Plasma HIV-1 RNA viral load is greater than 1,500 copies.
   d. CD4+T cell count: decreased to less than 750 cells/mm³. Clients with values less than 200 cells/mm³ have an 85% likelihood of progressing to AIDS within 3 years.
   e. CBC and platelets are decreased.
   f. Brain, lung, or CT scans may be abnormal.
5. Collaborative Care
   a. **Nursing Interventions**
      1) Prevention
         a) Teach about transmission routes.
         b) Emphasize need to use condoms with sexual encounters.
         c) Explain that risk is reduced by limiting sexual partners.
         d) Teach IV drug users to use clean needles or, if they reuse, to clean between each use with water and bleach.
         e) Emphasize need for pregnant women who are HIV-positive to begin or remain on antiviral therapy; infants should NOT be breastfed.
         f) Ensure consistent use of standard precautions by health care workers in clinical settings.
      2) Stages 1 and 2
         a) Teach about risk of transmission of HIV to others and ways to prevent.
         b) Emphasize importance of compliance with antiviral therapy, once initiated.
         c) Encourage healthy lifestyle habits.
         d) Provide psychological support.
      3) Stage 3
         a) Prevent infection.
         b) Enhance oxygenation.
         c) Provide comfort measures.
         d) Monitor weight, I&O, and calorie count; encourage high-calorie foods.
         e) Perform frequent oral care.
         f) Provide scrupulous skin care.
         g) Monitor mental status; reorient PRN; maintain consistent environment.
         h) Provide psychosocial support; include significant others.

   b. Medications
      1) Medication therapy: Highly active antiretroviral therapy guidelines (HAART) are devised by the World Health Organization and are updated as new research findings become available.

Point to Remember

It is crucial that, once a client begins HAART therapy, that doses must NOT be missed. Doing so contributes to medication resistance and reduces medication treatment options.

      2) Efavirenz, azidothymidine, and lamivudine
         a) Common adverse effects: neutropenia, gastrointestinal distress, anemia, insomnia
      3) Zidovudine recommended for protecting the unborn fetus of women who are HIV-positive
      4) Interferon
      5) Pneumocystis pneumonia prophylaxis: pentamidine
      6) Antifungals: metronidazole and amphotericin B
      7) Antituberculosis medications as needed
      8) Acyclovir herpes treatment
      9) Protease inhibitors: saquinavir, ritonavir
      10) Antivirals: zalcitabine, dideoxycytidine
   c. Client Education
      1) Transmission, control measures, and safe sex practices
      2) Nutritional needs, self-medication of prescribed medications, and potential adverse effects
      3) Symptoms that need to be reported immediately (e.g., infection, bleeding)
      4) Need for follow-up monitoring CD4+T cell and viral load counts
B. **Systemic lupus erythematosus (SLE):** a chronic inflammatory disease that occurs when the body's immune system attacks the tissues and organs. Inflammation caused by lupus can affect multiple organ systems such as the joints, skin, kidneys, blood cells, heart, and lungs.
   1. Contributing Factors
      a. Female gender
      b. Age between 15 and 40 years
      c. African American, Latino, or Asian ethnicity
      d. Exposure to sunlight
      e. Long-term use of certain medications
         1) Chlorpromazine
         2) Hydralazine
         3) Isoniazid
         4) Procainamide
      f. Exposure to mercury and/or silica

2. Manifestations

   a. Insidious onset characterized by remissions and exacerbations

   b. Erythematosus "butterfly rash" on both cheeks and across the bridge of the nose; rash deepens on exposure to sunlight

ERYTHEMATOSUS "BUTTERFLY RASH"

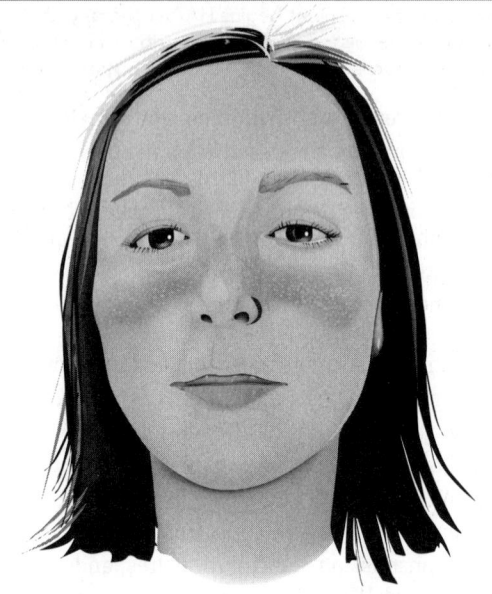

ALLEN CROSWHITE
ASSESSMENT TECHNOLOGIES INSTITUTE

   c. Polyarthralgia

   d. Fever, malaise, and weight loss

   e. Alopecia

   f. Anemia, lymphadenopathy

   g. Positive for antinuclear antibodies

   h. Depression

   i. Coin-like lesions (in discoid lupus)

   j. Pleural effusion, pneumonia

   k. Pericarditis

   l. Raynaud's phenomenon

   m. Neurological: psychosis, paresis, seizures, migraines

   n. Abdominal pain

   o. Edema

   p. Nephritis

3. Collaborative Care

   a. **Nursing Interventions**

     1) Monitor vital signs, especially related to cardiovascular function.

     2) Monitor urinary function.

     3) Provide comfort measures.

     4) Instruct to use sunscreen and cover skin and head when exposed to sunlight.

     5) Encourage rest periods during the day.

     6) Provide measures that promote restful sleep.

     7) Cleanse skin with mild soap and pat to dry; apply moisturizer.

     8) Monitor for infection and teach measures to avoid.

   b. Medications

     1) NSAIDs to reduce inflammation: contraindicated for clients with renal compromise

     2) Corticosteroids for immunosuppression and to reduce inflammation

     3) Immunosuppressant agents: methotrexate, azathioprine

     4) Antimalarial (hydroxychloroquine) for suppression of synovitis, fever, and fatigue

   c. Client Education and Referral

     1) Instruct the client to use sunscreen and wear protective clothing.

     2) Encourage small, frequent meals if anorexia is present.

     3) Limit salt intake for fluid retention secondary to steroid therapy and renal involvement.

     4) Refer to support groups as appropriate.

SECTION 13

Burns

A. **Overview**

1. Thermal, chemical, electrical, and radioactive agents can cause burns, resulting in cellular destruction of the skin layers and underlying tissue. The type and severity of the burn impact the treatment plan.

2. Burn injuries can result in the loss of temperature regulation, sweat and sebaceous gland function, and sensory and organ function.

3. Assessment and severity of the burn is based upon the following

   a. Percentage of total body surface area (TBSA)

   b. Depth of the burn

   c. Body location

   d. Client's age

   e. Causative agent

   f. Presence of other injuries

   g. Respiratory involvement and overall health of the client

B. **Burn Assessment**

1. Extent of body surface

2. Depth of burn and manifestations

C. **Maintain cardiac output and provide IV fluid replacement using Parkland formula.**

1. Give 4 mL/kg/% burn.

2. Give half of total fluids in first 8 hr.

3. Give second half over remaining 16 hr.

4. Deduct any fluid given prehospital from the amount to be infused in the first 8 hr.

Point to Remember

The Rule of Nines assesses the percentage of burn and is used to help guide treatment decisions, including fluid resuscitation; it is part of the guidelines to determine burn management.

RULE OF NINES

Estimating TBSA Affected by Burns	Example

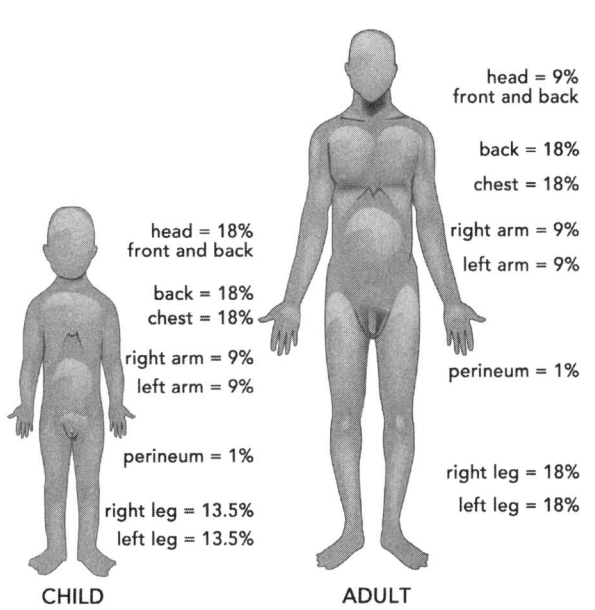

head = 9%
front and back

back = 18%

chest = 18%

right arm = 9%

left arm = 9%

perineum = 1%

right leg = 18%

left leg = 18%

ADULT

head = 18%
front and back

back = 18%
chest = 18%

right arm = 9%
left arm = 9%

perineum = 1%

right leg = 13.5%
left leg = 13.5%

CHILD

An adult client weighing 165 lb is brought to the emergency department with second-degree burns covering the anterior and posterior surfaces of both legs. Transport time was 1 hr, and the client received 1 L of fluid en route. Using the Parkland formula, what is the total amount of IV fluid that should be infused at the hospital during the next seven hours of treatment?

Step 1: Review the Parkland formula.

4 mL x kg body weight x % of total burned surface area = amount of fluid to be infused over 24 hr. Half that amount of fluid is to be infused in the first 8 hr, minus any fluid infused prehospital.

Step 2: Calculate the client's weight in kg.

165 lb / 2.2 = 75 kg

Step 3: Calculate the % of burn.

Anterior/posterior of right leg = 18%

Anterior/posterior of left leg = 18%

18% + 18% = 36%

Step 4: Calculate total fluids required in 24 hr.

4 mL x 75 kg x 36

4 x 75 = 300

300 X 36 = 10,800 mL/24 hr

Step 5: Calculate mL to be given in first 8 hr (1/2 of total fluid volume, minus amount of fluid given en route).

10,800 / 2 = 5,400

5,400 - 1,000 = 4,400

Total amount of IV fluid that should be infused at the hospital during the next 7 hr of treatment: 4,400 mL

BURN DESCRIPTIONS

CLASSIFICATION	DEGREE (OLD TERM)	LAYER INVOLVED	APPEARANCE	EXAMPLES	PAIN
Superficial	First degree	Epidermis	Pink to red, tender, no blisters, mild edema, no eschar	Sunburn, flash burns	Yes
Superficial Partial Thickness	Second degree	Epidermis and parts of dermis	Red to white with blisters, mild to moderate edema, no eschar	Flame or burn scalds	Yes
Deep Partial Thickness	Third degree	Epidermis and deep into dermis	Red to white with moderate edema, no blisters, soft/dry eschar	Flame and burn scalds Grease, tar, or chemical burns Exposure to hot objects for prolonged time	Yes
Full-Thickness	Third degree	Same as partial—may extend into subcutaneous tissue; nerve damage	Red to tan, black, brown, white. No blisters; severe edema, hard inelastic eschar	Burn scalds Grease, tar, chemical, or electrical burns Exposure to hot objects for prolonged time	May or may not be painful
Deep Full-Thickness	Fourth degree	All layers, plus muscles, tendons, bones	Black with no edema	Chemical	None

5. Diagnostic testing
   a. CBC, serum electrolytes, BUN, ABGs, fasting blood glucose, liver studies, urinalysis, clotting studies, and chest x-ray. Add creatinine and myoglobin for deep burns.
      1) Initial Fluid Shift (first 24 hr after injury)
         a) Hct/Hgb elevated due to fluid shifts into interstitial spacing and fluid loss
         b) Sodium decreased secondary to third spacing
         c) Potassium increased due to disruption of sodium-potassium pump, tissue destruction, and RBC hemolysis
      2) Fluid Mobilization (48 to 72 hr after injury)
         a) Hct/Hgb decrease due to fluid shift from interstitial back into vascular fluid
         b) Sodium remains decreased; potassium increases due to renal loss and movement back into the cells
   b. WBC count: initial increase, then decrease with a shift to the left (an increase in the percentage of neutrophils having only one or a few lobes)
      a) Blood glucose: elevated due to stress response
      b) ABGs: slight hypoxemia and metabolic acidosis
      c) Total protein and albumin: low due to fluid loss

D. **Collaborative Care**

1. **Nursing Interventions** for Moderate and Major Burns
   a. Maintain airway and ventilation.
   b. Provide humidified oxygen as prescribed.
   c. Monitor vital signs.
   d. Maintain cardiac output and provide IV fluid replacement using Parkland formula.
      1) Give 4 mL/kg/% burn.
      2) Give half of total fluids in first 8 hr.
      3) Give second half over remaining 16 hr.
      4) Deduct any fluid given prehospital from the amount to be infused in the first 8 hr.
   e. Maintain urine output of 30 to 50 mL/hr for a burn client.
   f. Monitor for manifestations of shock.
   g. Provide pain management.
   h. Assess for and prevent infection.
   i. Provide nutritional support.
      1) Client with a large burn injury will be in a hypermetabolic state and may exceed 5,000 calories/day.
      2) Increase protein intake to prevent tissue breakdown and promote healing.
      3) Enteral or total parenteral therapy is often necessary.
   j. Promote restoration of mobility.
   k. Provide psychological support to both client and family members.

2. Medications
   a. Antimicrobial Creams
      1) Silver nitrate 0.5% soaks
      2) Silver sulfadiazine 1% cream: broad-spectrum coverage; water soluble
      3) Mafenide acetate cream: broad-spectrum coverage; penetrates tissue wall; never use a dressing; breakdown of medication causes a heavy acid load, which may cause acidosis; painful
      4) Bacitracin
   b. Pain Management
      1) PCA infusion pump for continuous dosing
      2) Intravenous opioid analgesics, such as morphine sulfate, hydromorphone, and fentanyl

3. Treatments
   a. Wound care
   b. Biologic skin coverings
   c. Permanent skin coverings

4. Methods of Treating Burns
   a. Open-Exposure Method
      1) Allows for drainage of burn exudate
      2) Eschar forms hardened crust (may constrict circulation, requiring escharotomy).
      3) Use of topical therapy; asepsis crucial
      4) Skin easily visualized and assessed
      5) Range of motion easier
      6) Disadvantages
         a) Increases pain and heat loss
         b) Difficult to manage burns of hands and feet
   b. Closed Method
      1) Gauze dressing wrapped distal to proximal
      2) Decreased fluid and heat loss
      3) Limited mobility may result in contractures
      4) Wound assessment only during dressing changes
   c. Topical antimicrobials
   d. Biologic Dressings and Tissue Grafts
      1) Homograft or allograft (human tissue donors)
      2) Xenograft or heterograft (animal sources)
      3) Amniotic membrane
      4) Biosynthetic or synthetic (transparent film)

5. Client Education
   a. Skin Care Following Discharge
      1) Wear pressure garment 23.5 hr/day to reduce scarring and control swelling.
      2) Engage in regular exercise per physical therapy.
      3) Elevate affected areas as much as possible.
      4) Keep skin moisturized.
      5) Control itching with cool baths and loose, cotton fabric.
      6) Avoid sun exposure.
      7) Change in appearance of skin as scars fade from red to near natural coloration.
      8) Encourage the client to consume extra calories and protein.

End-of-Life Care

A. **Definition:** care and management of the client and caregivers facing end-of-life care issues with the outcome of providing "good death." A good death is free from avoidable suffering for patients and families in consideration with their preferences and consistent with practice standards.

B. **Contributing Factors**

1. Age
2. Chronic terminal illness
3. Hospice care
4. Palliative care

C. **Manifestations**

1. Anorexia
2. Decreased peripheral circulation (mottled skin)
3. Disorientation and somnolence
4. Change in breathing pattern; Cheyne-Stokes respirations
5. Increased respiratory secretions
6. Decreased metabolic function
7. Incontinence
8. Restlessness
9. Weakness and fatigue

D. **Collaborative Care**

1. **Nursing Interventions**

   a. Assess for an end-of-life care plan, advanced directives, and caregiver support.
   b. Do not force client to eat or drink.
   c. Talk to the client even if the client does not respond.
   d. Keep perineal area clean and dry.
   e. Position for comfort.
   f. Elevate head of bed.
   g. Administer medications to manage symptoms of pain, restlessness, excess secretions.
   h. Avoid noxious stimuli.

2. Symptom Management

   a. Pain is the symptom dying clients fear the most.
      1) Long-acting opioid narcotics (morphine 20 mg/mL)
      2) Massage
      3) Music therapy
      4) Aromatherapy
   b. Dyspnea and gurgling are the "most distressing" symptoms noted by caregivers.
      1) Morphine elixir
      2) Scopolamine, atropine sulfate ophthalmic drops 1% (oral or sublingual) or hyoscyamine drops (oral)
      3) Oxygen via nasal cannula (Offer oxygen for comfort, regardless of O_2 saturation.)
      4) Avoid deep suctioning

   c. Restlessness and Agitation
      1) Lorazepam
      2) Haloperidol
   d. Nausea and Vomiting
      1) Prochlorperazine
   e. Incontinence
      1) Keep perianal area clean and dry.
      2) Use disposable underpads or paper undergarments.
      3) Client may be more comfortable with urinary catheter.

E. **Referral and Follow-Up**

1. Hospice care
2. Chaplain
3. Social services

F. **Postmortem Care**

1. Notify provider, chaplain, and mortuary as defined by end-of-life care plan.
2. If no autopsy is planned, remove any tubes or lines.
3. Clean and prepare client for immediate viewing as desired by family or significant other.
4. Provide family or significant other the opportunity to participate in care as desired.
5. Be aware that patients differ in their needs at end of life based on gender and ethnicity.
6. Assess cultural values and religious beliefs of the patient and family for their influence on the dying experience.
7. Verify the completion of death certificate and required facility documents.
8. Prepare client for transport to morgue, funeral home, or mortuary per facility protocol (ensure client identification tags are present).

Nutrition: Therapeutic Diets

Overview

A. To a large degree, nutrients absorbed and utilized by the body determine the health of the body.

B. The process of ingestion, digestion, absorption, and metabolism of food and fluids is essential for life. Disease processes and altered clinical conditions involving the GI tract can prevent all or some of these processes from taking place.

C. The nurse reviews the medical history and conducts a nutritional assessment to determine the possibility of increased metabolic needs, and sources of potential problems with ingestion, digestion, or absorption.

D. Contributing factors may include chronic disease, trauma, recent surgery of the GI tract, drug and alcohol abuse, and altered cognitive and functional processes that may affect nutritional status.

E. The nurse assesses for
   1. Decreased appetite; weight loss
   2. History of recent illness
   3. Poor-fitting or no dentures, or poor dental health; poor eyesight; dry mouth or mucous membranes
   4. Cognitive or functional decline; chronic physical illness
   5. Acute or chronic pain; history of substance abuse
   6. Altered mental health conditions, economic, and/or environmental factors that may impact nutritional requirements
   7. Weight gain or subjective complaints of lack of satiety
F. Older adults in any health care or community setting are at increased risk for altered nutrition due to the physiologic changes of aging, cognitive and functional decline, environmental factors, and social isolation.

II Guidelines for Healthy Eating

A. **Protein:** 10% to 35% of total kcal/day
B. **Fat:** 20% to 35% of total kcal/day
C. **Carbohydrates:** 40% to 65% of total kcal/day
D. **Fluid recommendations:** 2 to 3 L/day for women; 3 to 4 L/day for men
E. **Fiber recommendations:** 25 g/day for women; 38 g/day for men
F. **Sodium recommendations:** Less than 2,300 mg under age 50, 1,500 mg/day or less for people older than 50 years; African Americans; history of diabetes mellitus, hypertension, or chronic kidney disease
G. Recommendations differ for pregnant/lactating women, children, and teens.
H. Consider cultural and religious influences on food preferences when planning diet.
I. **Older adult recommendations:** Drink 8 glasses of water, eat plenty of fiber, daily calcium, vitamins D and B12 supplements. Diet low in sodium and cholesterol.

FOODS WITH INCREASED LEVELS OF FAT AND WATER-SOLUBLE VITAMINS

Foods Rich in Fat-Soluble Vitamins

Vitamin A	Liver, egg yolk, whole milk, butter, green and yellow vegetables
Vitamin D	Fish oils, fortified milk and margarine, sunlight
Vitamin K	Egg yolks, liver, cheese, green leafy vegetables

Foods Rich in Water-Soluble Vitamins

Vitamin C	Citrus fruits, tomatoes, broccoli, cabbage
Thiamine (B$_1$)	Lean meats (e.g., beef, pork, liver), whole grain cereals, legumes
Riboflavin (B$_2$)	Milk, organ meats, enriched grains, green leafy vegetables
Niacin (B$_3$)	Meat, beans, peas, peanuts, enriched grains
Pyridoxine (B$_6$)	Products containing yeast, wheat, corn, organ meats
Cobalamin (B$_{12}$)	Lean meats, liver, kidneys
Folic acid (B$_9$)	Leafy green vegetables, eggs, liver

III Therapeutic and Modified Diets

A. **Overview**
   1. Therapeutic nutrition is often an essential component in the treatment of disease and clinical disorders.
   2. The diet becomes therapeutic when modifications are made to meet client needs. Modifications may include increasing or decreasing caloric intake, fiber, or other specific nutrients; omitting specific foods; and modifying the consistency of foods.
   3. Nurses often collaborate with or refer clients to the dietitian for nutritional or dietary concerns.
B. **Clear-Liquid Diet**
   1. Indications
      a. Rest GI tract.
      b. Maintain fluid balance.
      c. Immediate postoperative period
      d. Nausea, vomiting, diarrhea
      e. Prep for diagnostic testing.
      f. Short-term basis only; nutritionally inadequate
   2. Consists of products that are liquid at room temperature
      a. Primarily water
      b. Tea and coffee
      c. Broth
      d. Carbonated beverages
      e. Clear juices
      f. Gelatin
      g. Limit caffeine due to risk of dehydration.
C. **Full-Liquid Diet**
   1. Indications
      a. Advanced to this if tolerates clear liquids
      b. Intolerance to solid foods
      c. Febrile illness
      d. Acute gastritis
   2. Consists of
      a. Clear liquids
      b. Milk Products
         1) Milk
         2) Custard
         3) Pudding
         4) Creamed soups
         5) Ice cream/sherbet
      c. Strained fruits, vegetables, and cereal
D. **Pureed Diet**
   1. Indications
      a. Transition from full liquid to regular diet
      b. Swallowing or chewing difficulties; oral/facial surgery
   2. Consists of
      a. Food and fluids that have been pureed to a thick liquid form (e.g., scrambled eggs, pureed meats, vegetables, fruits).
      b. Consistency varies with client needs.
      c. Nutritional content varies with client needs.

E. **Soft Diet (bland or low-fiber)**
1. Indications
   a. Transition from liquid to regular diet
   b. Acute infections
   c. Chewing difficulties
   d. Gastric or duodenal ulcers by eliminating irritating foods
2. Consists of the following foods
   a. Low in fiber
   b. Lightly seasoned
   c. Easily digested
   d. Smooth and creamy
   e. Non-gas-forming; avoid cereals, beans, fruits, and vegetables

F. **Mechanical Soft Diet**
1. Indications
   a. Chewing or swallowing difficulty
   b. Head, neck, or mouth surgery
   c. Intestinal stricture
   d. Post CVA
2. Consists of foods that require minimal chewing
   a. Ground or finely diced meat
   b. Canned fruits
   c. Softly cooked vegetables
   d. Cheese
   e. Rice
   f. Light bread
3. Foods to Exclude
   a. Dried fruits
   b. Most raw fruits and vegetables
   c. Nuts and food with seeds

G. **Low-Protein Diet**
1. Indications
   a. Hepatic encephalopathy
   b. Hepatic coma
   c. Renal impairment
2. Limit high-protein foods.
   a. Meats
   b. Eggs
   c. Milk and milk products
   d. Beans
3. Other Dietary Considerations
   a. Increase carbohydrates to meet nutritional needs.
   b. Limit sodium in presence of edema and/or ascites.

H. **High-Protein Diet**
1. Indications
   a. Tissue repair and building
   b. Burns
   c. Malabsorption syndromes
   d. Pregnancy
2. Encourage high biological value (HBV) protein.
   a. Egg whites (gold standard)
   b. Soy products
   c. Milk products
   d. Fish and fowl
   e. Organ and meat sources
3. Encourage oral fluids to decrease damage to renal capillaries as a result of increased protein.

I. **Diet for Alteration in Amino-Acid Metabolism**
1. Use for phenylketonuria (PKU), galactosemia, and lactose intolerance.
2. Dietary restrictions are aimed at reducing or eliminating the offending enzyme.
3. Avoid milk and milk products for all three diets; include soy-based supplements.
4. For PKU, avoid high-protein foods such as meats, dairy products, and eggs. In addition, avoid aspartame (Nutrasweet) as it contains phenylalanine.
5. For galactosemia, the simple sugar in lactose must be avoided. Educate families to read labels carefully, as galactosemia can be life-threatening.
6. Supplement calcium and vitamin D in those with lactose-restricted or -eliminated diets.

J. **Low-Cholesterol Diet**
1. Indications
   a. Cardiovascular disease
   b. Diabetes mellitus
   c. Hyperlipidemia
2. Limit animal products that are high in low-density lipoproteins, saturated fats, and trans fats.
   a. Egg yolks
   b. Organ meats
   c. Fatty meats (such as bacon)
   d. Whole milk, butter
3. Encourage high-density lipoproteins, omega-3 fatty acids, and unsaturated fats.
   a. Sardines and salmon
   b. Olive and flaxseed oils
   c. Shellfish
   d. Walnuts
   e. Fruits and vegetables
   f. Lean meats
   g. Skinless fowl

K. **Modified-Fat Diet**
   1. Indications
      a. Gallbladder disease
      b. Hepatic disorders
      c. Cystic fibrosis
      d. Malabsorption syndrome
   2. Avoid the following foods
      a. Whole-milk products
      b. Gravies, creams
      c. Fatty meat and fish
      d. Nuts and chocolate
      e. Polyunsaturated oils
   3. Foods Allowed
      a. Two to three eggs per week
      b. Lean meat, fowl, fish
      c. Fruits and vegetables
      d. Bread and cereal
L. **Potassium-Modified Diets**
   1. High-Potassium Foods
      a. Bananas
      b. Oranges
      c. Milk
      d. Spinach
      e. Apricots and prunes
      f. Soy, lima, and kidney beans
      g. Baked potatoes (white and sweet)
   2. Low-Potassium Foods
      a. Breads
      b. Cereals
      c. Asparagus
      d. Cabbage
      e. Cherries
      f. Blackberries and blueberries
M. **Sodium-Restricted Diets**
   1. Indications
      a. Hypertension
      b. Heart failure
      c. Myocardial infarction
      d. Adrenal cortical diseases
      e. Kidney disease
      f. Liver cirrhosis
      g. Preeclampsia

   2. High-Sodium Foods
      a. Salty snack foods (such as potato chips)
      b. Canned soups and vegetables
      c. Baked goods that contain baking powder or baking soda
      d. Processed meats (e.g., bologna, ham, and bacon)
      e. Dairy products, especially cheese
      f. Pickles, olives
      g. Soy sauce, steak sauce
      h. Salad dressings
   3. Encourage clients to become "label savvy" for sodium.
N. **Iron Alterations**
   1. Increased iron intake is indicated for correction or prevention of iron deficiency anemia, which is most likely to occur in infants, toddlers, adolescents, and pregnant women.
   2. Food sources high in iron include fish, meats (particularly organ meats), green leafy vegetables, enriched breads, cereals and macaroni products, whole-grain products, dried fruits such as raisins and apricots, and egg yolks.
   3. Vitamin C enhances absorption of iron from the gastrointestinal tract.
   4. Oral iron supplementation can cause constipation and GI distress, so adequate iron intake through foods is ideal.
O. **Calcium Alterations**
   1. Increased calcium intake is indicated for growing children and adolescents, pregnant and lactating women, and postmenopausal women (to help prevent osteoporosis and osteopenia).
   2. Food sources high in calcium include milk and milk products such as yogurt and cheese; dark green vegetables such as collard greens, kale, and broccoli; dried beans and peas; shellfish and canned salmon; and antacids such as Tums, Rolaids, and Titralac.
   3. No more than 600 mg calcium can be absorbed at one time, so supplements should be taken 3 times daily; no more than 2,500 mg of calcium should be consumed per day.
   4. Vitamin D is required for absorption of calcium from the gastrointestinal tract.

"Need to Know" Laboratory Values

I Serum Electrolytes

A. **Sodium (Na⁺):** 136 to 145 mEq/L

B. **Potassium (K⁺):** 3.5 to 5 mEq/L

C. **Calcium total (Ca⁺⁺):** 9.0 to 10.5 mg/dL

D. **Magnesium (Mg⁺⁺):** 1.3 to 2.1 mEq/L

E. **Phosphorus (PO₄):** 3.0 to 4.5 mg/dL

F. **Chloride (Cl):** 98 to 106 mEq/L

II Arterial Blood Gases (ABGs)

A. **pH:** 7.35 to 7.45

B. **PaCO₂:** 35 to 45 mm Hg

C. **PaO₂:** 80 to 100 mm Hg

D. **HCO₃ (bicarbonate):** 21 to 28 mEq/L

III CBC

A. **RBCs:** males 4.7 to 6.1 million/uL; females 4.2 to 5.4 million/uL

B. **Hgb males:** 14 to 18 g/dL; females: 12 to 16 g/dL

C. **Hct males:** 42% to 52%; females 37% to 47%

D. **WBCs:** 5,000 to 10,000 mm³

E. **Erythrocyte sedimentation rate (ESR):** less than 20 mm/hr

IV Blood Lipid Levels

A. **Total serum cholesterol:** desirable less than 200 mg/dL; risk for cardiac or stroke event with levels greater than 150 mg/dL is the target range for therapy and has been shown to be the cut point to decrease cerebrovascular or arterial incidences.

B. **LDL (low-density lipids):** desirable less than 130 mg/dL

C. **HDL (high-density lipids):** males greater than 45 mg/dL; females greater than 55 mg/dL

D. **Triglycerides:** desirable less than 150 mg/dL; males 40 to 160 mg/dL; females 35 to 135 mg/dL

V Anticoagulant Therapy Coagulation Times

A. **PT:** 11 to 12.5 seconds. Therapeutic range for anticoagulant therapy is 1.5 to 2 times the normal or control value. Critical Value greater than 20 seconds.

B. **Activated Partial Thromboplastin Time (aPTT):** 30 to 40 seconds. Critical value greater than 70 seconds.

C. **Partial Thromboplastin Time (PTT):** 60 to 70 seconds greater than 100 seconds. Therapeutic range for anticoagulant therapy is 1.5 to 2 times the normal or control value.

D. **INR**

1. Normal INR is 0.8 to 1.1.

2. If the client requires anticoagulation, the desired value is increased to approximately 2 to 3. Critical value greater than 5.

3. The INR is a corrected ratio of a client's prothrombin time to normal.

4. Universal test is not affected by variations in laboratory norms.

E. **Platelets:** 150,000 to 400,000/mm³. Critical value less than 20,000 or greater than 1 million/mm³.

NOTE: Therapeutic ranges for the INR vary based on the indication for anticoagulation. Immediately report critical values to the provider.

VI Liver Function Tests

A. **Albumin:** 3.5 to 5 g/dL

B. **Ammonia:** 10 to 80 mcg/dL

C. **Total bilirubin:** 0.1 to 1.0 mg/dL

D. **Total protein:** 6 to 8 g/dL

VII Urinalysis

A. **Specific gravity:** 1.005 to 1.030

B. **Protein:** 0 to 8 mg/dL

C. **Glucose:** less than 0.5 g/day

D. **Ketones:** none

E. **pH:** 4.6 to 8

F. **WBC:** males 0 to 3 per high-power field; females 0 to 5 per high-power field

VIII Renal Function

A. **Serum creatinine:** males 0.6 to 1.2 mg/dL; females 0.5 to 1.1 mg/dL

B. **BUN:** 10 to 20 mg/dL

C. **Creatinine clearance test:** males 90 to 139 mL/min; females 80 to 125 mL/min. This is a calculation of glomerular filtration rate (GFR) and is the best indicator of overall renal function.

IX Therapeutic Medication Monitoring

A. **Digoxin level:** 0.8 to 2.0 ng/mL

B. **Lithium level:** 0.4 to 1.4 mEq/L

C. **Phenobarbital:** 10 to 40 mcg/mL

D. **Theophylline:** 10 to 20 mcg/mL

E. **Phenytoin:** 10 to 20 mcg/mL

X Blood Glucose Levels

A. **Glucose (fasting):** 70 to 105 mg/dL

B. **Glycosylated hemoglobin (HbA1c):** 4% to 6% is within the expected reference range. Greater than 8% indicates poor diabetes mellitus control.

NOTE: Normal laboratory value reference ranges can have slight variations depending on the facility or organization. To recognize deviations, candidates should know the laboratory value ranges. It is important to recognize values that are elevated or low.

UNIT SEVEN

Mental Health Nursing

Overview

ı Mental Health

A state of well-being in which each individual is able to realize his own potential, cope with the normal stresses of life, work productively and fruitfully, and contribute to the community.

ıı Mental Illness

Refers to all mental disorders with definable diagnoses and includes developmental, biological, and psychological disturbances in mental functioning.

ııı Mental Health Nursing

This type of nursing employs a purposeful use of self as its art and a wide range of nursing, psychosocial, and neurobiological theories and research evidence as its science.

MENTAL HEALTH-ILLNESS CONTINUUM

| Occasional stress with no impairment. | Mild to marked distress with moderate to chronic impairment. |

A. **Theoretical Models**
   1. Psychoanalytic
      a. **Sigmund Freud**
         1) Id, ego, superego
         2) 5 Stages of Development
            a) Oral: 0 to 1 year
            b) Anal: 1 to 3 years
            c) Phallic: 3 to 6 years
            d) Latency: 6 to 12 years
            e) Genital: 12 years to young adult
         3) Transference
         4) Countertransference

   b. **Erik Erikson**
      1) 8 Stages of Growth and Development
         a) Infancy: 0 to 1 year
            Trust vs. Mistrust
         b) Early Childhood: 1 to 3 years
            Autonomy vs. Shame and Doubt
         c) Preschooler: 3 to 6 years
            Initiative vs. Guilt
         d) School Age: 6 to 12 years
            Industry vs. Inferiority
         e) Adolescence: 12 to 20 years
            Identity vs. Role Confusion
         f) Young Adult: 20 to 35 years
            Intimacy vs. Isolation
         g) Middle Adult: 35 to 65 years
            Generativity vs. Stagnation
         h) Older Adult: 65 years and older
            Integrity vs. Despair
   2. Behavioral
      a. **Ivan Pavlov**
         Classical Conditioning
      b. **B. F. Skinner**
         Operant Conditioning
   3. Humanistic
      a. **Abraham Maslow**
         Hierarchy of Needs

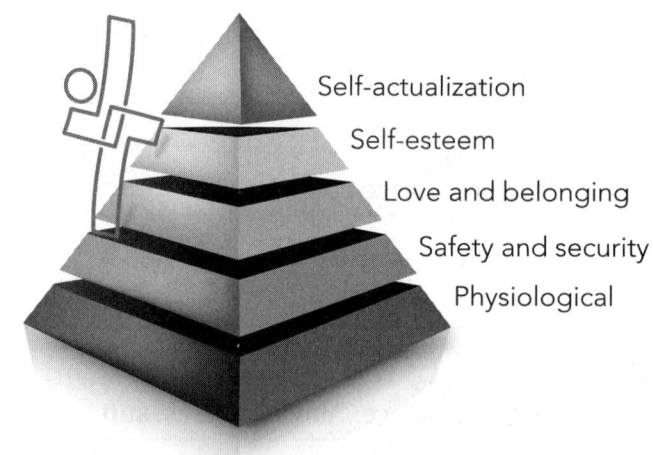

Self-actualization
Self-esteem
Love and belonging
Safety and security
Physiological

THEORISTS

MAJOR THEORETICAL CONTRIBUTIONS	MAJOR CONTRIBUTIONS USED IN NURSING

Psychoanalyst: Sigmund Freud

Interactive systems of the personality: Id, ego, and superego **5 Stages of Development**: Oral, anal, phallic, latency, and genital Erik Erikson later expanded upon these stages.	**Transference** develops when the client experiences feelings toward the nurse or therapist that were originally held toward significant others. **Countertransference** is the health care worker's unconscious, personal response to the client.

Psychoanalyst: Erik Erickson

8 Stages of Growth and Development	Erikson's developmental framework helps the nurse identify age-appropriate behaviors during assessment.
Infancy (0 to 1 year): Trust vs. Mistrust Behavior: Hopefulness, trusting vs. withdrawn, alienated	Success: Trust should be seen with the primary caregiver. Crisis: Infant is withdrawn and unresponsive.
Early Childhood (1 to 3 years): Autonomy vs. Shame and Doubt Behavior: Self-control and using willpower vs. uncertainty of doing anything at all	Success: A toddler shows signs of self-control in toilet training. Crisis: A toddler shows signs of doubt in being able to toilet train.
Preschooler (3 to 6 years): Initiative vs. Guilt Behavior: Ability to initiate activities vs. feeling conflicted about what was initiated	Success: A preschooler may initiate helping set the table for dinner. Crisis: A preschooler took candy without paying for it and knew it was wrong.
School Age (6 to 12 years): Industry vs. Inferiority Behavior: Feeling competent in activities and work vs. feelings of low self-esteem	Success: "I'm getting really good at piano since I started taking lessons." Crisis: "I'm dumb because I can't read as fast as everyone else."
Adolescence (12 to 20 years): Identity vs. Role Confusion Behavior: A sense of self vs. becoming confused about self	Success: "I am fine with who I am." Crisis: "I belong to a gang because I am nothing without them."
Young Adult (20 to 35 years): Intimacy vs. Isolation Behavior: Ability to love deeply and commit oneself in relationships vs. remaining uncommitted and alone	Success: "My partner has been my best friend for 10 years." Crisis: "No one is worthy of being in a relationship with me."
Middle Adult (35 to 65 years): Generativity vs. Stagnation Behavior: Ability to give and care for others vs. self-absorption and inability to grow as a person	Success: "I will be taking a leave of absence for 3 months to stay with my mother who is terminally ill." Crisis: "I just want to be by myself and watch television all night."
Older Adult (65 years and older): Integrity vs. Despair Behavior: Sense of accomplishment in life vs. feeling dissatisfied with life	Success: "I have led a happy and productive life." Crisis: "My life has been a waste."

Behaviorist: Ivan Pavlov

Classical conditioning: Pavlov discovered when a neutral stimulus (a bell) was repeatedly paired with another stimulus (food that triggered salivation), eventually the sound of the bell alone could elicit salivation in dogs.	Humans can also experience classically conditioned responses that are involuntary and not spontaneous choices.

Behaviorist: B.F. Skinner

Operant conditioning: Voluntary behaviors are learned through consequences and behavioral responses are elicited through reinforcement, which causes a behavior to occur more frequently.	Positive behavior can be encouraged to continue through positive reinforcement such as offering a reward or returning a privilege.

Humanistic: Abraham Maslow

The Hierarchy of Needs Pyramid	
Self-actualization	People strive to become everything they are capable of.
Self-esteem	People need to have a high self-regard, and have it reflected to them from others.
Love and belonging	This involves the need for intimate relationships and experiencing love and affection from others.
Safety and security	Once physiological needs are met, the safety needs emerge. These needs include security, protection, freedom from fear, and the need for structure, order, and limits.
Physiological	The most basic needs are food, oxygen, water, sleep, sex, and a constant body temperature. If all needs were deprived, this level would take priority.

THEORY REVIEW

List Erikson's (E) stage of growth and development and Maslow's (M) priority need for the following scenarios.

1. A teenager has been admitted to the emergency department for a drug overdose.

E:

M:

2. An elderly client who lives alone is being discharged following a total hip replacement.

E:

M:

3. An infant is born weighing 1 lb 4 oz (635 g).

E:

M:

4. A young college graduate who was recently engaged receives a diagnosis of tinea corporis.

E:

M:

5. A student who is in the fourth grade has been admitted to a psychiatric hospital for depression and suicidal ideation.

E:

M:

Answer Key: 1. Identity vs. Role Confusion, Physiological (The basic needs to sustain life are priority due to the drug overdose); 2. Integrity vs. Despair, Physiological (The basic needs to maintain life are priority because the client lives alone and is physically compromised); 3. Trust vs. Mistrust, Physiological (The basic needs to maintain life are priority); 4. Intimacy vs. Isolation, Love and Belonging (Physiological and Safety are not priority with tinea corporis because neither are threatened with this diagnosis. However, intimacy, love, and belonging are priority needs); 5. Industry vs. Inferiority, Safety (This pediatric client must have protective/safe measures taken to maintain life).

B. **Nursing Process**

1. **Assess** using the Mental Status Examination (MSE).

   a. Appearance: Grooming, dress, hygiene, facial expression

   b. Behavior: Excessive or reduced body movements, level of eye contact

   c. Speech: Slow, rapid, normal, loud, soft, disorganized, slurred

   d. Mood: Sad, labile, euphoric, flat, bland affect

   e. Thoughts: Disorganized, flight of ideas, obsessions

   f. Perceptual disturbances: Hallucinations, delusions

   g. Cognition: Orientation to time, place and person, level of consciousness, remote and recent memory, judgment

   h. Ideas of harming self or others: Presence of a plan, means and opportunity to carry out the plan

2. **Diagnose** with input from the treatment team.

   a. The problem should include related factors and defining characteristics with the probable cause and supporting data.

   b. Example: Hopelessness (problem) related to abandonment (related factor) as evidenced by client statement: "Nothing will change" (defining characteristic).

3. **Plan** interventions based on the following criteria:

   a. Safe for client, other clients, staff, and family

   b. Compatible with other therapies, client's personal goals, and cultural values

   c. Realistic and individualized with consideration given to the client's age, physical condition, willingness to change, and community resources

   d. Evidence-based, when available

4. **Implementation** should include:

   a. Coordination of care with all members of the treatment team

   b. Health teaching and promotion

   c. Milieu therapy

   d. Pharmacological and integrative therapies

5. **Evaluation** should be based on:

   a. Ongoing assessment of data for consideration of revisions in the treatment plan

   b. Realistic outcomes for each client

C. **Nurse–Client Relationship**

1. Orientation phase: This phase can last for a few meetings or longer.
   a. Rapport and trust is established.
   b. The nurse's role is clarified, and all roles are defined.
   c. Confidentiality is established.
   d. The terms of termination are introduced.
   e. The nurse becomes aware of transference and countertransference issues.
   f. Client problems are articulated, and mutually agreed-upon goals are established.
2. Working phase: This allows for a strong working relationship.
   a. Maintain client relationship.
   b. Share information and gather further data.
   c. Promote client's problem-solving skills.
   d. Facilitate behavioral change.
   e. Overcome resistance behaviors.
   f. Evaluate problems and goals.
   g. Promote practice and expression of alternative adaptive behaviors.
3. Termination phase: This is the final phase of the nurse-patient relationship.
   a. Summarize the goals achieved.
   b. Discuss new coping strategies.
   c. Review situations that occurred during the relationship.
   d. Exchange memories and validate experiences of the relationship to promote closure.
4. Factors that Promote Client Growth
   a. Communicating genuineness
   b. Expressing empathy
   c. Having positive regard for client

D. **Communication Techniques**

1. Therapeutic
   a. Active listening includes:
      1) Observing the client's nonverbal behaviors
      2) Understanding and reflecting on the client's verbal message
   b. **Clarifying techniques**
      1) **Restating** allows the nurse to mirror overt and covert messages.
         Client: "I can't focus."
         Nurse: "You are having problems focusing?"
      2) **Reflecting** provides a means to assist the client to better understand his thoughts and feelings.
         Client: "What should I do about my son's addiction?"
         Nurse: "What do you think you should do?"
      3) **Exploring** allows the nurse to examine ideas and experiences in more depth.
         "Tell me more about …"
   c. Ask open-ended questions to elicit client responses:
      "What do you perceive as your biggest stressor right now?"
   d. Offer self:
      "I would like to spend time talking with you."
   e. Offer general leads:
      "And then?"
   f. Focus:
      "You've mentioned many events. Let's talk about your wanting to end it all again."
2. Nontherapeutic
   a. Giving premature advice:
      "You should leave your home immediately."
   b. Minimizing feelings:
      "Things often get worse before they get better."
   c. False reassurance:
      "Everything is going to be fine."
   d. Disapproval:
      "I disagree with that."
   e. Making value judgments:
      "You wife is dying of lung cancer, and you smoke?"

COMMUNICATION REVIEW

Analyze the following communication scenarios and determine whether the nurse's responses are therapeutic or nontherapeutic and which communication technique is used.

		COMMUNICATION TECHNIQUE:
1. Client: "I wish I were dead." Nurse: "I know what you mean."	☐ THERAPEUTIC ☐ NONTHERAPEUTIC	
2. Client: "I am so worried." Nurse: "What specifically are you worried about?"	☐ THERAPEUTIC ☐ NONTHERAPEUTIC	
3. Client: "I haven't taken my medicine in 4 days." Nurse: "Why would you stop taking your medications?"	☐ THERAPEUTIC ☐ NONTHERAPEUTIC	
4. Client: "I wish everyone would leave me alone." Nurse: "You are going to do fine, you'll see."	☐ THERAPEUTIC ☐ NONTHERAPEUTIC	

Answer Key: 1. Nontherapeutic/minimizing feelings; 2. Therapeutic/clarifying with reflection; 3. Nontherapeutic/confrontational, asking "why";
4. Nontherapeutic/false reassurance

3. **Group therapy:** A group of individuals interacting together with a shared purpose.

   a. Phases of Group Development

      1) Orientation phase defines the purpose of the group.

      2) Working phase allows for a focus on problem solving.

      3) Termination phase promotes reflection on the progress that has been made, and identifies post-termination goals.

   b. Therapeutic Factors of Groups

      1) Instill hope: The leader promotes optimism about success of group treatment.

      2) Altruism: Members gain from giving support to others, allowing for an improvement of self-worth.

      3) Universality: Members realize that they are not alone with the problems they face.

SECTION 2

Anxiety and Anxiety Disorders

A. **Anxiety**

   1. Definition: A universal human experience that is considered the most basic of human emotions.

   2. Levels of Anxiety

      a. Mild: occurs in normal experience of everyday life, and promotes a sharp focus of reality.

      b. Moderate: narrows the perceptual field, and some details become excluded.

      c. Severe: severely narrows the perceptual field, and right amount of focus on detail is lost.

      d. Panic: the extreme level of anxiety; leaves a person unable to process the environment.

LEVELS OF ANXIETY

	SIGNS AND SYMPTOMS	NURSING INTERVENTIONS
Mild	Heightened perceptual field, alert and can grasp what is going on, restless, irritable or impatient, foot or finger tapping	Help the client identify the anxiety. Anticipate anxiety-provoking situations. Demonstrate interest in client by leaning forward and maintaining eye contact. Ask questions to clarify what is said. Encourage problem solving.
Moderate	Narrow perceptual field, voice tremors, difficulty concentrating, increased respiratory and heart rate, pacing, banging hands on table	

LEVELS OF ANXIETY (CONTINUED)

	SIGNS AND SYMPTOMS	NURSING INTERVENTIONS
Severe	Greatly reduced perceptual field, problem solving feels impossible, feelings of dread, confusion, chest discomfort, diaphoresis, loud and rapid speech, threats and demands	Maintain calm manner. Remain with client. Minimize environmental stimuli. Use clear, simple statements. Use low-pitched voice.
Panic	Unable to focus on the environment, may feel unreal, cannot process what is happening, hallucinations or delusions may occur, somatic reports increase.	Listen for themes in communication. Attend to physical and safety needs.

B. **Defense Mechanisms**

   1. Definition: Automatic coping styles that protect individuals from anxiety and maintain self-image.

   2. Adaptive use: Allows anxiety to be lowered and goals to be achieved.

   3. Maladaptive use: Occurs when one or several are used in excess, disallowing goals to be achieved.

   4. Defense Mechanisms

      a. Denial: Attempt to escape unpleasant realities.

         1) Adaptive use: Client states, "I don't believe you" when hearing news that a loved one died.

         2) Maladaptive use: A woman who lost her husband 3 years ago keeps his clothes hanging in the closet and talks about him in the present tense.

      b. Projection: Unconscious rejection of emotionally unacceptable features and attributing them to others.

         1) Adaptive use: This is considered an immature defense mechanism, and there is no adaptive example.

         2) Maladaptive use: A woman who has repressed an attraction toward other women refuses to socialize, fearing other women will make homosexual advances.

      c. Regression: Reverting to an earlier developmental level

         1) Adaptive use: A 5-year-old begins sucking his thumb when a new sibling is born.

         2) Maladaptive use: An employee who is not promoted begins missing appointments and showing up late for meetings.

      d. Sublimation: Directing unacceptable behaviors into a socially acceptable area. This is always adaptive.

         1) Example: A student who is angry with a faculty member writes a short story of a hero.

C. **Anxiety/Obsessive-Compulsive Disorders**

1. Clients who have anxiety disorders use ineffective behaviors to try to control their anxiety.

2. Types of Anxiety Disorders

   a. Phobias

      1) Definition: Persistent, irrational fear of a specific object, activity, or situation that leads to avoidance

      2) Examples

         a) Acrophobia: Fear of heights

         b) Social anxiety disorder: Social phobia characterized by severe anxiety or fear provoked by exposure to social or performance situations

         c) Claustrophobia: Fear of closed spaces

   b. Panic

      1) Definition: Panic attacks are the most commonly seen feature of this disorder. Panic attacks are characterized as a sudden onset of extreme apprehension or fear usually associated with impending doom.

   c. Obsessive-Compulsive Disorder (OCD)

      1) Definition: Obsessions are thoughts, impulses, or images that persist and cannot be dismissed from the mind even though the individual makes attempts to do so. Compulsions are ritualistic behaviors an individual feels driven to perform to attempt a reduction of anxiety. Obsessions and compulsions often occur together, and the rituals become time-consuming, interfering with normal routines and relationships.

   d. Generalized Anxiety Disorder (GAD)

      1) Definition: Characterized by excessive anxiety or worry about numerous situations, and the anxiety is out of proportion to the true impact of the event.

   e. Separation Anxiety Disorder

      1) This is a normal part of early development, but it can continue into adulthood, and inappropriate levels of concern over being away from a significant other can be exhibited.

ANXIETY/OBSESSIVE-COMPULSIVE DISORDERS

	SIGNS AND SYMPTOMS
Phobias	Irrational fear of an object or situation that persists.
Panic disorder	Recurrent episodes of panic attacks that can include palpitations, chest pain, breathing difficulties, nausea, and feelings of choking.
Obsessive-compulsive disorder (OCD)	Obsessions: persistent intrusive thoughts. Compulsions: repetitive behaviors that a client feels driven to perform (such as hand washing).
Generalized anxiety disorder (GAD)	Excessive anxiety/worry more days than not over 6 months associated with restlessness, fatigue, difficulty concentrating, sleep disturbances, and irritability.
Separation anxiety disorder	Adults exhibit worry, shyness, uncertainty, and lack of self-direction.

3. Medications for Anxiety Disorders

   a. Antidepressants

      1) Selective Serotonin Reuptake Inhibitors (SSRIs)

         a) Citalopram

         b) Fluoxetine

         c) Sertraline

      2) Serotonin Norepinephrine Reuptake Inhibitors (SNRIs)

      3) Venlafaxine

      4) Duloxetine

      5) Tricyclics

         a) Imipramine

         b) Amitriptyline

   b. Anti-anxiety Agents

      1) Benzodiazepines

         a) Alprazolam

         b) Clonazepam

         c) Diazepam

      2) Nonbenzodiazepine

         a) Buspirone

   c. Anticonvulsants

      1) Gabapentin

ANXIETY DISORDER REVIEW

Match the disorder with the correct nursing communication.

____ 1. Phobias

____ 2. Panic disorder

____ 3. Generalized anxiety disorder

____ 4. Obsessive-compulsive disorder

____ 5. Separation anxiety disorder

a. "Tell me more about how you feel since your mom has been away?"

b. "Tell me more about how your partner responds to your returning home each day to check the coffee pot."

c. "Where would you like to begin our discussion regarding your fear of flying?"

d. "What do you believe brings on your episodes of chest pain and difficulty breathing?"

e. "You have mentioned a lot of stressors that have been occurring for several months. Which situation is causing the greatest stress for you?"

Answer Key: 1. C; 2. D; 3. E; 4. B; 5. A

Schizophrenia

A. **Schizophrenia**

1. Definition: A complex brain disorder that affects thinking, language, emotions, social behavior, and the ability to perceive reality correctly.

2. Phases

   a. Acute: Onset or exacerbation of symptoms with loss of functional abilities.

   b. Stabilization: Symptoms diminish and client progresses toward previous level of functioning.

   c. Maintenance: The client is at or near baseline functioning.

3. Assessment

   a. Positive symptoms are the presence of something that is not normally present, such as:

      1) Alterations in thought include delusions that are false, fixed beliefs that cannot be corrected with reasoning.

      2) Alterations in speech can include word salad (i.e., meaningless jumble of words) or echolalia (i.e., pathological repeating of another's words).

      3) Alterations in perception include hallucinations that involve a sensory experience for which no external stimulus exists. Examples include hearing voices, seeing things, or experiencing tastes.

   b. Negative symptoms refer to the absence of something that should be present. Examples include flat or blunted affect and inappropriate emotional response.

   c. Cognitive symptoms are subtle changes in memory or thinking leading to an inability to cope and effectively make decisions.

4. **Nursing Interventions**

   a. Provide a structured, safe environment (i.e., milieu) for the client in order to decrease anxiety and to distract the client from constant thinking about hallucinations.

   b. Promote therapeutic communication to lower anxiety, decrease defensive patterns, and encourage participation in the milieu.

   c. Establish a trusting relationship with the client.

   d. Use appropriate communication to address hallucinations and delusions.

      1) Ask the client directly about hallucinations. The nurse should not argue or agree with the client's view of the situation.

      2) Do not argue with a client's delusions, but focus on the client's feelings and possibly offer reasonable explanations.

      3) Assess the client for paranoid delusions, which can increase the risk for violence against others.

      4) Attempt to focus conversations on reality-based subjects.

   e. First-Generation Antipsychotics (treat positive symptoms)

      1) Thioridazine

      2) Haloperidol

      3) Loxapine

   f. Second-Generation Antipsychotics (treat positive and negative symptoms)

      1) Clozapine

      2) Olanzapine

      3) Quetiapine

      4) Risperidone

   g. Therapy

      1) Cognitive behavioral therapy can assist in controlling symptoms.

SCHIZOPHRENIA REVIEW

Determine whether the following symptoms are positive or negative.

1. The client shows a flattened affect.	☐ POSITIVE ☐ NEGATIVE
2. The client states the CIA is spying on his every move.	☐ POSITIVE ☐ NEGATIVE
3. The client stops speaking to everyone.	☐ POSITIVE ☐ NEGATIVE
4. The client does not complete a task.	☐ POSITIVE ☐ NEGATIVE
5. The client states she feels spiders crawling all over her body.	☐ POSITIVE ☐ NEGATIVE

Answer Key: 1. Negative; 2. Positive; 3. Negative; 4. Negative; 5. Positive

---

Childhood Disorders

A. **Motor Disorders**

1. Stereotypic Movement Disorder

   a. Definition: A complex neurobiological and developmental disability that typically appears before 3 years of age.

2. Tourette Disorder

   a. Definition: Motor and verbal tics appearing between 2 and 7 years of age. These symptoms cause marked distress and impairment in social and occupational functioning. This disorder is usually permanent.

   b. Interventions include antipsychotics and behavioral techniques.

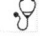

3. **Nursing Interventions**

   a. Motor Disorders

      1) Maintain safe environment (for example, a helmet may be required for head banging).

      2) Positive reinforcement for correct behavior response.

      3) Assess the parent's understanding of the motor disorder.

      4) Encourage participation in behavioral therapy and support groups.

B. **Intellectual Development Disorder (IDD)**

   1. Characterized by deficits in intellectual functioning, social functioning, and managing activities of daily living. Impairments can range from mild to severe.

   2. Interventions

      a. Assess cognitive and physical development and functioning.

      b. Care and teaching should be individualized to the client's needs.

      c. Make appropriate referrals (e.g., early intervention program, social work, speech therapy, physical therapy, occupational therapy).

      d. Add visual cues with verbal instruction.

      e. Give one-step instructions.

C. **Attention-Deficit Disorder (ADD)**
   Attention-Deficit/Hyperactivity Disorder (ADHD)

   1. Definition: Children with ADD show an inappropriate degree of inattention and impulsiveness. These symptoms are present for children with ADHD with the addition of hyperactivity.

   2. **Nursing Interventions**

      a. Observe for level of physical activity, attention span, talkativeness, frustration tolerance, and the ability to follow directions.

      b. Assess social skills, problem-solving skills, and school performance.

      c. Assess for comorbidities (e.g., anxiety, depression).

   3. Medications

      a. Stimulants

         1) Methylphenidate

         2) Amphetamine and dextroamphetamine

D. **Autism Spectrum Disorders (ASDs)**

   1. Definition: Complex neurobiological and developmental disabilities that typically appear during the first three years of life.

   2. Symptoms include deficits in social relatedness, including communication, nonverbal behavior, and interactions.

   3. Interventions should begin early within the second or third year of life through specialized treatment programs.

      a. Assist with behavior modification program.

      b. Promote positive reinforcement.

      c. Structure opportunities for small successes.

      d. Set clear rules.

      e. Decrease environmental stimulation.

      f. Introduce the child to new situations slowly.

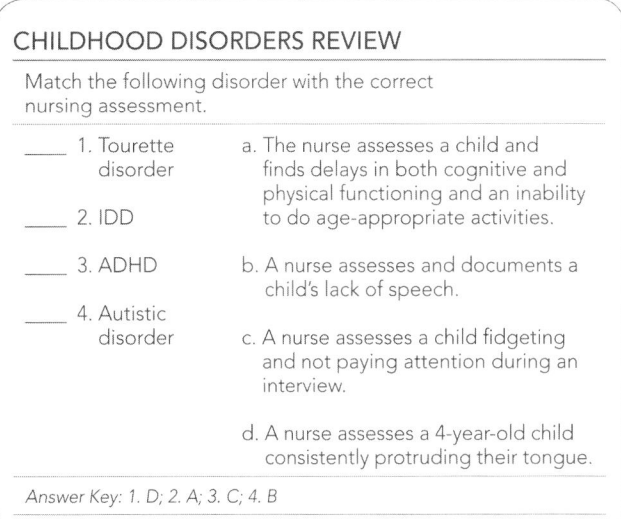

CHILDHOOD DISORDERS REVIEW

Match the following disorder with the correct nursing assessment.

_____ 1. Tourette disorder

_____ 2. IDD

_____ 3. ADHD

_____ 4. Autistic disorder

a. The nurse assesses a child and finds delays in both cognitive and physical functioning and an inability to do age-appropriate activities.

b. A nurse assesses and documents a child's lack of speech.

c. A nurse assesses a child fidgeting and not paying attention during an interview.

d. A nurse assesses a 4-year-old child consistently protruding their tongue.

Answer Key: 1. D; 2. A; 3. C; 4. B

SECTION 5

Depressive/Bipolar Disorders

A. **Major Depressive Disorder (MDD)**

   1. Definition: Persistently depressed mood lasting for a minimum of 2 weeks.

   2. Symptoms

      a. Fatigue

      b. Anhedonia

      c. Changes in appetite

      d. Insomnia or hypersomnia

      e. Anergia

      f. Feelings of worthlessness

      g. Persistent thoughts of suicide

   3. Primary Risk Factors

      a. Female gender

      b. Unmarried status

      c. Low socioeconomic class

      d. Early childhood trauma

      e. Family history of depression

      f. Postpartum period

      g. Medical illness

   4. Three Phases of Treatment and Recovery

      a. Acute is focused on reducing depressive symptoms and lasts 6 to 12 weeks.

      b. Continuation is focused on prevention of a relapse through pharmacotherapy, education, and psychotherapy, and lasts 4 to 9 months.

      c. Maintenance is focused on prevention of further episodes and lasts 1 year or more.

   5. **Nursing Interventions**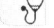

      a. Evaluate the client's risk of harm to self or others.

      b. Evaluate the client's use of drugs and alcohol.

      c. Assess client's history of depression.

      d. Assess client's support systems.

6. Medications
   a. SSRIs
      1) Citalopram
      2) Escitalopram
   b. Selective Serotonin Reuptake Inhibitor and Serotonin Receptor Agonist
      1) Vilazodone
   c. SNRIs
      1) Venlafaxine
      2) Duloxetine
   d. Norepinephrine Dopamine Reuptake Inhibitor (NDRI)
      1) Bupropion
   e. Tricyclic Antidepressants (TCAs)
      1) Imipramine
   f. Monoamine Oxidase Inhibitors (MAOIs)
      1) Phenelzine
      2) Tranylcypromine
7. Electroconvulsive Therapy (ECT)
   a. Induced seizure activity found to be helpful in treating clients who have MDD. Clients may experience temporary short-term memory loss after several ECT treatments.
8. Transcranial Magnetic Stimulation (TMS)
   a. Noninvasive treatment that uses magnetic pulses to stimulate the cerebral cortex. There have been no neurological deficits or memory problems noted.

B. **Suicide**
   1. Definition: The intentional act of killing oneself by any means.
   2. **Nursing Interventions**
      a. Assess for suicidal ideation with intent.
      b. Assess for lethal suicide plan.
      c. Assess for coexisting psychiatric or medical illness.
      d. Assess family history of suicide.
      e. Assess recent lack of support.
      f. Assess for feelings of hopelessness and helplessness.
      g. Assess for covert statements such as, "Things will never work out."
      h. Assess for overt statements such as, "I can't take it anymore."
   3. Environmental Guidelines for Suicide Prevention
      a. Meal trays must not contain glass or metal silverware.
      b. Hands should be in full view while patient is sleeping.
      c. Carefully observe patient swallow medication.
      d. Screen all potentially harmful gifts (such as flowers in a glass vase).
      e. Injury-proof rooms and bathrooms.
      f. Remove all possessions from client that could lead to injury.
      g. One-on-one constant supervision.

C. **Bipolar Disorder**
   1. Definitions
      a. Bipolar I: Mood disorder characterized by at least one week-long manic episode. Manic episodes may alternate with depression.
      b. Bipolar II: Low-level mania alternates with profound depression.
   2. Mania Characteristics
      a. Inflated sense of self-importance
      b. Extreme energy
      c. Excessive talking with pressured speech
      d. Indiscriminate spending, reckless sexual encounters, risky investments
   3. **Nursing Interventions**
      a. Assess whether client is a danger to self or others.
      b. Assess the need to protect client from uninhibited behaviors.
      c. Assess for coexisting medical conditions such as substance use disorder.
   4. Medications
      a. Mood Stabilizer: Lithium
      b. Anticonvulsants: Valproic acid
      c. Atypical Antipsychotics
         1) Aripiprazole
         2) Risperidone
      d. Anti-anxiety Agents: Clonazepam

REVIEW OF DEPRESSIVE/BIPOLAR DISORDERS

Place a check by the nursing interventions that are considered therapeutic for a client experiencing the following.

Depression

☐	1. Encourage exercise.
☐	2. Encourage overgeneralizations.
☐	3. Encourage problem solving.
☐	4. Encourage formation of supportive relationships.

Mania

☐	1. Provide long explanations.
☐	2. Use firm, calm approach.
☐	3. Provide frequent high-calorie fluids.
☐	4. Maintain low-level stimuli.

Answer Key:

Depression/Therapeutic: 1, 3, & 4. Overgeneralizations, such as "She always" or "He never," lead to negative appraisals, making 2 incorrect.

Mania/Therapeutic: 2, 3, & 4. Long explanations could be poorly understood by a client experiencing mania; short statements are preferred, making 1 incorrect.

Personality Disorders

A. **Personality Disorders**

1. All personality disorders share characteristics of inflexibility and difficulties in interpersonal relationships that impair social or occupational functioning.

2. Cluster A
   a. Paranoid
   b. Schizoid
   c. Schizotypal

3. Cluster B
   a. Antisocial
   b. Borderline
   c. Narcissistic
   d. Histrionic

4. Cluster C
   a. Dependent
   b. Obsessive-compulsive
   c. Avoidant

B. **Medications**

1. Depending on the disorder:
   a. Antidepressants
   b. Anti-anxiety agents
   c. Antipsychotics

PERSONALITY DISORDERS

DISORDER	NURSING INTERVENTIONS
Cluster A (Odd/Eccentric)	
Paranoid Distrust, suspiciousness of others, and hypervigilance	Avoid being too nice or too friendly. Give clear explanations. Warn about changes in treatment plan and explain reasons for delays.
Schizoid Emotional detachment, isolates self, few close relationships Content being an observer	Not impacted by approval or rejection of others. Do not try to increase socialization.
Schizotypal May exhibit extreme anxiety in social situations related to severe social and interpersonal deficits	Respect client's need for social isolation. Be aware of client's suspicious behavior. Be aware that superstition and magical thinking are common.

PERSONALITY DISORDERS (CONTINUED)

DISORDER	NURSING INTERVENTIONS
Cluster B (Dramatic/Emotional)	
Antisocial Disregard for the rights of others, impulsive risk-taking behaviors common, lacks empathy	Be aware of and assess for substance abuse. Set clear limits on specific behavior. Be cautious of manipulation through guilt when client doesn't get what he wants.
Borderline Extreme emotional lability, impulsivity, and self-image distortions that severely impair functioning	Provide clear and consistent boundaries. Use clear communication. Review therapeutic goals and boundaries when behavior issues are evident. Assess for self-mutilating behaviors.
Narcissistic Lack of empathy impairs relationships, may appear arrogant due to over-inflated sense of self, difficulty with criticism	Remain neutral and avoid power struggles. Convey unassuming self-confidence.
Histrionic Attention seeking, frustrates easily, often melodramatic and seductive	Understand seductive behavior as a response to distress. Assess for suicidal behavior if admiration is withdrawn. Model concrete, descriptive vs. vague language.
Cluster C (Anxious/Fearful)	
Dependent Excessive clinging and need to be taken care of, submissive	Be aware of countertransference that can occur due to client's clinging behavior. Identify current stresses. Satisfy client's needs when setting limits.
Obsessive-Compulsive Preoccupied with orderliness, perfectionism, and control, rigid and inflexible, fears failure	Guard against power struggles with client as the need to control is high. Assess for client's use of intellectualization, rationalization, and reaction formation as defense mechanisms. Be aware of client's critical nature toward self and others.
Avoidant Social inhibition and feelings of inadequacy, hypersensitive to negative evaluation	Maintain a friendly, accepting, reassuring approach. Do not push client into social situations.

SECTION 7

Addictive Disorders

A. Definitions

1. Substance use disorder: Pathologic and disordered use of a substance that may lead to intoxication and withdrawal if the substance is removed.

2. Codependency: Over-responsible for the behaviors of others, often ignoring own needs and desires. Self-worth is defined in terms of caring for others.

   a. Behaviors may include finding excuses for the person's substance use or destroying the person's drug or alcohol supply.

CENTRAL NERVOUS SYSTEM DEPRESSANTS

DRUG	Barbiturates Benzodiazepines Alcohol
INTOXICATION	Slurred speech, unsteady gait, drowsiness, impaired judgment
WITHDRAWAL	Nausea and vomiting, tachycardia, diaphoresis, tremors, grand mal seizures, restlessness and irritability

CENTRAL NERVOUS SYSTEM STIMULANTS

DRUG	Cocaine Amphetamines Methamphetamines
INTOXICATION	Tachycardia, dilated pupils, elevated blood pressure, grandiosity, impaired judgment, paranoia with delusions
WITHDRAWAL	Fatigue, depression, agitation, apathy, anxiety, craving, increased appetite

OPIATES

DRUG	Heroin Meperidine Fentanyl Hydromorphone
INTOXICATION	Constricted pupils, decreased respirations, decreased heart rate, decreased blood pressure, initial euphoria followed by dysphoria
WITHDRAWAL	Yawning, insomnia, panic, diaphoresis, cramps, nausea and vomiting, chills, fever, diarrhea

B. **Nursing Interventions**

1. Assess vital signs.
2. Assess for dehydration.
3. Assess for low self-worth.
4. Provide for client safety.
5. Assess toxicology screen/blood alcohol level.
6. Assess for severe withdrawal syndrome.
7. Assess for an overdose that warrants immediate medical attention.
8. Assess for suicidal thoughts and behaviors.
9. Assess family members for codependency.
10. Explore the client's interests in participating in a 12-step program such as Alcoholics Anonymous or Narcotics Anonymous.
11. Explore the family's interest in participating in self-help groups such as Al-Anon or Alateen.

SECTION 8

Neurocognitive Disorders

A. **Delirium and Dementia**

1. **Delirium** is characterized by a disturbance of consciousness and a change in cognition that develop over a short period of time.

2. **Dementia** is a progressive deterioration of cognitive functioning and global impairment of intellect with no change in consciousness.

COGNITIVE DISORDERS

	Delirium	Dementia
ONSET	Sudden, over hours to days	Slowly, over months to years
CONTRIBUTING FACTORS	Fever, hypotension, infection, hypoglycemia, adverse drug reaction, head injury, emotional stress, seizures	Alzheimer's disease, neurological disease, vascular disease, alcohol use disorder, head trauma
COGNITION	Impaired memory, judgment, and attention span that can fluctuate	Impaired memory, judgment, and attention span; abstract thinking
SPEECH	Rapid, inappropriate, incoherent	Incoherent, slow, inappropriate
PROGNOSIS	Reversible with treatment	Not reversible

3. **Alzheimer's disease** is the most common cause of dementia in older adults. It is marked by impaired memory and thinking skills. This disease is classified into three stages:

   a. Stage 1: Mild
      1) Memory lapses
         a) Losing or misplacing items
         b) Difficulty concentrating and organizing
         c) Unable to remember material just read
         d) Still able to perform ADLs
         e) Short-term memory loss noticeable to close relations
   b. Stage 2: Moderate
      1) Forgetting events of one's own history
         a) Difficulty performing tasks that require planning and organizing (e.g., paying bills, managing money)
         b) Difficulty with complex mental arithmetic
         c) Personality and behavioral changes: appearing withdrawn or subdued, especially in social or mentally challenging situations; compulsive, repetitive actions
         d) Changes in sleep patterns
         e) Can wander and get lost
         f) Can be incontinent
         g) Clinical findings that are noticeable to others

   c. Stage 3: Severe
      1) Losing ability to converse with others
         a) Assistance required for ADLs
         b) Incontinence
         c) Losing awareness of one's environment
         d) Progressing difficulty with physical abilities (e.g., walking, sitting, and eventually swallowing)
         e) Eventually loses all ability to move; can develop stupor and coma
         f) Death frequently related to choking or infection

4. Medications for Clients who have Alzheimer's Disease
   a. Cholinesterase Inhibitors
      1) Donepezil
      2) Galantamine
   b. NMDA Antagonist
      1) Memantine
   c. SSRIs
      1) Citalopram
      2) Paroxetine
   d. Anti-anxiety Agents
      1) Lorazepam
      2) Oxazepam

5. **Nursing Interventions** for Dementia
   a. Evaluate the client's level of cognitive and daily functioning.
   b. Identify any threats to client's safety.
   c. Review all medications the client is taking.
   d. Interview family members to obtain a full history.
   e. Use short, simple words and phrases.
   f. Speak slowly.
   g. Have clocks, calendars, and personal items in clear view.
   h. Explore how well the family understands the disease progression.
   i. Review resources available to the family.
   j. Maintain consistent routine.

6. **Nursing Interventions** for Delirium
   a. Establish the client's baseline level of consciousness by interviewing family members.
   b. Assess vital signs and perform neurological checks.
   c. Assess for acute onset and fluctuating levels of consciousness.
   d. Assess the client's ability to function in the immediate environment.
   e. Determine the physiologic reason delirium is occurring.
   f. Maintain safety.

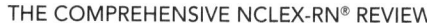

SECTION 9

Eating Disorders

A. Anorexia Nervosa

1. An eating disorder characterized by an extreme fear of gaining weight and altered perception of one's own body weight.

2. Presenting Signs and Symptoms
   a. Describes self as "fat"
   b. Preoccupation with thoughts of food
   c. Judges self-worth by body weight
   d. Low body weight
   e. Amenorrhea
   f. Cold extremities
   g. Constipation
   h. Hypotension, bradycardia
   i. Impaired renal function
   j. Hypokalemia

3. **Nursing Interventions**
   a. Develop a supportive relationship with client.
   b. Monitor electrolytes and vital signs.
   c. Monitor food and fluid intake.
   d. Set achievable weight goals.
   e. Limit exercise regimen to promote weight gain.
   f. Explore client's feelings of self-worth.
   g. Assist in the development of effective coping strategies.
   h. Encourage client attendance in behavior modification therapy.
   i. Encourage family support groups.
   j. Administer antidepressants as prescribed.
   k. Provide positive reinforcement for weight gain.

B. Bulimia Nervosa

1. An uncontrollable compulsion to consume large amounts of food in a short period (binge eating), followed by a compensatory need to rid the body of the calories consumed.
   a. Purging: Client uses self-induced vomiting, laxatives, diuretics, and enemas to lose or maintain weight.
   b. Nonpurging: Client may also compensate for binge eating through other means, such as excessive exercise.

2. Presenting Signs and Symptoms
   a. Bradycardia, hypotension
   b. Electrolyte imbalances
   c. Erosion of teeth
   d. Esophageal tears from vomiting
   e. Normal to slightly low body weight
   f. Muscle weakening
   g. Calluses/scars on hand from self-induced vomiting

3. **Nursing Interventions**
   a. Develop a supportive relationship with client.
   b. Monitor electrolytes and vital signs.
   c. Monitor food and fluid intake.
   d. Monitor the client 30 to 60 min after a meal.
   e. Monitor exercise regimen.
   f. Explore client's feelings of self-worth.
   g. Observe teeth for erosion and caries.
   h. Observe room for food hoarding.
   i. Encourage client attendance in behavior modification therapy.
   j. Encourage family support groups.
   k. Administer antidepressants as prescribed.

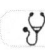

SECTION 10

Anger/Violence, Abuse, and Assault

A. **Anger and Violence**

1. Feelings that can precipitate anger: Discounted, embarrassed, guilty, humiliated, hurt, ignored, unheard, rejected, threatened, tired, and vulnerable

2. Definitions

   a. Anger is an emotional response to frustration of desires and can be expressed in a healthy way. Problems begin to occur when anger is expressed through violence.

   b. Violence is always an objectionable act that involves intentional use of force that can result in injury or death.

3. Predictors of Violence

   a. Loud voice

   b. Intense avoidance of eye contact

   c. Verbal abuse

   d. Pacing and restless

   e. Jaw clenching, rigid posture

   f. Stone silence

   g. Alcohol or drug intoxication

4. **Cycle of Violence**

   a. **Tension-Building Stage** is characterized by minor incidents by the abuser, such as pushing and verbal abuse. The victim often accepts blame.

   b. **Battering Stage** is characterized by the abuser releasing built-up tension by beating the victim brutally. The victim may try to cover the injury or look for help.

   c. **Honeymoon Stage** is characterized by kindness and loving behaviors such as flowers given by the abuser. The victim is hopeful and wants to believe the abuser will change.

CYCLE OF VIOLENCE

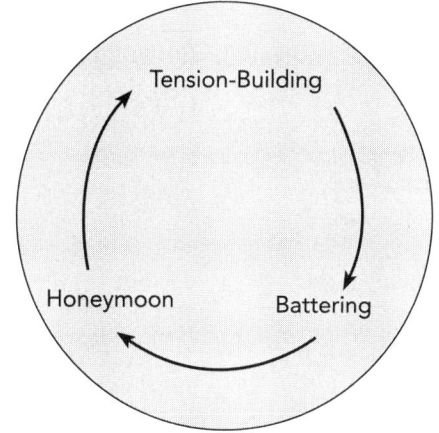

5. **Nursing Interventions**

   a. De-escalation

      1) Maintain a calm approach.

      2) Use short, simple sentences.

      3) Avoid verbal struggles/conflict.

      4) Identify patient's perceived need.

      5) Assess for stressors.

      6) Use a nonaggressive posture.

      7) Maintain client's self-esteem/dignity.

      8) Maintain a large personal space.

   b. Medications

      1) Anti-anxiety Agents

         a) Lorazepam

         b) Alprazolam

         c) Diazepam

      2) Antipsychotics

         a) Haloperidol

         b) Chlorpromazine

   c. Restraints and Seclusion

      1) Restraints are a manual method to prevent client movement with the intention to protect the client from self-harm or assaulting others.

      2) Seclusion is the involuntary confinement of a client alone in a room. The goal is always centered around the safety of the client and others and is never punitive.

B. **Abuse**

1. **Physical abuse** is the infliction of physical pain or bodily harm (e.g., hitting, choking).

2. **Sexual abuse** is any form of sexual contact or exposure without consent. This is often referred to as assault when referring to adults.

3. **Emotional abuse** is the infliction of mental anguish such as threatening or intimidating.

4. **Neglect** can be physical or emotional and includes failure to meet the needs of education and appropriate medical care.

5. **Economic abuse** is the withholding of financial support or illegal use of funds for one's personal gain.

THE VICTIM INTERVIEW

DO	DO NOT
Conduct the interview in private.	Try to prove abuse.
	Display horror, anger, or shock.
Be direct, honest, and professional.	Place blame or make judgments.
Be understanding and attentive.	Force anyone to remove clothing.
Assess for client safety.	

c. **Sexual Assault**

1. Any type of sexual activity to which the victim does not consent, ranging from inappropriate touching to penetration.

2. Rape is nonconsensual vaginal, anal, or oral penetration obtained by force or by threat of bodily harm, or when consent is unobtainable.

   a. Drugs associated with date rape

      1) Gamma-hydroxybutyrate (GHB) produces relaxation, euphoria, and disinhibition.

      2) Flunitrazepam causes sedation, muscle relaxation, and amnesia.

      3) Ketamine causes a dreamlike state and compliance of the victim.

3. Rape Trauma Syndrome

   a. This is a variant of PTSD that can last for weeks following rape. Symptoms can include feelings of numbness, disbelief, fear, denial, flashbacks, and emotional lability.

4. **Nursing Interventions**

   a. Use a nonjudgmental and empathic approach.

   b. Assess, treat, and document all injuries.

   c. Provide a private environment and limit personnel who examine the client.

   d. Assess client emotions and provide support.

REVIEW FOR ANGER/VIOLENCE, ABUSE, AND ASSAULT

Match the following.

____ 1. A nonpunitive intervention used to protect the client from harming self or others

____ 2. A stage of violence in which gifts and apologies are administered

____ 3. Anti-anxiety agent

____ 4. The failure to make educational provisions for a child

____ 5. Intense eye contact

____ 6. Antipsychotic

a. Lorazepam

b. Seclusion

c. Predictor of violence

d. Honeymoon

e. Haloperidol

f. Neglect

Answer Key: 1. B; 2. D; 3. A; 4. F; 5. C; 6. E

Trauma- and Stressor-Related Disorders

A. **Acute Stress Disorder (ASD)**

1. Definition: Diagnosed 3 days to 1 month after exposure to a highly traumatic event. May cause change in mood, sleep patterns, and physiologic reactivity.

B. **Posttraumatic Stress Disorder (PTSD)**

1. Definition: Diagnosed after 1 month to months or years after a traumatic event. Persistent re-experiencing of a highly traumatic event that involved actual or threatened death or serious injury to self or others to which the individual responded with intense fear, helplessness, or horror.

2. **Nursing Interventions** (ASD and PTSD):

   a. Establish therapeutic relationship.

   b. Assess for persistent re-experiencing of a highly traumatic event through dreams, flashbacks, thoughts, and images.

   c. Assess for suicidal ideation or violence.

   d. Assess family and social support.

   e. Assess for current life stressors and social withdrawal.

   f. Assess for insomnia.

   g. Assess for agitation and restlessness.

   h. Maintain stable, nonthreatening environment.

3. Medications (ASD and PTSD):

   a. SSRIs: fluoxetine, paroxetine

   b. SNRIs: venlafaxine

   c. Tricyclic antidepressants: amitriptyline

   d. Alpha agonists: clonidine, prazosin

   e. Beta blocker: propranolol

Legal Aspects of Mental Health Nursing

A nurse who works in a mental health setting is responsible for providing ethical, competent, and safe care consistent with local, state, and federal laws.

A. **Types of Admissions**
   1. Voluntary
      a. Admits self
      b. Consents to all treatment
      c. Can refuse treatment, including medications, unless a danger to self or others
      d. Can demand and receive discharge
   2. Involuntary
      a. Client deemed by lawful authority to be a danger to self or others
      b. At the end of a specified time, the client must have a hearing or be released

B. **Informed consent required for:**
   1. Electroconvulsive therapy
   2. Medications
   3. Seclusion
   4. Restraints

C. **Client Rights**
   1. Clients diagnosed and/or hospitalized with a mental health disorder are guaranteed the same civil rights as any other citizens.
      a. Right to plan of care
      b. Right to receive or refuse treatment
      c. Access to stationery and postage
      d. Receipt of unopened mail
      e. Visits by health care provider, attorney, or clergy
      f. Daily interaction with visitors or phone access
      g. Right to have and/or spend money
      h. Storage space for personal items
      i. Right to own property, vote, and marry
      j. Right to make wills and contracts
      k. Access to educational resources
      l. Right to sue, or be sued, including challenging one's hospitalization

Point to Remember

A nurse's priority is to promote and provide care to a client in the least restrictive environment possible.

Maternal and Newborn Nursing

Female Reproductive System

I Reproduction

A. **Reproductive Organs**

1. Ovaries
2. Fallopian tubes
3. Uterus
4. Cervix
5. Vagina

B. **Fertilization and Fetal Development**

1. Conception (i.e., fertilization): union of sperm and ovum
2. Conditions necessary for fertilization
   a. Mature egg and sperm
   b. Timing
      1) Lifetime of ovum is 24 hr.
      2) Lifetime of sperm in female genital tract is 72 hr.
      3) Menstruation begins approximately 14 days after ovulation if conception has not occurred.
   c. Vaginal and cervical secretions
      1) Less acidic during ovulation (sperm cannot survive in a highly acidic environment)
      2) Thinner during ovulation (sperm can penetrate more easily)
   d. Process of fertilization (7 to 10 days)
      1) Ovulation occurs.
      2) Ovum travels to fallopian tube.
      3) Sperm travels to fallopian tube.
      4) One sperm penetrates the ovum.
      5) Zygote forms (i.e., fertilized egg).
      6) Zygote migrates to uterus.
      7) Zygote implants in uterine wall.
      8) Progesterone and estrogen are secreted by the corpus luteum to maintain the lining of the uterus and prevent menstruation until the placenta starts producing these hormones. (Progesterone is a thermogenic hormone that raises body temperature, an objective sign that ovulation has occurred.)
3. Placental development
   a. Chorionic villi
      1) Secrete human chorionic gonadotropin (hCG), which stimulates production of estrogen and progesterone from the corpus luteum.
         a) Production of hCG begins on the day of implantation and can be detected by day 6.
      2) Burrow into the endometrium, forming the placenta.
   b. Placental hormones
      1) hCG
      2) Human chorionic somatomammotropin (hCS): acts as growth hormone and insulin antagonist
      3) Estrogen and progesterone

4. Fetal membranes develop and surround the fetus.
   a. Amnion: inner membrane
   b. Chorion: outer membrane
5. Umbilical cord
   a. Two arteries carry deoxygenated blood to the placenta.
   b. One vein carries oxygenated blood to the fetus.
   c. No pain receptors
   d. Encased in Wharton's jelly (thick substance that surrounds the umbilical cord and acts as a buffer, preventing pressure on the vein and arteries in the umbilical cord)
   e. Covered by chorionic membrane
6. Amniotic fluid
   a. Replaced every 3 hr
   b. 800 to 1,200 mL at end of pregnancy
   c. Functions: temperature regulation, protection, and promotes musculoskeletal development of the fetus

Pregnancy

I Prenatal Period

Begins with conception and ends before birth.

A. **Anatomy and Physiology**

1. **Female anatomy**: hormones, ovulation, organs
2. **Male anatomy**: sperm, vas deferens, seminal fluid
3. **Fetal/maternal circulation**: fetal and maternal blood do not mix

PSYCHOLOGICAL AND PHYSIOLOGICAL ADAPTATIONS OF PREGNANCY

TRIMESTER	NURSING INTERVENTIONS
Ambivalence	
1st	Assess meaning of pregnancy to the client/partner and socioeconomic supports; refer if needed.
Accepting	
2nd	Assess if ambivalence is increased and how the client views the fetus.
Preparing for birth	
3rd	Teach manifestations of onset of labor, newborn care, feeding methods, birth control, and home preparations for baby. Review birthing plan.
Skin: striae, linea nigra, chloasma	
2nd, 3rd	Discuss that commercial treatments are not useful; pigmentation usually disappears after pregnancy; striae may fade.
Breasts: size, striae, tenderness	
1st	Teach that fullness and sensitivity are hormone-related. Instruct about supportive bra and that over-the-counter products do not reduce stretch marks.

TRIMESTER	🩺 NURSING INTERVENTIONS

Breasts: colostrum

2nd, 3rd	Teach that colostrum may be expressed as early as 16 weeks. Discuss breast care: pads; nipple care: keep dry.

Respiratory: dyspnea

2nd, 3rd	Sleep propped or sitting up. Lightening (fetus begins descent into pelvis) between 38 to 40 weeks; can breathe easier.

Cardiovascular: faintness and syncope

2nd	Encourage moderate exercise, deep breathing, side-lying position; avoid sudden changes in position.

Cardiovascular: varicose veins

2nd, 3rd	Assess activity: sitting/standing, constrictive clothing, crossing legs. Teach leg elevation, position changes, support hose, exercise.

GI: nausea/vomiting

1st	Teach diet: dry crackers, five to six small meals, ginger, raspberry. Avoid fried, odorous, spicy foods and foods with strong smells. Assess weight, urine output (UO), and signs of hyperemesis. Teach to call if cannot eat/drink for more than 24 hr, urine becomes scant and dark, heart pounds, or client becomes dizzy.

GI: constipation

2nd, 3rd	Teach about activity, fluids, fiber.

GI: heartburn

2nd, 3rd	Encourage small meals; sit upright for 30 min or more after eating; avoid spicy, fatty foods. Drink hot herbal tea.

GU: frequency

1st, 3rd	Assess for urinary tract infection (UTI). Teach frequent voiding; do not decrease fluids. Urinate after intercourse. Call provider if dysuria, cloudy or foul-smelling urine, flank pain. Kegel exercises.

GU: leukorrhea

2nd, 3rd	Teach that this is normal; do not douche; maintain good hygiene; wear perineal pads; report if accompanied by pruritus, foul odor, or change in character.

GU: Braxton Hicks

2nd, 3rd	Teach difference between Braxton Hicks and true labor. (See the table on false vs. true labor in this unit.)

Nutrition

1st, 2nd, 3rd	Assess/teach weight gain patterns; average weight gain 25 to 35 lb; caloric increase 300 to 400 kcal/day; protein increase by 25 g/day; iron intake 30 mg/day; folate intake 600 mcg/day; prenatal vitamins. Limit caffeine intake.

SIGNS/SYMPTOMS OF PREGNANCY

Presumptive — Subjective signs/symptoms

Amenorrhea

Fatigue

Nausea and vomiting

Urinary frequency

Breast changes: darkened areola, enlarged Montgomery's tubules

Quickening: slight fluttering movements of the fetus felt by the client, usually between 16 to 20 weeks of gestation

Probable — Objective signs

Cervical changes

Hegar's sign: softening and compressibility of lower uterus

Chadwick's sign: deepened violet-bluish color of vaginal mucosa secondary to increased vascularity of the area

Goodell's sign: softening of cervical tip

Ballottement: rebound of unengaged fetus

Braxton Hicks contractions: false contractions, painless, irregular, and usually relieved by walking

Positive pregnancy test

Positive — Signs related to presence of fetus

Fetal heart tones

Visualization of fetus by ultrasound

Fetal movement palpated by an experienced examiner

B. **Verifying Pregnancy**

1. Serum and urine tests provide an accurate assessment for the presence of human chorionic gonadotropin (hCG).

2. hCG can be detected 6 to 11 days in serum and 26 days in urine after conception following implantation.

   a. Production begins with implantation, peaks at about 60 to 70 days of gestation, and then declines until around 80 days of pregnancy, when it begins to gradually increase until term.

   b. Higher levels can indicate multifetal pregnancy, ectopic pregnancy, hydatidiform mole (gestational trophoblastic disease), or a genetic abnormality such as Down syndrome.

   c. Lower blood levels of hCG may suggest a miscarriage or ectopic pregnancy. Some medications (e.g., anticonvulsants, diuretics, tranquilizers) can cause false–positive or false–negative pregnancy results.

C. **Calculating Delivery Date**

1. Nägele's rule: Formula for calculating estimated date of confinement (EDC) or estimated date of birth (EDB). To calculate EDB, subtract 3 months and add 7 days to the first day of the last menstrual period.

2. McDonald's rule: Measure uterine fundal height in centimeters from the symphysis pubis to the top of the uterine fundus. Between 18 and 32 weeks of gestation, the fundal height measurement should approximate gestational age.

D. **Antepartum Fetal Assessment**

1. Ultrasound

   a. Indications for Use

      1) Confirm pregnancy and location (i.e., uterine vs. ectopic).

      2) Evaluate fetus: number, heartbeat, gestational age, abnormalities, growth and development, activity (BPP).

      3) Evaluate placenta: location (i.e., previa or abruptio), grading.

      4) Evaluate amniotic fluid volume.

   b. **Nursing Interventions**

      1) Preparation of a client

         a) Explain the procedure.

         b) Ensure client has a full bladder.

2. Nonstress Test (NST)

   a. Most widely used test for evaluating fetal well-being

   b. Noninvasive

   c. Monitors response of the fetal heart rate (FHR) to fetal movement

   d. Indications for Use

      1) Assess for fetal well-being and an intact CNS during the third trimester.

   2) Assess fetus of clients with high-risk pregnancies (e.g., maternal diabetes mellitus, hypertension, heart disease, IUGR, postdates, history of previous stillbirth, or decreased fetal movement).

   e. Interpretation of Findings

      1) Reactive NST (normal)

         a) Two or more fetal heart rate accelerations (increase in FHR of at least 15/min above the baseline and last 15 seconds) within a 20-min period.

         b) Before 32 weeks gestation, acceleration is defined as increase of at least 10 beats/min lasting at least 10 seconds in FHR.

      2) Nonreactive NST (abnormal)

         a) Does not produce two or more qualifying accelerations in 20 min.

         b) If does not meet criteria in 40 min, additional testing is indicated: contraction stress test (CST) or biophysical profile (BPP).

   f. **Nursing Interventions**

      1) Seat the client in a reclining chair or place in a semi-Fowler's or left-lateral position.

      2) Apply two belts and transducers to the client's abdomen.

REACTIVE NST

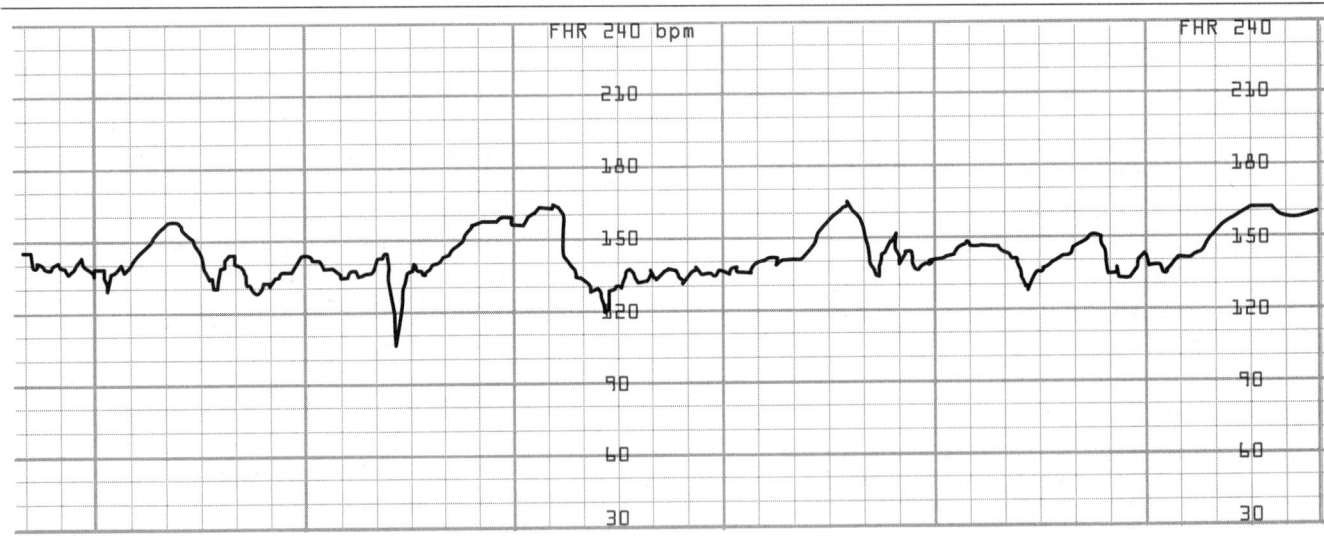

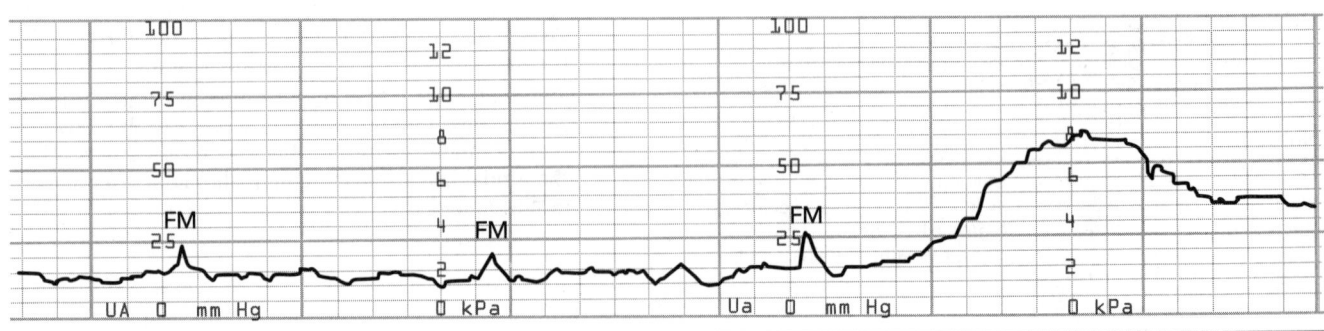

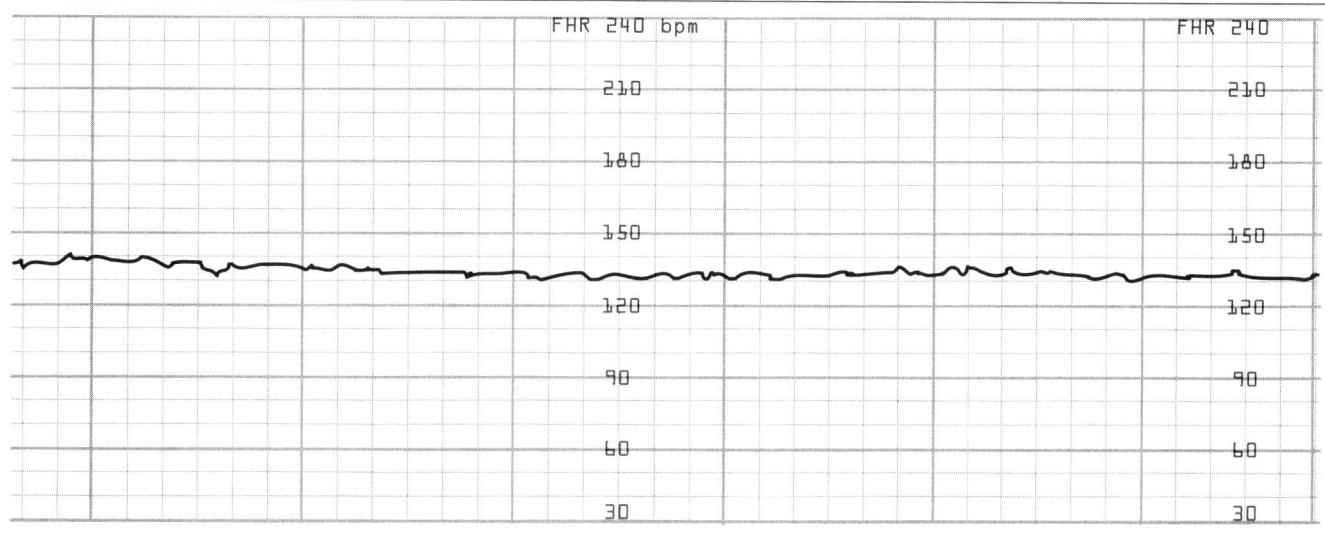

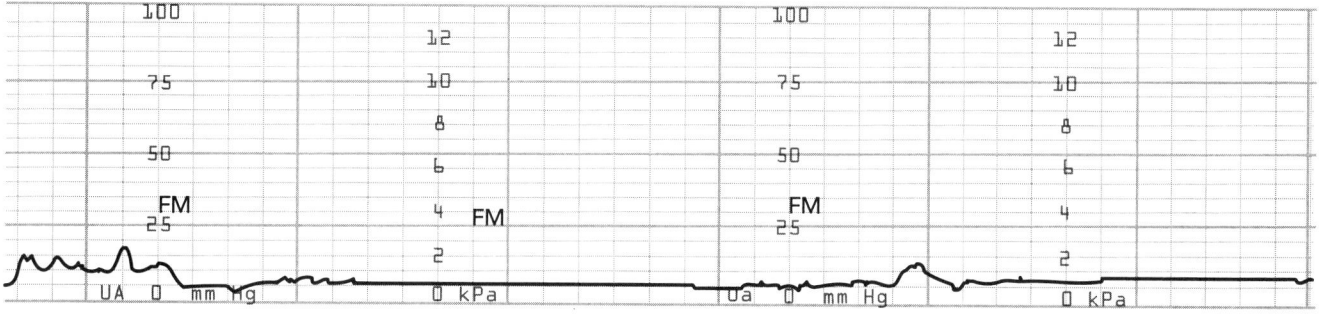

3. Contraction Stress Test (CST)

a. Method

1) Nipple stimulation

2) Oxytocin (Pitocin) IV

b. Indications for Use

1) Nonreactive NST

2) High-risk pregnancies; same as indications for NST

c. **Nursing Interventions**

1) Explain procedure and obtain informed consent.

2) Obtain baseline FHR, fetal movement, and contraction pattern 10 to 20 min before and 30 min afterward.

3) Initiate method and observe for uterine tachysystole (hyperstimulation).

4) Obtain at least three contractions in a 10-min period, each lasting 40 to 60 seconds.

5) Maintain bed rest during the procedure.

d. Interpretation of Findings

1) Test results are either negative, positive, equivocal, suspicious, or unsatisfactory.

2) Negative CST (normal)

a) At least three uterine contractions in 10 min, with no late decelerations

b) Reassuring finding

3) Positive CST (abnormal)

a) Late decelerations occur with 50% or more of contractions

b) Nonreassuring finding

c) Suggestive of uteroplacental insufficiency

4. Biophysical Profile (BPP)

   a. Uses real-time ultrasound to visualize physiological characteristics of the fetus.

   b. Assesses five variables: fetal breathing movements, gross body movements, fetal heart rate, reactive FHR (NST), amniotic fluid volume.

   c. Award score of 0 (abnormal finding) or 2 (normal finding) to each variable.

BIOPHYSICAL PROFILE

Fetal breathing movements

NORMAL SCORE:	2	At least 1 episode of 30 seconds in 30 min
ABNORMAL SCORE:	0	Absent or less than 30 seconds duration

Gross body movements

NORMAL SCORE:	2	At least 3 body or limb extensions with return to flexion in 30 min
ABNORMAL SCORE:	0	Less than 3 episodes

Fetal tone

NORMAL SCORE:	2	At least 1 episode of extension with return to flexion
ABNORMAL SCORE:	0	Slow extension and flexion, lack of flexion, or absence of movement

Reactive FHR

NORMAL SCORE:	2	Reactive NST
ABNORMAL SCORE:	0	Nonreactive NST

Amniotic fluid volume

NORMAL SCORE:	2	At least 1 pocket of fluid equal to or greater than 2 cm, or more than 5 cm total fluid
ABNORMAL SCORE:	0	Pockets absent or less than 5 cm total

Total Score

The score will be even numbers only ranging from 0 to 10.
Normal = 8 to 10
Equivocal/borderline = 6
Abnormal = 0 to 4

5. Amniocentesis

   a. Early Pregnancy

      1) Genetic work-up for fetal anomalies (e.g., Down syndrome, trisomy 18, trisomy 13)

      2) Detect presence of AChE in neural tube defects (NTDs)

      3) Performed at 14 to 16 weeks

   b. Late in Pregnancy

      1) Assess fetal lung maturity and fetal well-being.

      2) L:S ratio of 2:1 indicates fetal lung maturity.

   c. **Nursing Interventions** for Amniocentesis

      1) Preprocedure: Explain procedure and risks to client and obtain informed consent.

      2) Ensure client has a patent IV.

      3) Postprocedure

         a) Monitor FHR, fetal activity.

         b) Assess for signs of labor.

         c) Assess for vaginal bleeding or hemorrhage.

         d) Administer Rho(D) immune globulin (RhoGAM) if client is Rh-negative.

      4) Education on complications to report

         a) Bleeding

         b) Contractions

         c) Signs and symptoms of infection

NOTE: According to the NCLEX® scope of practice, only RNs may administer RhoGAM IM. It is a blood product!

6. Percutaneous Umbilical Blood Sampling (PUBS)

   a. Also referred to as cordocentesis

   b. Direct access to fetal circulation

   c. Used for fetal blood sampling and transfusion

   d. Performed in high-risk centers

   e. In many centers, replaced by placental biopsy

7. Chorionic Villi Sampling

   a. Obtain sample of chorionic villi (i.e., placental) tissue.

   b. Assess fetal genetic abnormalities.

   c. Performed transcervical or transabdominal.

   d. Performed during the first trimester.

   e. Similar risk and nursing interventions as amniocentesis.

8. Maternal Serum Alpha-Fetoprotein Screening (MSAFP)

   a. Screening tool for NTDs

   b. Ideally performed at 16 to 18 weeks

   c. Lower than normal levels—follow up for Down syndrome

   d. Higher than normal levels—follow up for neural tube defects

E. **Fetal Assessment**

   1. FHR normal range is 110 to 160/min.

   2. Fundal height used to evaluate gestational age and growth of fetus.

   3. Fetal activity: kick counts or daily fetal movement counts.

      a. Contact provider if fetal movement decreases or ceases entirely for 12 hr.

      b. Contact if less than 10 kicks/2 hr.

      c. Try to do at the same time each day.

      d. Most active after meals and in the evening.

      e. Fetal movement may be decreased by drugs, including alcohol and cigarette smoke.

      f. Obesity may hinder the sensation of fetal activity.

II Obstetrical Terminology

A. **Pregnancy Outcome**

1. Gravidity: number of pregnancies

2. Parity: number of pregnancies that reach viability (20 weeks),

3. Five-digit system (GTPAL)

   a. **G** – Gravidity (i.e., number of pregnancies including this pregnancy)

   b. **T** – Term births (38 weeks or more)

   c. **P** – Preterm births (from 20 weeks up to 37 completed weeks)

   d. **A** – Abortions/miscarriages (prior to viability)

   e. **L** – Living children

III Collaborative Care

A. **Prenatal Care**

1. Initial Exam

   a. Psychosocial assessment

   b. Complete history, including medications, pertinent history from partner, family history of genetic concerns

   c. Complete physical

   d. Baseline laboratory values

      1) CBC

      2) Blood type and Rh

      3) Urinalysis

      4) STI screen, including:

         a) HIV

         b) Rubella titer

         c) Hepatitis B

   e. Nutritional counseling (See the table on psychological and physiological adaptations of pregnancy in this unit.)

   f. Teratogens: Fetus especially vulnerable during first trimester

      1) Drugs

         a) Category C and D medications such as warfarin, lithium, methimazole, phenytoin, tetracycline, and antipsychotics

         b) Illegal drugs

      2) Cigarettes and alcohol

         a) Smoking increases incidence of abortion, prematurity, SGA, and SIDS.

         b) Quantity of alcohol to produce fetal effects is unclear: IUGR, CNS malformation, neurologic problems.

      3) Thermal risks and radiation

         a) Avoid hot tubs, long baths, or excessively hot showers.

      4) Infections

         a) Group B Strep

            (1) Culture obtained at 35 to 36 weeks.

            (2) Treat positive culture with PCN IVPB every 4 hr during labor.

            (3) Monitor newborn for infection.

         b) TORCH

            (1) **T** – Toxoplasmosis

            (2) **O** – Other (e.g., syphilis, varicella, parvovirus)

            (3) **R** – Rubella

            (4) **C** – Cytomegalovirus

            (5) **H** – Herpes infections

         c) See the table on sexually transmitted infections in this unit.

2. Initial and Subsequent Exams

   a. Weight

   b. Fundal height

   c. FHR

   d. Fetal activity (include date of quickening)

   e. Urine check for glucose and protein

   f. Anticipatory guidance. (See the table on psychological and physiological adaptations of pregnancy in this unit.) Review when to contact provider.

      1) Rupture of membranes prior to 37 weeks

      2) Abdominal or back pain (contractions) before 37 weeks

      3) Vaginal bleeding

      4) Elevated temperature

      5) Dysuria, oliguria

      6) Severe headache with vision changes

3. 16 to 22 weeks

   a. Screen for NTDs with maternal serum alpha-fetoprotein.

4. 28 weeks

   a. Screen for diabetes mellitus.

   b. Administer Rho(D) immune globulin (RhoGAM) if Rh-negative.

   c. Begin NST testing twice a week for any pregnancy at risk for intrauterine fetal death.

5. 35 weeks

   a. Test for group B strep.

B. **Anticipatory care:** Do not assume symptoms are normal adaptations of pregnancy—assess.

   1. Physiological Changes

      a. Physiological changes in pregnancy are the result of hormone production and the enlarging uterus.

PHYSIOLOGICAL CHANGES

SYSTEM	CHANGES
Reproductive	Uterus increases in size, shape, position Ovulation and menses cease
Cardiovascular	Increased cardiac output and blood volume Increased heart rate Increased coagulation
Respiratory	Increased maternal oxygen needs Uterine enlargement displaces diaphragm, causing increased respiratory rate and decreased total lung capacity
Musculoskeletal	Pelvic joint relaxation Body alterations require adjustment in posture Separation of rectus abdominis muscles
Gastrointestinal	Nausea and vomiting, slowed digestive processes, constipation
Renal	Increased glomerular filtration, urinary frequency
Endocrine/Metabolic	Increased hormone production (hCG, progesterone, estrogen, hCS, and prostaglandins) Increased thyroid and parathyroid activity; insulin resistance
Integument	Hyperpigmentation causing chloasma, linea nigra, striae gravidarum, and palmar erythema

      b. Changes in physical appearance may lead to a negative body image. The client may make statements of resentment toward the pregnancy and express anxiousness for the pregnancy to be over soon.

   2. Expected Vital Signs

      a. Blood pressure

         1) Within the prepregnancy range during first trimester

         2) Decreases 5 to 10 mm Hg during second trimester

         3) Position affects blood pressure; supine position may cause supine hypotensive syndrome or vena cava syndrome. Signs and symptoms include dizziness, lightheadedness, and pale, clammy skin. Interventions include left-lateral side, semi-Fowler's position, or wedge under one hip if supine.

      b. Pulse

         1) Increases by 10 to 15/min around 20 weeks

      c. Respirations

         1) Increases by 1 to 2/min due to elevation of the diaphragm

   3. Fetal Heart Tones

      a. Normal baseline rate 110 to 160/min

      b. Accelerations are reassuring, indicate intact fetal CNS

Complications of Pregnancy

I Medical Problems

Preexisting conditions may complicate pregnancy. Some medical conditions develop during pregnancy and cause complications.

> **NOTE:** Remember that only the RN may care for or assess high-risk or unstable clients, according to the NCLEX® scope of practice.

A. **Cardiac Disease**

   1. Contributing Factors

      a. Preexisting heart condition

      b. Increased maternal plasma volume

   2. Greatest Risks for Heart Failure

      a. End of second trimester (28 to 32 weeks)

      b. During labor

      c. After delivery (first 48 hr)

   3. Manifestations

      a. Subjective data

         1) Dizziness

         2) Shortness of breath

         3) Weakness

         4) Fatigue

         5) Chest pain on exertion

         6) Anxiety

      b. Objective data: physical assessment findings

         1) Arrhythmias

         2) Irregular heart rate

         3) Tachycardia

         4) Heart murmur

         5) Distended jugular veins

         6) Cyanosis of nails or lips

         7) Pallor

         8) Generalized edema

         9) Diaphoresis

         10) Increased respirations

         11) Moist, frequent cough

         12) Hemoptysis

         13) Crackles at base of lungs

         14) Intrauterine growth restriction

         15) Decreased amniotic fluid

         16) FHR with decreased variability

   4. Laboratory and Diagnostic Testing

      a. Laboratory tests

         1) Hgb

         2) Hct

         3) WBC

         4) Chemistry profile

         5) Sedimentation rate

         6) Maternal ABGs

         7) Clotting studies

b. Other diagnostic procedures
   1) Echocardiogram
   2) Holter monitoring
   3) Chest x-ray
   4) Ultrasound
   5) Pulse oximetry
   6) NST
   7) Biophysical profile
5. Collaborative Care
   a. **Nursing Interventions**
      1) Assess for signs and symptoms of fatigue, anemia, weight gain more than 1 to 2 lb/week, pulmonary edema, peripheral edema, palpitations, tachycardia, angina.
      2) Prevent infection.
      3) Provide nutritional counseling; well-balanced diet with iron and folic acid.
   b. **Medications**: Pharmacological management is determined by the client's cardiac diagnoses and clinical presentation.
      1) Propranolol: beta blocker; used to treat tachyarrhythmias and to lower maternal blood pressure
      2) Ampicillin antibiotic; prophylaxis given to prevent endocarditis
      3) Heparin sodium: anticoagulant used in treating clients with pulmonary embolus, deep-vein thrombosis, prosthetic valves, cyanotic heart defects, and rheumatic heart disease
      4) Digoxin: cardiac glycoside; used to increase cardiac output during pregnancy, and may be prescribed if fetal tachycardia is present
      5) Anticoagulant therapy (heparin)
         a) Teach bleeding precautions
         b) Report any bleeding

B. **Hypertension in pregnancy:** Hypertensive disease in pregnancy is divided into clinical subsets: gestational hypertension; mild and severe preeclampsia; eclampsia; hemolysis, elevated liver enzymes, and low platelets (HELLP) syndrome.

1. **Vasospasm** contributing to poor tissue perfusion is the underlying mechanism for the signs and symptoms of pregnancy hypertensive disorders.
2. **Gestational hypertension (GH)**
   a. Begins after the 20th week of pregnancy.
   b. Presents with elevated blood pressure of 140/90 mm Hg or greater on two occasions, at least 4 hr apart, within 1 week.
   c. There is no proteinuria.
   d. Blood pressure returns to baseline by 6 weeks postpartum.
3. **Mild preeclampsia is GH** with the addition of proteinuria of 1 to 2+.

4. **Severe preeclampsia**
   a. Blood pressure 160/110 mm Hg or greater on two separate occasions 6 hr apart on bed rest
   b. Proteinuria greater than 3+ (dipstick)
   c. Oliguria
   d. Serum creatinine greater than 1.1 mg/dL
   e. Cerebral or visual disturbances (e.g., headache and blurred vision)
   f. Hyperreflexia with possible ankle clonus
   g. Pulmonary or cardiac involvement
   h. Extensive peripheral edema
   i. Hepatic dysfunction (elevated liver function tests)
   j. Epigastric and right upper-quadrant pain
   k. Thrombocytopenia
5. **Eclampsia**
   a. Severe preeclampsia, plus seizure activity
   b. Usually preceded by persistent headache, blurred vision, severe epigastric or right upper quadrant abdominal pain, and altered mental status
6. **HELLP** syndrome is a variant of GH in which hematologic conditions coexist with severe preeclampsia involving hepatic dysfunction. HELLP syndrome is diagnosed by laboratory tests, not clinically.
   a. **H** – hemolysis resulting in anemia and jaundice
   b. **EL** – elevated liver enzymes resulting in elevated ALT and AST, epigastric pain, and nausea and vomiting
   c. **LP** – low platelets (less than 100,000/mm³), resulting in thrombocytopenia, abnormal bleeding and clotting time, bleeding gums, petechiae, and possibly DIC

NOTE: Gestational hypertensive disease and chronic hypertension may occur simultaneously. Gestational hypertensive diseases are associated with placental abruption, acute renal failure, hepatic rupture, preterm birth, and fetal and maternal death.

7. Contributing Factors
   a. No single profile identifies risks for gestational hypertensive disorders, but some high risks include:
      1) Maternal age younger than 20 or older than 40
      2) First pregnancy
      3) Morbid obesity
      4) Multifetal gestation
      5) Chronic renal disease
      6) Chronic hypertension
      7) Familial history of preeclampsia
      8) Diabetes mellitus
      9) Rh incompatibility
      10) Molar pregnancy
      11) Previous history of GH

8. Manifestations of Preeclampsia (vary depending upon severity)

 a. Hypertension

 b. Proteinuria: 1+ or greater on dipstick, or 300 mg in 24-hr urine specimen

 c. CNS irritability: headaches, hyperreflexia, positive ankle clonus

 d. Visual disturbances: scotoma, blurred or double vision

 e. Decreased liver perfusion: elevated liver enzyme (LDH, AST, ALT), epigastric or right-upper quadrant pain

 f. Decreased renal perfusion: proteinuria, oliguria

 g. Decreased plasma colloid osmotic pressure: elevated Hct, tissue edema with weight gain, pulmonary edema

 h. Elevated plasma uric acid

9. Laboratory and Diagnostic Testing

 a. Blood pressure elevation

 b. Urine studies: urinalysis for proteinuria, 24-hr urine protein

 c. Liver enzymes, serum creatinine, BUN, uric acid

10. Collaborative Care

 a. **Nursing Interventions**

 1) Monitor blood pressure.

 2) Administer medications.

 3) Discuss nutrition (balanced diet; 60 to 70 g protein, 1,200 mg calcium, 600 mcg folic acid; limit salty foods; eat foods with roughage; avoid alcohol and tobacco; and limit caffeine intake).

 4) Perform maternal assessments: daily weight, I&O, reflexes, CNS.

 5) Obtain fetal assessments: serial ultrasound, Doppler blood flow analysis; NST, CST, BPP; fetal kick count.

 6) Encourage bed rest on left side.

 7) Initiate seizure precautions (preeclampsia/eclampsia).

 8) Provide quiet environment: private room not next to nurses' station, dim lights.

 9) Monitor for HELLP and DIC (severe preeclampsia/eclampsia).

NOTE: Immediately after a seizure, client may be confused and combative. Restraints may be temporarily needed. Do not leave client alone.

 b. Medications

 1) Antihypertensive medications to keep blood pressure less than 160/110 mm Hg

 2) Magnesium sulfate: anticonvulsant

 a) Administer IV magnesium sulfate, which is the medication of choice for prophylaxis or treatment. Reduces seizure threshold (depression of the CNS); secondary side effect is decreased blood pressure as it relaxes smooth muscles.

 b) **Nursing Interventions**

 (1) Use an infusion control device to maintain a regular flow rate.

 (2) Inform the client that she may initially feel flushed, hot, and sedated with the magnesium sulfate bolus. Nausea/vomiting may occur.

 (3) Monitor vital signs; blood pressure, pulse, respirations; CNS; level of consciousness, headache or visual disturbances, reflexes; renal perfusion; output (of indwelling urinary catheter); epigastric pain; FHR.

 (4) Place the client on fluid restriction of 100 to 125 mL/hr, and maintain a urinary output of 30 mL/hr or greater.

 (5) Monitor the client for signs of magnesium sulfate toxicity.

 (a) Absence of patellar deep tendon reflexes

 (b) Urine output less than 30 mL/hr

 (c) Respirations less than 12/min

 (d) Decreased level of consciousness

 (e) Cardiac dysrhythmias

NOTE: If magnesium toxicity is suspected, discontinue magnesium infusion immediately. Administer calcium gluconate and notify provider. Take actions to prevent respiratory or cardiac arrest.

C. **Diabetes Mellitus**

 1. Types

 a. Pregestational diabetes mellitus: Client had diabetes prior to pregnancy.

 b. Gestational diabetes mellitus: An impaired tolerance to glucose with the first onset or recognition during pregnancy. The ideal blood glucose level during pregnancy is 70 to 110 mg/dL. Client develops diabetes mellitus during pregnancy, usually in the second or third trimester.

 2. Contributing Factors

 a. Obesity

 b. Maternal age older than 25 years

 c. Family history of diabetes mellitus

 d. Previous delivery of an infant who was large or stillborn

 3. Manifestations

 a. Hypoglycemia (nervousness, headache, weakness, irritability, hunger, blurred vision, tingling of mouth or extremities)

 b. Hyperglycemia (thirst, nausea, abdominal pain, frequent urination, flushed dry skin, fruity breath)

4. Laboratory Testing and Diagnostic Procedures
   a. Routine urinalysis with glycosuria
   b. Glucose tolerance test (50 g oral glucose load, followed by plasma glucose analysis 1 hr later performed at 24 to 28 weeks of gestation—fasting not necessary; a positive blood glucose screening is 140 mg/dL or greater; additional testing with a 3-hr glucose tolerance test is indicated)
      1) A 3-hr glucose tolerance test (following overnight fasting, avoidance of caffeine, and abstinence from smoking for 12 hr prior to testing; a fasting glucose is obtained, a 100 g glucose load is given, and serum glucose levels are determined at 1, 2, and 3 hr following glucose ingestion)
   c. Monitor HbA1c.
   d. Monitor for ketones.
   e. BPP to ascertain fetal well-being
   f. Amniocentesis with alpha-fetoprotein
   g. NST to assess fetal well-being
5. Collaborative Care
   a. Risks to newborn increase with poor glucose control.
      1) Congenital anomalies
      2) Spontaneous abortions
      3) Macrosomia: birth trauma and dystocia
      4) Death
      5) Hypoglycemia after birth
   b. **Nursing Interventions**
      1) Diet
      2) Exercise
      3) Blood glucose monitoring
      4) Insulin if medication required
   c. Medications
      1) Oral hypoglycemic, such as glyburide, is occasionally used for gestational diabetes.
         a) May require insulin
         b) Insulin needs decrease during the first trimester.
         c) Insulin needs increase during the second and third trimester due to an increase in hormones such as hCS (insulin antagonist).

D. **Hyperemesis gravidarum:** Excessive pregnancy-related nausea and/or vomiting. Hospitalization may be necessary because of dehydration and weight loss.
   1. Begins first or second month of pregnancy
   2. Contributing factors
      a. High levels of human chorionic gonadotropin (hCG) and estrogen
   3. Decreased gastric motility and gastroesophageal reflux
   4. Manifestations
      a. Loss of 5% or more of prepregnancy body weight
      b. Dehydration, causing ketosis and constipation
      c. Nutritional deficiencies
      d. Metabolic imbalances

5. Collaborative Care
   a. **Nursing Interventions**
      1) Assess psyche; refer as needed.
      2) Assess weight.
      3) Assess for dehydration, electrolyte imbalance, and metabolic alkalosis.
      4) Monitor I&O.
      5) Administer IV fluids.
      6) Small meals per client preference.
   b. Medications
      1) Antiemetics such as ondansetron
      2) Vitamin B$_6$, no more than 100 mg daily used solo or in combination with doxylamine
   c. Therapeutic Measures
      1) Acupressure; relaxation techniques
   d. Client Education
      1) Nausea and vomiting usually peak between 2 and 12 weeks of pregnancy and go away by the second half of pregnancy.
      2) **Eat small, frequent meals**; eating dry foods such as crackers may help relieve uncomplicated nausea.
      3) Increase fluid intake to prevent dehydration; teach to increase fluids during the times of the day when the client feels the least nauseated; seltzer, ginger ale, or other sparkling waters may be helpful.

Placental and Cervical Problems

A. **Abruptio Placentae**
   1. Contributing Factors
      a. Trauma
      b. Preeclampsia
      c. Multiparity
      d. Cocaine use

B. **Placenta Previa**
   1. Contributing Factors
      a. Placenta implants completely or partially over cervical os.

PLACENTA PREVIA AND ABRUPTIO PLACENTAE

	PLACENTA PREVIA	ABRUPTIO PLACENTAE
Vaginal bleeding	Usually bright red in color. Can range from minimal to severe and life-threatening.	Usually dark red in color. Can range from absent to moderate dependent on the grade of abruption.
Pain	Often none	Abdomen "boardlike" and very tender
Maternal effect	Hemorrhage, shock, death	
Fetal effect	Anoxia, CNS trauma, death	
Treatment	Partial previa might be treated with bed rest. Complete previa will be treated as with abruptio placentae.	Emotional support; immediate cesarean birth; blood transfusions, monitor for DIC.

NOTE: Vaginal exams are contraindicated with vaginal bleeding.

C. **Hydatidiform mole/molar pregnancy:** Benign abnormal growth of chorionic villi. Appears as avascular transparent grapelike clusters. May develop choriocarcinoma (rare).

1. Contributing Factors
   a. Previous use of ovulation-stimulating drugs
   b. Age extremes: early teens or over 40
   c. History of spontaneous abortion
   d. Poor nutrition
   e. Often unknown
2. Manifestations
   a. Vaginal bleeding; brown, grapelike clusters; anemia
   b. Rapid uterine growth (i.e., increase in fundal height); cramping
   c. Extreme nausea
   d. Hyperthyroidism
   e. Preeclampsia prior to 24 weeks
3. Diagnostic Testing
   a. Ultrasound
   b. Persistent, high, hCG levels
4. Collaborative Care
   a. Assess psyche
   b. Spontaneous expulsion
   c. Elective expulsion
      1) Curettage
      2) Induction not recommended
      3) RhoGAM postexpulsion if Rh-negative
      4) Postexpulsion
         a) Follow postpartum protocol.
         b) Continue to monitor hCG levels.
         c) Follow up to rule out choriocarcinoma.
         d) Discuss contraception; should avoid pregnancy for 1 year or until hCG levels return to normal.

D. **Abortion:** expulsion of the fetus prior to viability
1. Types
   a. Spontaneous
   b. Therapeutic
   c. Elective
2. Collaborative Care
   a. Provide psychological support.
   b. Assist with ultrasound.
   c. Save all passed tissue for examination.
   d. Monitor for signs of hemorrhage (perform pad count, monitor Hgb and Hct).
   e. Assess for signs of shock.
   f. Prepare for D&C.
   g. Administer Rho(D) immune globulin (RhoGAM) to Rh-negative clients.
3. Discharge Teaching
   a. Notify provider if signs of infection occur, bleeding increases, or signs of depression develop.
   b. Discuss future pregnancy plans, birth control.
   c. Provide follow-up exam.

E. **Cervical insufficiency (incompetent cervix):** premature dilation of the cervix, usually in second trimester
1. Contributing Factors
   a. Congenital
   b. Acquired
      1) History of cervical trauma
      2) Previous spontaneous delivery in second trimester
2. Manifestations
   a. Increase in pelvic pressure
   b. Pink-stained vaginal discharge or bleeding
   c. Uterine contractions
3. Diagnostic and Therapeutic Procedures
   a. Ultrasound showing short cervix (i.e., less than 25 mm in length)
   b. Prophylactic cervical cerclage; removed at 36-37 weeks
4. Collaborative Care
   a. Emotional support
   b. If able to maintain pregnancy:
      1) Bed rest
      2) Monitor client and fetus
      3) Tocolytics
      4) Hydration
      5) Cerclage (i.e., purse string suture)

F. **Ectopic pregnancy:** fertilized ovum implants outside of uterus (pelvis, abdomen, often fallopian tubes)
1. Contributing Factors
   a. Narrowing or scarring of fallopian tube: previous STI or PID; IUD; endometriosis; tubal surgery
2. Manifestations
   a. Delayed or missed irregular menses
   b. Unilateral stabbing pain and tenderness in lower abdomen
   c. Bleeding
   d. Shock (symptoms: hypotension, tachycardia, pallor).
3. Collaborative Care
   a. Provide psychological support.
   b. Replace fluids.
   c. Administer methotrexate (MTX).
   d. Prepare for surgery and postoperative care.

Labor and Delivery

Labor and Delivery

Labor and delivery include the period during which the baby and placenta are delivered and up to 1 to 2 hr after delivery.

A. **Labor and delivery processes**—Six major factors: "P's" of labor and delivery process.

1. **Psyche**—the mother's psychological response to labor

2. **Powers**—uterine contractions

   a. Uterine contractions: act to dilate and efface the cervix

      1) Frequency—From the beginning of one contraction to the beginning of the next contraction. Contraction frequency closer than 2 min is considered hyperstimulation.

      2) Duration—From the beginning to end of the same contraction. Contraction duration greater than 90 seconds is considered hyperstimulation.

      3) Intensity—Strength of the uterine contraction. Can only be accurately measured with an internal uterine pressure catheter (IUPC).

   b. Effacement—Shortening and thinning of the cervix. The goal is 100% effacement.

   c. Dilation—Opening of the cervix. The diameter of the cervix ranges from 0 cm (closed) to 10 cm (fully dilated).

3. **Passenger**—the fetus and placenta

4. **Presentation**—the part of the fetus that enters the pelvic inlet first

   a. The three primary presentations are cephalic, breech, and shoulder. Breech and shoulder presentations are indications for cesarean birth.

   b. Station—the relationship of the presenting part to the maternal ischial spines that measures the degree of descent of the fetus

      1) Negative stations are above ischial spines (−1, −2).

      2) Zero station is at the ischial spines, or engaged (0).

      3) Positive stations are below the ischial spines (+1, +2, +3). Delivery is typically sooner.

5. **Position**—Relationship of presenting part (e.g., occiput, mentum, sacrum) to the maternal pelvic inlet. Clients with fetus in persistent occiput posterior position (POP) have increase back (labor) pain and longer labors.

6. **Passageway**—the birth canal, pelvis, cervix, pelvic floor and vagina

   a. Cephalopelvic disproportion—When the fetus has a head size, shape, or position that does not allow for passage through the pelvis. This can also occur secondary to maternal pelvic structure or associated problems.

B. **Manifestations of False vs. True Labor**

FALSE VS. TRUE LABOR

FALSE LABOR	TRUE LABOR
Uterine contractions	
Braxton Hicks, irregular, do not increase in frequency or intensity. Usually felt in the lower back or the abdomen above the umbilicus. Decrease with walking or position changes. Often cease with sleep, comfort measures, oral hydration, and emptying of bladder.	May begin irregularly but become regular in frequency, become stronger and last longer. Walking can increase contraction intensity. Contractions continue despite comfort measures. Usually felt in the lower back radiating to the abdomen.
Cervical dilation and effacement	
No significant change in dilation or effacement. Cervix often stays in posterior position.	Cervical dilation and effacement steadily progress.
Bloody show	
Usually not present	Present as cervix dilates
Fetus	
Presenting part not engaged in pelvis	Presenting part engages in pelvis

C. **Nursing Care During Labor and Delivery**

1. Admission assessment includes prenatal and medical and surgical history.

2. Obtain informed consents.

3. Review birth plan.

4. Active labor is considered an emergency medical condition by the Emergency Medical Treatment and Active Labor Act (EMTALA).

5. Monitor maternal and fetal status:

   a. Vital signs and physical assessment

   b. FHR

      1) Normal rate is 110 to 160/min; varies with fetal age

      2) Variability best indicator of fetal well-being. Moderate = 6 to 25/min

      3) External: auscultation, ultrasound transducer

      4) Internal: spiral electrode

         a) Requires ruptured membranes

NOTE: Any internal monitoring increases the risk of infection.

   c. Uterine contractions

      1) External: manual or tocotransducer

      2) Internal: intrauterine pressure catheter (IUPC)

   d. Vaginal discharge

   e. Cervix

      1) Cervical exams are done with sterile gloves.

      2) Limit exams, especially if a vaginal infection is suspected or if ROM has occurred.

NOTE: Try to limit the frequency of vaginal exams secondary to the risk of infection.

NURSING CARE: STAGES OF LABOR

First Stage

Cervix dilates from 0 to 10 cm.

Three phases:

› Latent Phase: 0 to 3 cm
  » Contractions:
    › Irregular, mild-moderate
    › Frequency 5 to 30 min
    › Duration 30 to 45 seconds
  » Client talkative and excited
› Active Phase: 4 to 7 cm
  » Contractions:
    › Regular, moderate-strong
    › Frequency 3 to 5 min
    › Duration 40 to 70 seconds
  » Client anxious and in pain
› Transitional Phase: 8 to 10 cm
  » Contractions:
    › Regular, very strong
    › Frequency 2 to 3 min
    › Duration 45 to 90 seconds
  » Client may have nausea/vomiting and may become irritable.

 NURSING INTERVENTIONS

Admission assessment. Teach, review birth plan; determine pain goals. In all stages, include maternal/fetal assessments, fluid intake, frequent urination.

Assess amniotic fluid status; nitrazine paper used if suspect ROM. It will turn blue in the presence of alkaline amniotic fluid (pH 6.5 to 7.5).

Continue assessing maternal and fetal status. Assist with nonpharmacologic pain management. Provide analgesia if requested.

Second Stage

Pushing stage. From complete dilation through delivery of baby.

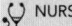 **NURSING INTERVENTIONS**

Assess FHR at least every 15 min.

Assist with pushing, breathing (prevent hyperventilation), comfort.

Record delivery time, medications, episiotomy/laceration.

Third Stage

After delivery of baby until delivery of placenta. Contractions are usually mild; client is usually focused on her baby.

 NURSING INTERVENTIONS

Assess vital signs, bleeding, fundus.

Provide immediate care of newborn: ABC, Apgar score, warm environment, safety measures, infection control.

Fourth Stage

1 to 2 hr after delivery of the placenta.

 NURSING INTERVENTIONS

Encourage breastfeeding and promote bonding.

Assess vital signs, fundus, and lochia every 15 min x 4; every 30 min x 2; and in 60 min.

Hemorrhage is priority concern.

D. **Fetal Assessment During Labor**

1. Indications for Assessment of FHR

    a. On admission and regular intervals as indicated by hospital protocol

    b. Before and after any procedure (e.g., medication, anesthesia, ROM, vaginal exam, ambulation)

    c. Throughout labor (in cases of high-risk pregnancy, use of oxytocic agents, fetal distress)

2. Interpretation of Findings

    a. FHR Classification System

        1) Category I tracings are normal (reassuring).

        2) Category III tracings are abnormal and associated with fetal hypoxemia.

THREE-TIER FHR CLASSIFICATION SYSTEM

Category I (normal)

Baseline FHR of 110 to 160/min

Baseline FHR variability: moderate heart rate beat fluctuations (6 to 25/min)

Accelerations: present or absent

Early decelerations: present or absent

Variable or late decelerations: absent

Category II

All FHR tracings not categorized as Category I or III

Category III (abnormal)

Sinusoidal pattern

Absent baseline FHR variability and any of the following:

› Recurrent variable decelerations
› Recurrent late decelerations
› Bradycardia

    b. Periodic FHR changes

        1) Accelerations (reassuring) 15 beats/min change lasting 15 seconds (term fetus)

        2) Decelerations; early, late, variable

PERIODIC FHR CHANGES

Name: VEAL	Cause: CHOP	Management: MINE
Variable	Cord compression	Move client
Early	Head compression	Identify labor progress
Acceleration	Other (okay)	No action needed
Late	Placental insufficiency	Execute actions immediately

EARLY DECELERATION

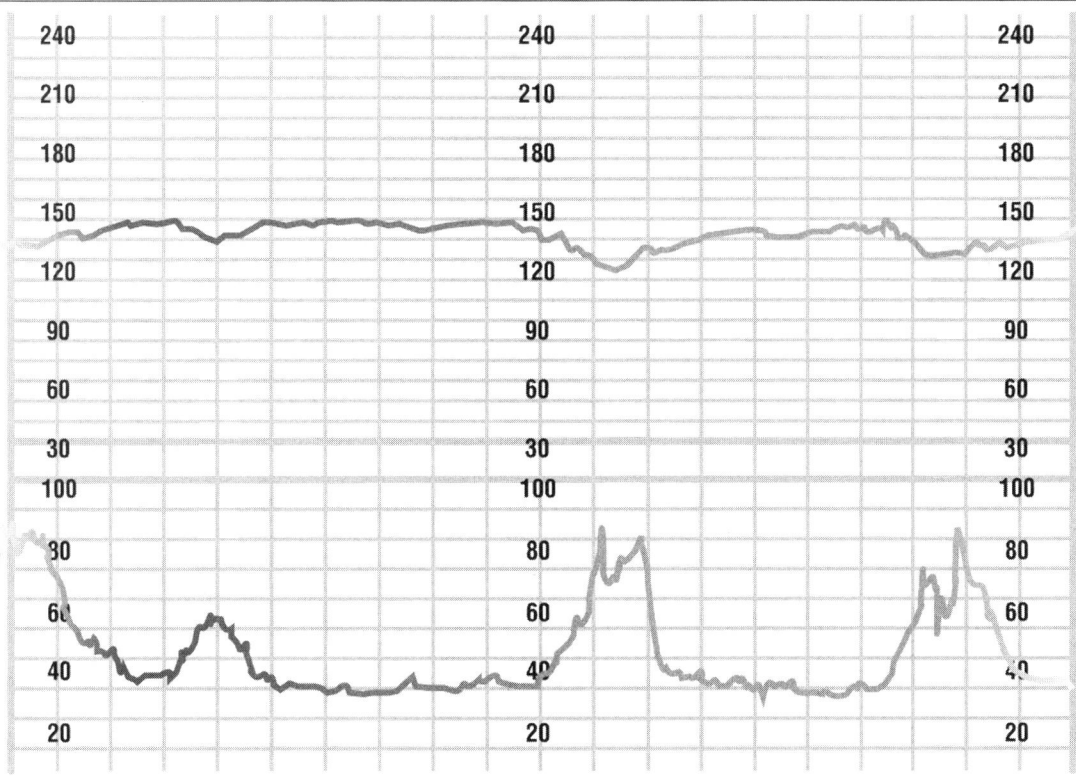

VARIABLE DECELERATION

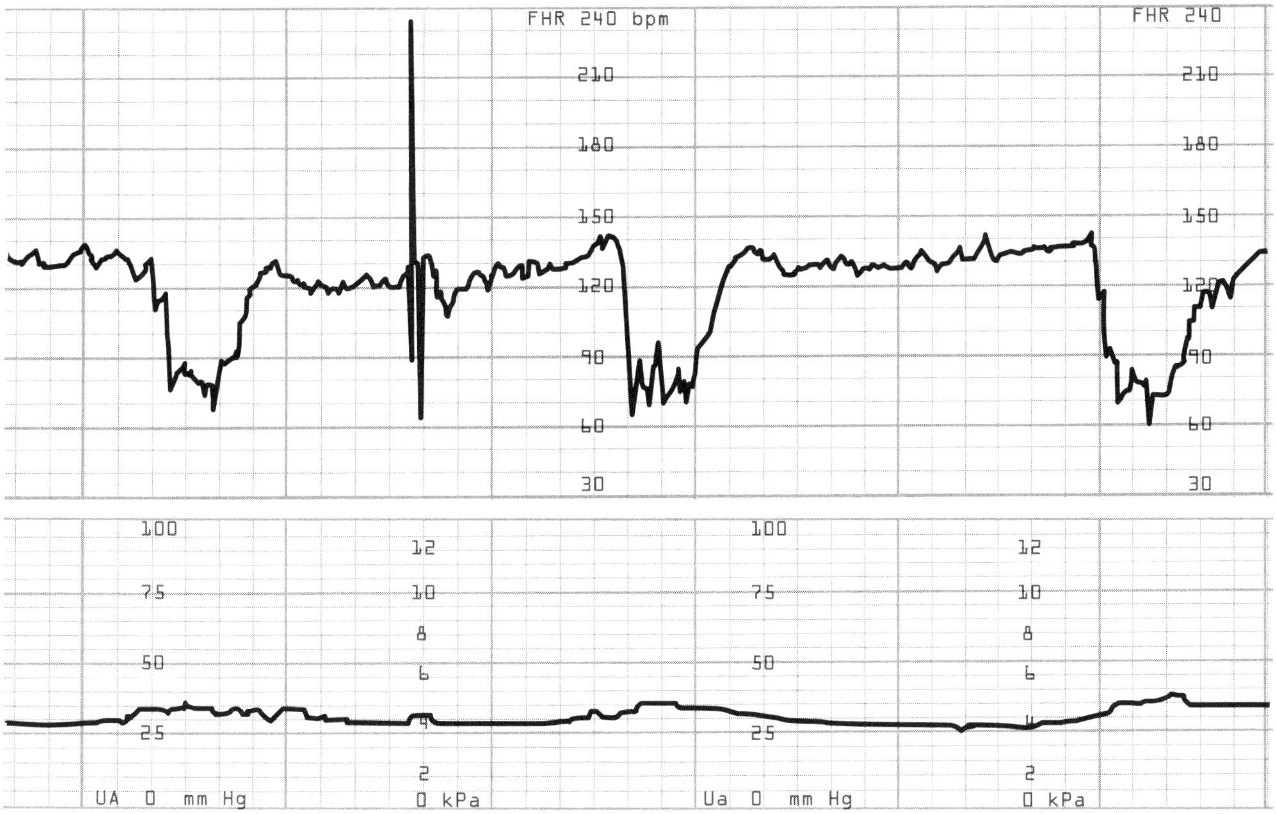

LATE DECELERATION

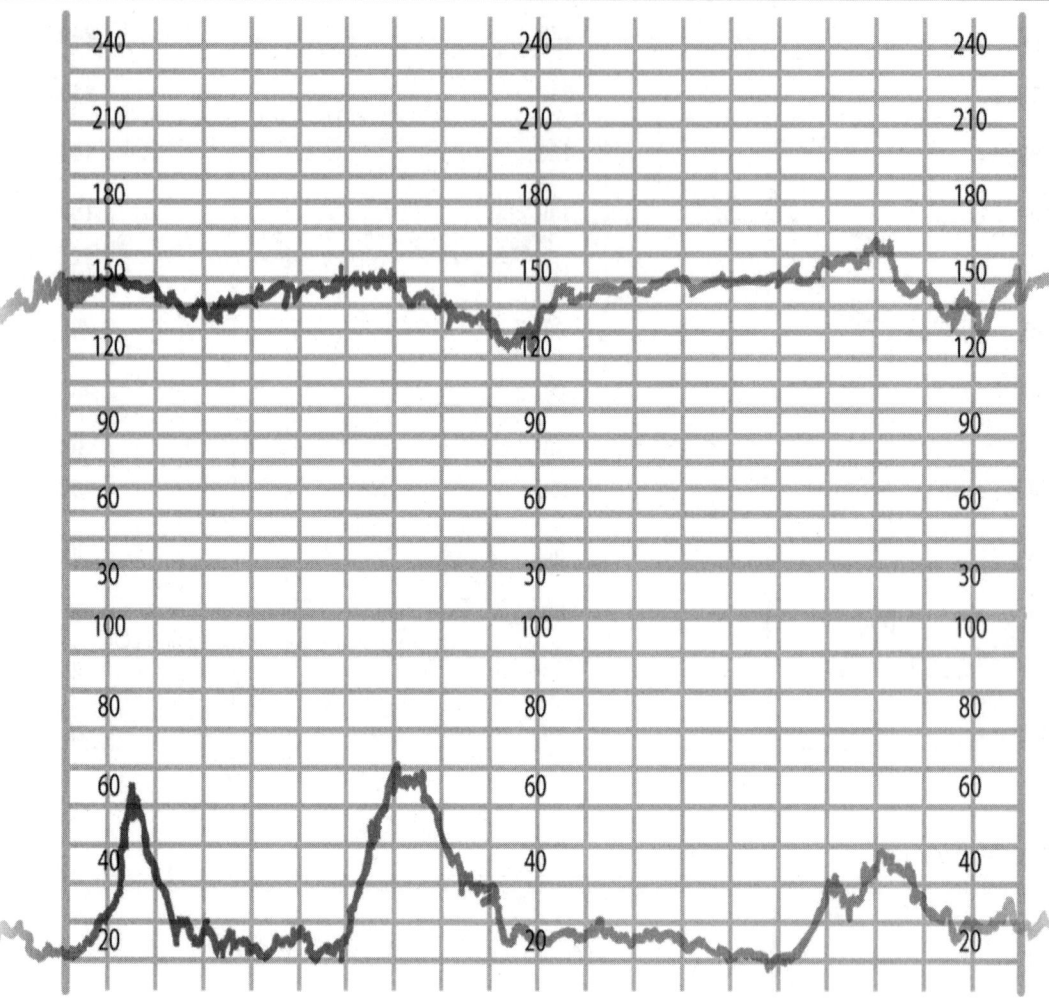

E. **Medications Used in Labor and Delivery**

MEDICATIONS USED IN LABOR AND DELIVERY

MEDICATION	USE	NURSING INTERVENTIONS
Oxytocin	Stimulate uterine contractions May be used in all stages of labor	Monitor contractions and FHR. Monitor vital signs. Administer by IV infusion pump through secondary line. Stop immediately for late decelerations or tachysystole (hyperstimulation). Have tocolytic (such as terbutaline) immediately available for tachysystole.
Methylergonovine maleate	Stimulate uterine contractions after delivery Treat postpartum hemorrhage	Monitor bleeding and uterine tone. Obtain baseline blood pressure. Massage fundus. Administer 0.2 mg IM or PO as prescribed.
Calcium gluconate	Antidote for magnesium sulfate toxicity	Administer calcium gluconate 1 g (10 mL 10% solution) IV for signs of toxicity. Dilute with equal amounts of NS and administer 0.5 to 1 mL/min.

MEDICATION	USE	NURSING INTERVENTIONS
Terbutaline, ritodrine HCl	Tocolytic used for preterm labor	Monitor contractions and FHR.
		Monitor vital signs.
		Administer terbutaline subcutaneous 0.25 mg every 20 min as needed.
		Monitor for adverse effects: tremors, dizziness, headache, tachycardia, hypotension, anxiety.
		Do not administer if client reports chest pain.
		Notify provider if: blood pressure less than 90/60 mm Hg; pulse rate greater than 130/min; signs of pulmonary edema; FHR greater than 180/min.
		Administer beta blocking agent as antidote.
Indomethacin	May be used as tocolytic for preterm labor	Monitor contractions and FHR.
		Monitor vital signs (can mask maternal fever).
		Administer with food to decrease side effect of GI distress.
		Only administer if gestational age is less than 32 weeks.
Magnesium sulfate	Tocolytic used for preterm labor CNS depressant to prevent seizure in preeclampsia	Preterm Labor › Monitor contractions and FHR. › Monitor fetal movement and FHR variability. › Monitor vital signs and urine output. Preeclampsia › Monitor vital signs, urine output, DTRs, and LOC. › Monitor magnesium levels (therapeutic range 4 to 8 mg/dL). › Administer via infusion pump in diluted form. › Use indwelling catheter to monitor urinary elimination. › Stop immediately if: respirations less than 12, altered LOC, magnesium levels above 10 mEq/L or 9 mg/dL. › Administer calcium gluconate 1 g (10 mL of 10% solution) for signs of toxicity. › Observe neonate for signs of respiratory depression, hypotonia, lethargy, and hypocalcemia. › Contraindicated for women with myasthenia gravis.
Naloxone HCl	Antidote for opioid-induced respiratory depression Reverse pruritus from epidural opioid	Monitor respiratory effort. Do not administer if mother is opioid-dependent. Newborn: Administer 0.1 mg/kg IV, IM, SQ, or ET tube. Adult: Administer 0.4 to 2 mg IV, may repeat IV at 2 to 3 min intervals up to 10 mg, can also administer IM or SQ.
Betamethasone	Preterm labor (24 to 32 weeks) › Prevent or reduce neonatal respiratory distress syndrome in preterm infants › Stimulate production or release of lung surfactant in preterm fetus	Assess for signs of preterm labor. Administer 12 mg deep IM for two doses 24 hr apart. Monitor blood glucose levels and lung sounds.
Misoprostol, dinoprostone	Preinduction cervical ripening (Bishop score 4 or less)	Obtain informed consent. Monitor contractions and FHR. Monitor vital signs. Evaluate Bishop score. Use cautiously in women with history of asthma, glaucoma, renal, hepatic, or cardiovascular disorders. Contraindicated in presence of fetal distress or vaginal bleeding.

LABOR AND DELIVERY MEDICATIONS WORKSHEET

Match the medication in the first column with the related statement in second column.

_____ 1. oxytocin

_____ 2. misoprostol

_____ 3. penicillin G

_____ 4. methylergonovine

_____ 5. terbutaline sulfate

_____ 6. betamethasone

_____ 7. methotrexate

_____ 8. indomethacin

A. Contracts the uterus after delivery, used to treat postpartum hemorrhage. Need baseline blood pressure before administering.

B. Induces labor or contracts the uterus after delivery. Stop immediately in the presence of late decelerations.

C. Stimulates fetal lung maturation between 24 to 32 weeks gestation.

D. Softens and thins the cervix.

E. Prostaglandin synthetase inhibitor. Can be used as tocolytic in preterm labor.

F. Used during labor when client is positive for group B strep.

G. May be used with ectopic pregnancy to stop the growth of the embryo to save the tube.

H. Beta adrenergic agonist. Last resort for preterm labor. Call provider for HR greater than 130.

Answer key: 1. B; 2. D; 3. F; 4. A; 5. H; 6. C; 7. G; 8. E

F. **Pain Management in Labor and Delivery**

1. Nonpharmacologic pain management

    a. Childbirth preparation methods (e.g., Lamaze, Bradley, Dick-Read, and/or pattern breathing methods) are used to promote relaxation and pain relief.

    b. Sensory stimulation strategies (based on the gate-control theory) to promote relaxation and pain relief.

        1) Aromatherapy

        2) Breathing relaxation techniques

        3) Visual imagery and use of focal points

        4) Music

    c. Cutaneous strategies (based on the gate-control theory) to promote relaxation and pain relief

        1) Back rubs, massage, and counterpressure

        2) Effleurage: light, gentle, circular stroking of the client's abdomen with fingertips

        3) Acupressure and acupuncture

        4) Water therapy

    d. Frequent maternal position changes

        1) Semi-sitting

        2) Squatting

        3) Kneeling

        4) Rocking

        5) Supine (must have wedge under one hip to tilt the uterus to avoid supine hypotension syndrome)

2. Pharmacologic pain management: analgesia and anesthesia

    a. When given early in labor, may slow or stop labor

    b. Opioid analgesics given late in labor may cause newborn respiratory depression

    c. Butorphanol tartrate and nalbuphine hydrochloride should not be given to opioid-dependent clients.

    d. Fentanyl citrate and sufentanil citrate have a short duration of action. Commonly administered with epidural and intrathecal anesthesia.

    e. Naloxone should be available as an antidote. Should not be given to client or newborn if woman is opioid-dependent.

    f. **Regional blocks** are most commonly used. They include pudendal, epidural, and intrathecal blocks.

    g. **Pudendal block** provides local anesthesia to the perineum, vulva, and rectal areas during delivery. It is administered 10 to 20 min before delivery.

    h. **Epidural block** consists of a local anesthetic along with an analgesic morphine or fentanyl injected into the epidural space at the level of the fourth or fifth lumbar vertebra. Continuous infusion or intermittent injections may be administered through an indwelling epidural catheter. Client-controlled epidural analgesia is a favored method of acute pain relief management for labor and birth. Hypotension is most common adverse effect.

        1) **Nursing Interventions**

            a) Administer 1 liter IV fluid bolus before epidural anesthesia.

            b) Assess platelet count prior to initiation of epidural.

            c) Assist in sitting or side-lying position.

            d) Monitor blood pressure frequently.

            e) Monitor for bladder distention.

            f) Continue to assess level of pain.

            g) Assist client to turn side to side every hour.

            h) Promote safety.

            i) Keep catheter insertion site clean and dry.

            j) Monitor return of sensation in legs.

            k) Assist with standing and walking first time after sensation returns.

        2) Contraindications to subarachnoid and epidural blocks.

            a) Maternal hypotension

            b) Coagulopathy (receiving anticoagulant therapy, or history of bleeding disorder)

            c) Infection at injection site

            d) Increased intracranial pressure

            e) Maternal inability to cooperate

G. **Therapeutic Procedures to Assist with Labor and Delivery**

1. **Amniotomy**: The artificial rupture of the amniotic membranes (AROM) to initiate or improve contractions. Labor typically begins within 12 hr after the membranes rupture. The client is at an increased risk for cord prolapse or infection.

    a. **Nursing Interventions**

    1) Record baseline FHR prior to, continuously during, and after the procedure.

    2) Observe for changes in FHR: bradycardia, variable decelerations, or late decelerations (cord compression or prolapse).

    3) Assess the amount, color, consistency, and odor of the amniotic fluid.

    4) Implement comfort measures such as peri care and clean pads.

    5) Monitor temperature every 2 hr.

2. **Amnioinfusion**: Intrauterine infusion of an isotonic solution (0.9% sodium chloride or lactated Ringer's) to reduce severity of variable decelerations caused by cord compression.

    a. **Nursing Interventions**

    1) Explain the procedure to the client.

    2) Assist with the amniotomy and insertion of IUPC if not already present.

    3) Warm fluid using a blood warmer prior to infusion.

    4) Maintain comfort and dryness of the client.

        a) Monitor the client continuously to prevent uterine overdistention and increased uterine tone.

        b) Continually assess intensity and frequency of the client's uterine contractions.

        c) Continually monitor FHR.

3. **Induction/augmentation of labor**: the process of chemically or mechanically initiating or strengthening uterine contractions

    a. Indications

    1) Maternal issues: history of rapid labors, preeclampsia, diabetes mellitus, severe Rh isoimmunization, chronic renal disease, and pulmonary disease

    2) Fetal/placental issues: IUGR, PROM, chorioamnionitis, postdates, fetal demise

    3) Inadequate uterine contractions (Pitocin used to augment labor)

    b. Contraindications for Induction of Labor

    1) Cephalopelvic disproportion (CPD)

    2) Nonreassuring FHR

    3) Placenta previa or vasa previa

    4) Prior classical uterine incision or uterine surgery

    5) Active genital herpes

    6) HIV

    7) Cervical cancer

    c. Medications

    1) Chemical Methods Used to Soften Cervix

        a) Prostaglandin E2, (placed transvaginally near cervix). Client must remain supine with wedge or in side-lying position for 30 min after insertion of gel. Delay Pitocin use for 6 to 12 hr after last gel insertion.

        b) Prostaglandin E1 administered intravaginally or PO tabs.

    2) Medication Used to Initiate Induction

        a) IV oxytocin

    3) **Nursing Interventions**

        a) Obtain informed consent. Monitor FHR and uterine activity every 15 min and with every change in dose.

        b) Observe for and report uterine tachysystole (i.e., more than 5 contractions in 10 min) or fetal distress.

        c) Obtain vital signs every 30 min and with every oxytocin change in dose.

        d) Administer pain management.

        e) Prior to administration of oxytocin vaginal exam performed for effacement, dilation, and station (fetus must be engaged at 0 station).

        f) Oxytocin should be connected "piggyback" to the main IV line at closest infusion port to the client.

        g) Discontinue oxytocin with signs of fetal distress or uterine tachysystole (hyperstimulation):

            (1) Contraction frequency more often than one every 2 min or 5 in 10 minutes

            (2) Contraction duration longer than 90 seconds

            (3) Contraction intensity greater than 90 mm Hg with IUPC

            (4) No relaxation of uterus between contractions

            (5) Prepare to administer terbutaline 0.25 mg subcutaneously, to decrease uterine activity.

4. **Vacuum-assisted delivery:** attachment of a vacuum cup to the fetal head to assist in birth of the head

    a. Indications

    1) Maternal exhaustion and ineffective pushing

    2) Fetal distress during second stage of labor

    b. **Nursing Interventions**

    1) Place in lithotomy position and support with pushing.

    2) Assess and record FHR before and during vacuum application.

    3) Assess for bladder distention before application.

    4) Document number of pulls, pressure, and pop offs.

    5) Observe neonate for bruising and caput succedaneum.

    6) Inform parents caput may resolve within 24 hr or could last up to 5 days.

5. **Forceps**: Obstetric instrument used to aid in delivery of the fetal head
   a. Indications
      1) Poor progress during second stage
      2) Fetal distress
      3) Persistent occiput posterior position
      4) Abnormal presentation
    b. **Nursing Interventions**
      1) Assess the neonate for intracranial hemorrhage, facial bruising, and facial palsy.
      2) Check FHR before traction is applied.
   c. Complications
      1) Lacerations to cervix or vagina
      2) Bladder or urethral injury
      3) Urine retention resulting from bladder or urethral injuries
      4) Hematoma formation in the pelvic soft tissues
6. **Episiotomy**: an incision that is made into the perineum to enlarge the vaginal outlet during delivery
   a. **Nursing Interventions**
      1) Monitor for pain, healing, infection, laceration of the anal sphincter (fourth-degree tear), and hemorrhage.
      2) Encourage Kegel exercises to improve and restore perineal muscle tone.
      3) Apply ice packs.
      4) Educate client on perineal care and use sitz baths.
7. **Cesarean birth**: birth of fetus through a transabdominal incision of the uterus
   a. Types
      1) Low transverse: decrease chance of uterine rupture with future pregnancies; less bleeding after delivery
      2) Classic: rarely used
   b. Indications
      1) Previous cesarean birth
      2) Failure to progress in labor
      3) Fetal factors: malpresentation, fetal distress, cephalopelvic disproportion, multiple fetuses, macrosomia, prolapsed cord
      4) Maternal factors: positive HIV, active genital herpes, complete placenta previa or abruption
   c. **Nursing Interventions**
      1) Obtain informed consent.
      2) Perform preoperative assessment and surgical checklist.
      3) Administer preoperative medications.
      4) Insert IV and Foley catheter.
      5) Perform postoperative and postpartum assessment.
      6) Assess for bleeding at site and lochia.
      7) Obtain routine postoperative vital signs.
      8) Monitor effects of anesthesia.
      9) Assess need for pain management.
      10) Assess for thrombophlebitis.

NCLEX ALERT: LABOR AND DELIVERY

1. It is never good to be late. (Late decelerations are bad.)
2. Absent variability (a straight line) for FHR is critical.
3. Never place laboring client flat on her back (supine hypotension/vena cava syndrome).
4. Unexplained pain in a labor and delivery client is not good (preterm labor, abruptio placentae, amniotic fluid embolism, uterine rupture).
5. Never provide fundal pressure with shoulder dystocia (suprapubic pressure okay, also assist with McRoberts maneuver).
6. OB client with tachycardia: Think hemorrhage first.
7. Medications for postpartum hemorrhage include: oxytocin, methylergonovine, and carboprost tromethamine.
8. Quick onset of epigastric pain is often the aura to seizure activity (implement safety precautions).
9. Oxygen administration should be at 8-10 L/min via nonrebreather face mask.
10. Nonpharmacologic measures should be used in combination with pharmacologic interventions.

SECTION 5

Complications During Labor and Delivery

A. **Preterm labor:** uterine contractions with cervical changes that occur between 20 and 37 weeks of gestation
   1. Contributing Factors
      a. Demographic factors
         1) Age less than 15 and greater than 35
         2) Low socioeconomic status
      b. Biophysical factors
         1) Previous preterm labor or birth
         2) Multifetal pregnancy
         3) Second trimester bleeding
         4) Infection
      c. Behavioral factors
         1) Lack of prenatal care
         2) Poor nutrition
         3) Substance abuse
   2. **Nursing Interventions**
      a. Obtain vaginal swab for fetal fibronectin testing.
      b. Assist with collection of cervical cultures.
      c. Activity restriction (e.g., bed rest with bathroom privileges, left-lateral position).
      d. Ensure hydration.
      e. Assess for signs of infection: UTI, vaginal drainage including odor.

f. Monitor maternal vital signs including temperature.

g. Monitor FHR and contraction pattern.

h. Administer tocolytic medications and betamethasone.

B. **Fetal Distress**

1. FHR baseline below 110 or above 160

2. Absent FHR variability

3. Category III FHR pattern (See the table on the FHR Classification System in this unit.)

4. Fetal blood pH less than 7.2

5. Contributing Factors

a. Uteroplacental insufficiency

1) Acute uteroplacental insufficiency

a) Excessive uterine activity associated with use of oxytocin

b) Maternal hypotension: epidural, vena caval compression, supine position, hemorrhage

c) Placental separation: abruptio, placentae previa

2) Chronic uteroplacental insufficiency

a) Gestational hypertension

b) Chronic hypertension

c) Smoking or illicit drug use

d) Diabetes mellitus

e) Postmaturity

6. **Nursing Interventions**

a. Stop oxytocin.

b. Administer oxygen at 8 to 10 L/min by nonrebreather face mask.

c. Reposition client.

d. Increase IV fluids.

e. Notify the provider.

f. Perform fetal scalp stimulation or vibroacoustic stimulation per protocol.

C. **Umbilical Cord Problems**

1. Contributing Factors

a. Cord compression: pressure on the umbilical cord during pregnancy, labor, or delivery that reduces blood flow from the placenta to the fetus

1) Causes: abnormal presentation, inadequate pelvis, presenting part at high station, multiple gestations, prematurity, premature rupture of membranes, and/or polyhydramnios

2) Complications: fetal asphyxia

b. Nuchal cord (cord around neck)

c. Prolapsed cord

2. **Nursing Interventions**

a. Prolapsed cord

1) Call for assistance immediately.

2) Notify care provider.

3) Use sterile-gloved hand, insert two fingers into the vagina, and apply finger pressure on either side of the cord to the fetal presenting part to elevate it off of the cord.

4) Reposition in a knee-chest or Trendelenburg position.

5) Administer oxygen at 8 to 10 L/min by nonrebreather face mask.

6) If cord is protruding from the vagina, wrap it loosely in a sterile saline-soaked towel.

7) Closely monitor FHR for variable decelerations and bradycardia.

8) Prepare for immediate birth: vaginal or cesarean.

b. Cord compression

1) Position change is priority.

2) Administer oxygen at 8 to 10 L/min by nonrebreather face mask.

3) Prepare to assist with amnioinfusion.

D. **Emergency Childbirth**

1. Contributing Factors

a. Precipitous delivery

2. **Nursing Interventions**

a. Encourage mother to pant, unless the fetus is in breech presentation.

b. Support the perineum.

c. Rupture the membranes if they have not yet ruptured.

d. Feel for the cord around the neonate's neck, and gently slip it over his head.

e. Keep the neonate dry and warm.

f. Do not cut the cord.

g. Deliver the placenta. Expect a gush of blood and a lengthening of the cord.

h. Save the placenta.

i. Massage fundus. Encourage breastfeeding to contract uterus.

E. **Amniotic Fluid Emboli** (anaphylactoid syndrome of pregnancy)

1. Rupture in the amniotic sac or maternal uterine veins accompanied by a high intrauterine pressure.

2. Amniotic fluid enters maternal circulation and travels to and obstructs pulmonary vessels, which causes respiratory distress and circulatory collapse.

3. Manifestations

a. Respiratory distress (e.g., restlessness, cyanosis, dyspnea, pulmonary edema, respiratory arrest)

b. Circulatory collapse (e.g., tachycardia, hypotension, shock, cardiac arrest)

c. Hemorrhage (e.g., bleeding from incisions and venipuncture sites, petechiae and ecchymosis, uterine atony)

d. Seizure activity

4. **Nursing Interventions**
   a. Administer 10 L oxygen via face mask.
   b. Prepare client for intubation.
   c. Initiate and/or assist with CPR.
   d. Administer IV fluids.
   e. Administer blood or blood products.
   f. Prepare for an emergency birth.
   g. Prepare for an emergency cesarean birth if fetus is not yet delivered.

F. **Dystocia:** Dysfunctional, Abnormal Labor
   1. Contributing Factors
      a. Dysfunction of uterine contractions
      b. Abnormal position
      c. Fetopelvic disproportion
      d. Maternal exhaustion
      e. Macrosomia
   2. **Nursing Interventions**
      a. Assess fetus and status of labor.
      b. Encourage to void and ambulate regularly.
      c. Assist in positioning and coaching during contractions.
      d. Prepare for a possible forceps, vacuum-assisted, or cesarean birth.
      e. Shoulder dystocia: McRoberts maneuver and suprapubic pressure (not fundal pressure).

NCLEX ALERT: STANDARDS OF CARE FOR THE OBSTETRIC CLIENT

1. Never perform a vaginal exam in the presence of unexplained vaginal bleeding.
2. Client bleeding should have IV access.
3. RhoGAM is given to Rh-negative mothers after a miscarriage, at 28 weeks gestation, and within 72 hr after delivery if baby is Rh-positive and RhoGAM is indicated.
4. Unstable clients should be assigned rooms close to nurses' station.

SECTION 6

Postpartum

ı Postpartum/Puerperium

A. **Approximate duration:** 6 weeks
B. **Main goal:** prevent postpartum hemorrhage
C. **Greatest risks:** hemorrhage, shock, and infection
D. **Includes physiological and psychological adjustments**
E. **Changes after delivery of the placenta:** hormones (e.g., estrogen, progesterone, and placental enzyme insulinase [hCS]) decrease, causing decreased blood glucose (hCS), diaphoresis, and diuresis (estrogen). Oxytocin increases (contractions, breast milk, and involution).

F. **Physical Assessment**
   1. Vital signs, Hgb, Hct, CBC, estimated blood loss in delivery
   2. Pain
      a. Monitor location, intensity of pain.
      b. Examine location of pain.
      c. Implement nonpharmaceutical measures.
      d. Implement pharmaceutical measures.
         1) Consider safety of medications related to breastfeeding.
            a) Hydrocodone/acetaminophen
            b) Ibuprofen
            c) PCA such as morphine sulfate or fentanyl
   3. Breasts
      a. Colostrum
         1) Transitions to milk 48 to 96 hr
         2) High nutrition
      b. Milk production occurs about day 2 or 3
         1) Sucking stimulates uterine contractions, promotes uterine involution and increased milk production.
         2) Supplementing with formula may decrease production.
         3) Breast milk actively supports the immune system. Protects against many bacterial, viral, and protozoal infections; IgA is major immunoglobulin in human milk that provides passive immunity.
      c. Engorgement
         1) About 48 hr postpartum
         2) May cause slight rise in temperature
         3) Nonlactating clients
            a) Avoid nipple stimulation
            b) Cold compress
            c) Pain medication
            d) Supportive bra
         4) Lactating clients
            a) Manually express some milk to facilitate latch
            b) Frequent feeding or pumping
            c) Warm shower
            d) Breast massage
            e) Supportive bra
            f) Maternal medications immediately after to minimize crossover to breast milk

NOTE: For engorgement, breastfeed every 2 to 3 hr. Encourage a warm shower immediately prior to breastfeeding. Immediately after and between feedings, apply cold compresses or ice-cold green cabbage leaves to breasts.

NOTE: Know the differences between mastitis and engorgement.

4. Uterus
   a. Involution
      1) Firm
      2) Fundus near umbilicus after delivery
      3) Descends approximately 1 cm/day
      4) Breastfeeding enhances
      5) Full bladder impedes involution
   b. Subinvolution
      1) Massage
      2) Frequent voiding
      3) Oxytocin
   c. Lochia: Note color, amount (scant to moderate), presence of clots, and odor (fleshy).
      1) Color
         a) Rubra—bright red, may contain small clots, transient flow increases during breastfeeding and upon rising. Lasts 1 to 3 days.
         b) Serosa—brownish red or pink. Lasts from day 4 to day 10.
         c) Alba—yellowish, white creamy color. Lasts from day 11 up to and beyond 6 weeks postpartum.
   d. Teach about return of menses.
      1) Ovulation may occur prior to first menses.
      2) Nonlactating client: 6 to 8 weeks.
      3) Breastfeeding exclusively: may be up to 6 months.
      4) Need for birth control.
5. Perineum
   a. Assess perineum using REEDA:
      1) **R** – Redness
      2) **E** – Edema
      3) **E** – Ecchymosis
      4) **D** – Drainage
      5) **A** – Approximation
   b. Comfort and healing
      1) Cold compress first 24 hr
      2) Sitz bath
      3) Positioning
      4) Perineal hygiene
      5) Kegel exercises
      6) Medication

NOTE: Saturation of one perineal pad in 15 min or less, numerous large clots, or pooling of blood under the buttocks are indicators of excessive blood loss.

6. Bladder
   a. Potential problem due to effects of anesthesia and hormones.
      1) Distended bladder increases potential for uterine atony and bleeding. Fundus will deviate to the side and above umbilicus.
      2) Assist with frequent urination.
      3) Provide noninvasive measures to promote urination.
      4) Perform bladder scan.
      5) Catheterize if retention persists.
7. Bowel
   a. Bowel movement in 1 to 2 days.
   b. Assess for hemorrhoids.
      1) Promote fiber, activity, fluids.
      2) Administer stool softener.
      3) Provide sitz bath.
      4) Apply topical anesthetic.
8. Edema and DTRs
   a. Assess for pitting edema.
   b. Excessive use of oxytocin increases risk for edema.
   c. 2+ DTRs normal.
9. Deep-Vein Thrombosis
   a. Prevention is key: early ambulation.
   b. Assess for pain, redness, or swelling of lower extremities.
10. Infection
   a. Temperature normally elevated to 38° C (100.4° F) first 24 hr after delivery.
   b. WBCs may be elevated to 20,000 to 25,000/mm³ the first 10 to 14 days.
   c. Do not assume "normal."
   d. Assess possible sources of infection.

G. **Psychologic Adaptations**
   1. Support systems
   2. Self-concept
   3. Bonding
      a. Initial contact within 30 to 60 min after birth
      b. Client exploration of infant
         1) Fingertips, then palms
         2) Extremities, then trunk
         3) En face
      c. Collaborative Care
         1) Minimize pain, fatigue, and hunger to enhance bonding.
         2) Describe newborn behaviors.

4. Maternal Role Adaptation

PHASES OF MATERNAL ADJUSTMENT

	CHARACTERISTICS	COLLABORATIVE CARE
Taking in	24 to 48 hr after birth: dependent, passive; focuses on own needs; excited, talkative	Assist with care; provide comfort, nutrition, hygiene; listen; review labor and delivery
Taking hold	Second to tenth day postpartum, or up to several weeks: focuses on maternal role and care of newborn; eager to learn; may develop blues	Provide teaching, written material, follow-up appointments, community resources; assess emotional status, discuss blues
Letting go	Focuses on family and individual roles	Assess progress; discuss community resources

5. Postpartum Blues and Depression

POSTPARTUM BLUES AND DEPRESSION

	Postpartum Blues	Postpartum Depression
CONTRIBUTING FACTORS	Fatigue, hormonal changes, role change, family tension, finances	History of depression*; poverty; unwanted pregnancy; lack support systems; newborn health problems
OCCURRENCE	50% to 60% of postpartum clients	10% to 15% of postpartum clients
ONSET	1 to 10 days postpartum	Up to 1 year or more after delivery; may persist for years
SIGNS/ SYMPTOMS	Emotionally labile	Persistent depression; overwhelmed; anxious; hopeless; unable to care for self and/or infant; thoughts of suicide
COLLABORATIVE CARE	Teaching; need for sleep, exercise, adequate nutrition; seek support and assistance with newborn care; community resources	Use depression screening tools; teaching; recognize signs and symptoms, seek assistance, needs rapid intervention

*Note: Medications used to treat depression, such as SSRIs, are frequently Category C or D drugs and may be discontinued during pregnancy. A nurse ensures that the medications are resumed as needed after delivery.

H. **Provide focused assessment:** BUBBLE HERV
1. **B** – Breasts
2. **U** – Uterus (fundal height, uterine placement, and consistency)
3. **B** – Bowel and GI function
4. **B** – Bladder function
5. **L** – Lochia (color, odor, consistency, and amount [COCA])
6. **E** – Episiotomy (redness, edema, ecchymosis, drainage, approximation [REEDA])
7. **H** – Hemorrhoids
8. **E** – Emotions
9. **R** – Rubella (prevent pregnancy at least 1 month after receiving), RhoGAM
10. **V** – Vaccines (influenza, pneumonia, Tdap [needed only once as adult, to prevent pertussis, not given if received tetanus–diphtheria vaccine within 2 years])

NOTE: Women who receive rubella immunization should prevent pregnancy for 1 month. Women who receive both RhoGAM and rubella vaccine should have a titer drawn at 3 months to verify immunity.

Complications During Postpartum

A. **Hemorrhage:** blood loss of greater than 500 mL with vaginal delivery or greater than 1,000 mL with cesarean birth
1. Contributing Factors
   a. Uterine atony
   b. Lacerations and hematomas
   c. Complications during pregnancy (e.g., placenta previa, abruptio placentae)
   d. Complications during labor (e.g., prolonged labor, rapid labor, administration of magnesium sulfate, use of forceps, retained placenta)
   e. Overdistended uterus (e.g., macrosomia, multiple fetuses)
   f. Coagulopathies (DIC)
2. Manifestations
   a. Saturation of one pad or more in 15 min
   b. Large clots (uterine atony) or spurting of bright red blood (cervical or vaginal laceration)
   c. Formation of hematomas
   d. Boggy uterus (uterine atony)
   e. Persistent lochia rubra beyond day 3 (retained placental fragments)
   f. Change in level of consciousness
   g. Signs and symptoms of shock
3. **Nursing Interventions**
   a. Assess source of bleeding.
      1) Fundus (massage if boggy)
      2) Perineum (laceration, episiotomy site, or hematomas: notify provider)
   b. Monitor vital signs and oxygen saturation.
   c. Assess bladder.
   d. Maintain or initiate isotonic IV fluids.
   e. Administer oxytocin.
   f. Administer other medications as needed (e.g., methylergonovine, misoprostol, carboprost tromethamine).

B. **Rh Incompatibility**

RHOGAM

MOTHER	BABY	MATERNAL COOMBS	RHOGAM GIVEN?
Rh⁺	Rh⁺	Not checked	No
Rh⁺	Rh⁻	Not checked	No
Rh⁻	Rh⁺	Negative	Yes
Rh⁻	Rh⁺	Positive	No
Rh⁻	Rh⁻	Not checked	No

1. **Nursing Interventions**
   a. Observe newborn for hyperbilirubinemia.
   b. Teach mother about Rh, RhoGAM.
      1) Prevents, does not reverse, formation of antibodies
      2) Given prenatally with any invasive procedure at 28 weeks and after delivery
   c. Administer RhoGAM.
      1) Rho(D) immune globulin
      2) IM
      3) Given within 72 hr after delivery

C. **Thromboembolic Disorder**
   1. Contributing Factors
      a. Venous stasis and hypercoagulation
      b. Immobility
      c. Pelvic pressure during labor/delivery
      d. History of thrombosis, varicosities, heart disease
   2. Manifestations
      a. Pain, heat, redness, swelling in lower leg or extremity
   3. **Nursing Interventions**
      a. Assess extremities including peripheral pulses, measuring and comparing circumferences of both legs.
      b. Homan's sign is not recommended.
      c. Venous Doppler to rule out DVTs. If DVT is suspected:
         1) Bed rest and analgesia
         2) Elevation of affected extremity
         3) Antithrombolytic stockings
         4) Anticoagulant therapy

D. **Puerperal Infections** (endometritis, mastitis, and wound infections)
   1. Elevated temperature of at least 38° C (100.4° F) for 2 or more consecutive days, excluding the first 24 hr.
   2. Endometritis usually begins on the second to fifth day postpartum.
      a. More common after cesarean birth
      b. Pelvic pain, uterine tenderness, foul smelling or profuse lochia, plus fever, tachycardia, elevated WBC and RBC sedimentation rate
   3. Mastitis usually unilateral occurring 2 to 4 weeks after delivery.
      a. Symptoms include chills, fever, malaise, and local breast tenderness and erythema.

Newborn

Neonatal Period: From Birth Through 28 Days

A. **Initial Care:** immediately after birth
   1. Airway, Breathing, Circulation (ABCs)
   2. Thermoregulation
   3. Umbilical Cord
      a. Inspect for two arteries and one vein. Observe for any bleeding from the cord, and ensure that the cord is clamped securely to prevent hemorrhage.
   4. Apgar
      a. Assess at 1 and 5 min

APGAR: FIVE CATEGORIES

	0	1	2
Heart rate	Absent	Slow, less than 100	Greater than 100
Respiratory effort	Absent	Slow, weak cry	Good cry
Muscle tone	Flaccid	Some flexion of extremities	Well-flexed extremities
Reflex irritability	No response	Grimace	Cry
Color	Blue, pale	Centrally pink with blue extremities	Completely pink

   b. Ratings
      1) 7 to 10 is within normal limits
      2) 4 to 6 is moderately distressed
      3) 0 to 3 is severely distressed
   5. Vital Signs

VITAL SIGN ASSESSMENTS

Heart Rate

NORMAL FINDINGS	100 to 160/min
NORMAL VARIATIONS	100/min sleeping 180/min when crying
DEVIATIONS FROM NORMAL	Persistent tachycardia 160/min or greater Persistent bradycardia 100/min or lower
NURSING INTERVENTIONS	Assess all pulses bilaterally; they should be equal and strong. Assess apical pulse for 1 min. Assess for murmurs.

Respirations

NORMAL FINDINGS	40 to 60/min
DEVIATIONS FROM NORMAL	Bradypnea: less than 25/min Tachypnea: greater than 60/min
NURSING INTERVENTIONS	Assess rate, rhythm, and adventitious breath sounds. Respirations will often be shallow and irregular in the newborn. Note any signs of distress. Nasal flaring, grunting, intercostal retractions, or see-saw breathing.

Temperature

NORMAL FINDINGS	Axillary 37° C
NORMAL VARIATIONS	36.5° to 37.2° C (97.7° to 98.9° F) axillary
DEVIATIONS FROM NORMAL	Temperature not stabilized after 10 hr
☿ NURSING INTERVENTIONS	Prevent heat loss: dry infant thoroughly; cover head; place in warm, dry environment; skin to skin contact with mother is encouraged.

Blood Pressure

NORMAL FINDINGS	60 to 80 systolic; 40 to 50 diastolic
NORMAL VARIATIONS	Variations occur with crying or sleeping
DEVIATIONS FROM NORMAL	**Hypotension** = potential sepsis or hypovolemic **Hypertension** in upper extremities = potential coarctation of aorta
☿ NURSING INTERVENTIONS	Assess in all four extremities on admission to nursery if problem suspected. Check arm and leg for significant differences between the lower and upper extremities; can be an indication of coarctation of the aorta.

NOTE: Rectal temperatures are contraindicated.

6. Safety
   a. Footprints and identification bands are applied in presence of parents and before infant leaves delivery room. Security system explained and initiated.
B. **Ongoing Newborn Care:** Admission to Discharge
   1. Physical Assessment

PHYSICAL ASSESSMENT

	FINDINGS
Posture	General flexion Spontaneous movement
Head	Circumference 2 to 3 cm greater than chest circumference Fontanels Posterior: Triangle shape, closes at 8 to 12 weeks Anterior: Diamond shape, closes at 18 months, pulse visible Observe for bulge or depression Shape Molding Caput succedaneum Cephalohematoma
Eyes	Vision best within 12 inches Strabismus; pseudostrabismus Subconjunctival hemorrhage Congenital cataracts
Ears	Responds to voice and other sounds Assess for low-set ears

	FINDINGS
Nose	Patent nares Preferential nose breather
Skin	Pink Acrocyanosis Erythema Jaundice Hyperpigmentation Milia Café au lait spots; giraffe spots Nevus flammeus (port wine stains) Telangiectasia nevi (stork bites) Vernix Lanugo
Mouth	Symmetry of lip movement Soft/hard palate intact Epstein pearls
Chest	Symmetrical chest movement Nipples prominent, well-formed Nipple buds are sign of maturity
Abdomen	Umbilical cord Liver may be palpable
Musculoskeletal	Evaluate joints for full range of motion Note presence of asymmetrical gluteal folds Spine straight and easily flexed Clavicles intact
Genitalia	Female: prominent labia, pseudomenstruation Male: scrotum large, palpable testes on each side, meatus at tip of penis, foreskin
GI/GU	Voiding within 24 hr; void 6 to 10 times a day after 4 days of life Meconium passed 24 to 48 hr after birth Breastfed babies have more frequent stools that appear yellow and seedy

REFLEXES

	EXPECTED FINDING	EXPECTED AGE
Sucking and rooting	Elicited by stroking the newborn's cheek or edge of his mouth. Normal response: newborn turns head toward the side that is touched and starts to suck.	Birth to 4 months
Palmar grasp	Elicited by placing an object in the newborn's palm. Normal response: Newborn grasps the object.	Present at birth and until 3 to 6 months
Plantar grasp	Elicited by touching the sole of the newborn's foot. Normal response: Newborn curls toes downward.	Birth to 8 months

	EXPECTED FINDING	EXPECTED AGE
Moro reflex (startle)	Elicited by striking a flat surface that the newborn is lying on, or allowing the head and trunk of the newborn in a semisitting position to fall backward to an angle of at least 30°. Normal response: Newborn's arms and legs extend and abduct symmetrically; fingers form a "C."	Birth to 4 months
Tonic neck reflex (fencer position)	The newborn will extend the arm and leg on the side when the head is turned to that side with flexion of the arm and leg of the opposite side.	Birth to 3 to 4 months
Babinski	Elicited by stroking outer edge of sole of foot toward toes. Normal response: Toes fan upward and out.	Birth to 1 year

2. Reactivity
   a. Observe for periods of reactivity in the newborn.
      1) **First period of reactivity**: The newborn is alert and exhibits exploring activity, makes sucking sounds, and has a rapid heartbeat and respiratory rate; lasts 15 to 30 min after birth.
      2) **Period of relative inactivity**: Sleep. Heart rate and respirations decrease; lasts from 30 min to 2 hr after birth.
      3) **Second period of reactivity**: Reawakens, often gags and chokes on mucus that has accumulated in his mouth. This period usually occurs 2 to 8 hr after birth and may last 10 min to several hr.

C. **Gestational Age Assessment:** New Ballard Score
   1. Provides maturity rating. Performed within 48 hr after birth.
   2. Components of Gestational Age Assessment
      a. Physical Components
         1) Skin
         2) Lanugo
         3) Plantar surfaces
         4) Breast
         5) Eye/ear
         6) Genitals
      b. Neuromuscular
         1) Posture
         2) Square window
         3) Arm recoil
         4) Popliteal angle
         5) Scarf sign
         6) Heel to ear

3. Medications
   a. Eye Prophylaxis
      1) Erythromycin or tetracycline administered within 1 hr after birth.
   b. Vitamin K IM administered within 1 hr of birth.
   c. Hepatitis vaccine administered within 12 hr of birth
4. Diagnostic and Therapeutic Procedures
   a. Cord blood: ABO blood type and Rh status if the mother's blood type is "O" or she is Rh-negative.
   b. CBC (anemia, polycythemia, infection, or clotting problems)
   c. Glucose level
   d. Serum bilirubin
   e. Newborn metabolic screen
   f. PKU
   g. Newborn hearing screen
   h. Pulse oximetry
5. Collaborative Care
   a. **Nursing Interventions**
      1) Monitor for signs and symptoms of respiratory distress.
      2) Promote patent airway.
         a) Perform oral and nasal suction only if needed.

NOTE: When using bulb syringe, remember M before N.

NOTE: Newborns delivered by cesarean birth are more susceptible to fluid remaining in the lungs than newborns who were delivered vaginally.

      3) Promote thermoregulation.
         a) Maintain body temperature of 36.5°C (97.7°F) axillary.
         b) Prevent heat loss.
      4) Monitor glucose levels.

NOTE: Identify potential risks and prevent heat loss by evaporation, conduction, convection, or radiation.

   b. Monitor Nutrition.
      1) Initiate feedings immediately after birth (breast or formula).
         a) Maintain a fluid intake of 100 to 140 mL/kg/24 hr.
         b) Monitor for normal weight gain (both breast milk and formula provide 20 kcal/oz).
   c. **Nursing Interventions** to Promote Successful Breastfeeding
      1) Explain breastfeeding techniques to the mother. Have the mother wash her hands, get comfortable, and have fluids to drink during breastfeeding.
      2) Offer the newborn the breast immediately after birth and feed every 2 to 3 hr.
      3) Explain the let-down reflex (i.e., stimulation of maternal nipple releases oxytocin that causes the letdown of milk).

4) Reassure the mother that uterine cramps are normal during breastfeeding, resulting from oxytocin.

5) Express a few drops of colostrum or milk and spread it over the nipple to lubricate the nipple and entice the newborn.

6) Show the mother the proper latch-on position.

d. Formula Feeding

1) Feed every 3 to 4 hr.

2) **Nursing interventions** to promote successful formula feeding

a) Always hold the bottle and never prop it.

b) Avoid supine position during feeding (danger of aspiration).

c) Hold newborn close and at 45° angle during feeding.

d) Teach how to prepare formula, bottles, and nipples.

e) Check the flow of formula from the bottle to ensure it is not coming out too slowly or quickly.

f) Place the nipple on top of the newborn's tongue.

g) Keep the nipple filled with formula to prevent the newborn from swallowing air.

h) Burp several times during a feeding, usually after each ½ to 1 oz of formula.

i) Discard unused formula when the newborn is finished feeding and after opened for 1 hr because of an increased possibility of bacterial contamination.

e. Monitor Elimination

1) Document number of voidings and stools.

2) Keep the perineal area clean and dry. Should have first void and stool within 24 hr.

f. Provide Skin Care

1) Cord care: Cleanse with neutral pH cleanser and sterile water. The cord should be kept clean and dry to prevent infection.

NOTE: The Association of Women's Health, Obstetric and Neonatal Nurses (2013) recommendations for cord care include cleaning the cord with water (using cleanser sparingly if needed to remove debris) during the initial bath of the newborn.

2) First bath after temperature stabilizes.

NOTE: When handling the newborn, gloves should be worn by providers until after the first bath.

g. Promote Bonding

1) Encourage mothers and family to hold the newborn.

h. Promote Safety and Security for the Newborn and Family

1) Verify that identification bands are correctly placed according to facility protocol.

2) Identity verification protocol should be followed each time the newborn is taken to the parent.

3) All facility staff who assist in caring for the newborn are required to wear identification badges.

i. Provide Circumcision Care

1) Before procedure, assess for family history of bleeding tendencies; hypospadias or epispadias; ambiguous genitalia; illness or infection.

2) Obtain informed consent.

3) Monitor for complications: bleeding or swelling with urine retention.

4) Teach parents to change diaper at least every 4 hr; clean penis with warm water; with clamp procedures, apply petroleum jelly with each diaper change for at least 24 hr; expect a yellowish mucus over the glans by day 2 and do not wash it off; avoid premoistened towelettes (contain alcohol) to clean the penis, which heals within 2 weeks.

6. Client Education

a. Safety

1) Position on back to sleep

2) Thermoregulation

3) Nutrition and weight gain (healthy newborn needs 100 to 140 mL/kg/24 hr, no water supplement; loss of 5% to 10% immediately after birth normal: regain in 10 to 14 days)

4) Elimination (voiding 6 to 8 diapers a day)

5) Avoid submerging in water until cord falls off—around 10 to 14 days after birth

6) CPR

7) Newborn behaviors

8) Car seat regulations

9) Oral and nasal suctioning

10) Sudden infant death syndrome (no exposure to secondhand smoke)

11) Signs of illness to report

12) Newborn follow-up care and immunization schedule

13) Crib safety: Space between mattress and sides of crib should be less than 2 fingerbreadths; slats on crib should be no more than 2.5 inches apart.

Q&A

1. What would be included in discharge teaching about bathing newborn?

2. Identify priority nursing intervention postcircumcision.

Answer Key: 1. Should be performed before feeding; use mild soap without hexachlorophene; no lotions, oils, or powders; and no tub bath until cord falls off and is healed. 2. Observe the newborn for bleeding. Check site every 15 min for 1 hr and then every hour for at least 12 hr. Also check for voiding and swelling.

Complications of the Newborn

It is essential for a nurse to immediately identify complications and implement appropriate interventions.

A. **Maternal Substance Abuse**

1. General Information

   a. Intrauterine alcohol and drug exposure can cause anomalies, neurobehavioral changes, and signs of withdrawal in the neonate.

   b. Response is dependent on specific drug, dosage, metabolism, and excretion by the mother and fetus, timing of exposure, and length of exposure.

2. Fetal Alcohol Syndrome (FAS)

   a. Contributing Factors

      1) Amount and duration of consumption (i.e., chronic or periodic intake)

      2) Daily intake increases the risk of FAS

   b. Manifestations—will have signs in three categories:

      1) Growth restriction

      2) CNS alterations such as intelligence deficit, attention deficit disorder, diminished fine motor skills, poor speech

      3) Craniofacial features such as microcephaly, small eyes or short palpebral fissures, thin upper lip, flat midface.

      4) Other signs

         a) Feeding problems

         b) Increased wakefulness

         c) Hearing loss

3. Tobacco Use During Pregnancy

   a. Manifestations

      1) Prematurity, low birth weight

      2) Increased risk for sudden infant death syndrome

      3) Increased risk for asthma, pneumonia

      4) Developmental delays

4. Drug and Alcohol Withdrawal Syndrome in the Newborn

   a. Objective data: Use a neonatal abstinence scoring system.

      1) CNS

         a) Increased wakefulness

         b) High-pitched, shrill cry, incessant crying

         c) Irritability, tremors

         d) Hyperactive with an increased Moro reflex. Heroin withdrawal will see decreased Moro reflexes and hypothermia or hyperthermia.

         e) Increased deep-tendon reflexes, increased muscle tone

         f) Seizures

      2) Skin

         a) Abrasions and/or excoriations on the face and knees

      3) Metabolic, vasomotor, and respiratory findings

         a) Nasal congestion with flaring

         b) Frequent yawning, skin mottling

         c) Tachypnea greater than 60/min

         d) Sweating and a temperature greater than 37.2°C (99°F)

      4) Gastrointestinal

         a) Poor feeding, regurgitation (projectile vomiting)

         b) Diarrhea and excessive, uncoordinated, and constant sucking

      5) Vital organ anomalies

         a) Heart defects, including atrial and ventricular septal defects, tetralogy of Fallot, and patent ductus arteriosus

   b. Medications

      1) Phenobarbital: anticonvulsant

         a) It is prescribed to decrease CNS irritability and control seizures for neonates who have alcohol or opioid addiction.

   c. Diagnostic Procedures

      1) Laboratory tests: Blood tests should be done to differentiate between neonatal drug withdrawal and central nervous system irritability.

         a) CBC

         b) Blood glucose

         c) Calcium and magnesium

         d) TSH, T_4, T_3

         e) Drug screen of urine or meconium to reveal the agent abused

         f) Hair analysis

      2) Diagnostic Procedures

         a) Chest x-ray to rule out congenital heart defects

   d. Collaborative Care

      1) **Nursing interventions** will include normal newborn care, plus:

         a) Perform a neonatal abstinence scoring system assessment.

         b) Assess newborn reflexes.

         c) Monitor ability to feed and digest intake.

         d) Monitor fluid and electrolytes, skin turgor, fontanelles, and I&O.

         e) Observe behavior, including crying, sleep patterns, tremors.

         f) Maintain IV.

         g) Reduce external stimuli: swaddle, do not place next to nurses' desk.

         h) Small, frequent feedings with high-calorie formula—may need gavage feedings.

         i) If sucking is a problem, use preterm nipples and nipples with larger holes.

         j) Have suction immediately available (risk for aspiration).

k) For newborns who are addicted to cocaine, avoid eye contact and use vertical rocking and a pacifier.

l) Initiate a consult with child protective services.

m) Consult lactation services to evaluate if breastfeeding is desired and not contraindicated.

B. **Hypoglycemia:** A serum glucose level of less than 40 mg/dL.

1. Contributing Factors

   a. Maternal diabetes mellitus

   b. Preterm infant

   c. LGA or SGA

   d. Stress at birth, such as cold stress and asphyxia

2. Manifestations

   a. Objective Data: Physical Assessment Findings

      1) Poor feeding

      2) Jitteriness/tremors

      3) Hypothermia

      4) Diaphoresis

      5) Weak cry

      6) Lethargy

      7) Flaccid muscle tone

      8) Seizures/coma

3. Diagnostic Laboratory Tests and Procedures

   a. Two consecutive plasma glucose levels less than 40 mg/dL in a newborn who is term, and less than 25 mg/dL in a newborn who is preterm

4. Collaborative Care

   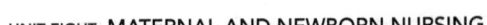

   a. **Nursing Interventions**

      1) Perform heel stick for blood glucose within 2 hr of birth.

      2) Provide frequent oral and/or gavage feedings.

      3) Monitor the neonate's blood glucose level closely per facility protocol.

      4) Monitor IV if the neonate is unable to orally feed.

C. **Respiratory Distress Syndrome (RDS)**

1. RDS occurs as a result of surfactant deficiency in the lungs and is characterized by poor gas exchange and ventilatory failure.

2. Surfactant is a phospholipid that assists in alveoli expansion.

3. Surfactant keeps alveoli from collapsing and allows gas exchange to occur.

4. Contributing Factors

   a. Preterm gestation

   b. Perinatal asphyxia (meconium staining, cord prolapse, and nuchal cord)

   c. Stress/asphyxia during labor (maternal hypotension, UPI)

5. Manifestations: Physical Assessment

   a. Objective Data

      1) Tachypnea (respiratory rate greater than 60/min)

      2) Nasal flaring

      3) Expiratory grunting

      4) Intercostal and substernal retractions

      5) Labored breathing

      6) Fine rales on auscultation

      7) Cyanosis

      8) Unresponsiveness, flaccidity, and apnea with decreased breath sounds (signs and symptoms of worsened RDS)

6. Diagnostic Procedures and Laboratory Tests

   a. Culture and sensitivity of the blood, urine, and cerebrospinal fluid (rule out sepsis)

   b. Blood glucose and serum calcium

   c. ABGs reveal hypercapnia (excess of carbon dioxide in the blood) and respiratory or mixed acidosis.

   d. Chest x-ray

7. **Nursing Interventions**

   a. Administer lung surfactant—beractant (preterm infant)

   b. Avoid suctioning ET tube for 1 hr after administration of medication.

D. **Preterm newborn:** Birth occurs after 20 weeks of gestation and before 38 weeks gestation.

1. Contributing Factors

   a. Maternal gestational hypertension

   b. Multiple pregnancies

   c. Adolescent pregnancy

   d. Lack of prenatal care

   e. Substance abuse

   f. Smoking

   g. Previous history of preterm delivery

   h. Abnormalities of the uterus or cervix

   i. Premature rupture of the membranes

2. Manifestations: Physical Assessment

   a. Objective Data

      1) New Ballard assessment shows a physical and neurological assessment totaling less than 37 weeks of gestation.

      2) Episodes of apnea

      3) Signs of increased respiratory effort and/or respiratory distress.

      4) Physical characteristics: Typically has low birth weight; minimal subcutaneous fat; head large in comparison to body; wrinkled features; weak grasp reflex; before 34 weeks, has inability to coordinate suck and swallow; and weak or absent gag, suck, and cough reflex.

3. **Nursing Interventions**
   a. Perform rapid initial assessment.
   b. Transfer to high-risk nursery.
   c. Maintain thermoregulation.
   d. Administer respiratory support.
   e. Administer parenteral or enteral nutrition and fluids (less than 34 weeks).
   f. Provide nonnutritive sucking.
   g. Minimize stimulation (cluster care, smooth and light touch, dim lighting, and noise reduction).

E. **Postterm Infant**
   1. Contributing Factors
      a. Gestational age of more than 42 weeks
   2. Manifestations: Physical Assessment
      a. Dry, parchment-like skin
      b. Longer, harder nails
      c. Profuse scalp hair
      d. Absent vernix
      e. Hypoglycemia
   3. Complications
      a. Progressive aging of placenta
      b. Difficult delivery
      c. High perinatal mortality
      d. Jaundice (hyperbilirubinemia)

   4. **Nursing Interventions**
      a. Early and frequent heel sticks (glucose testing)
      b. Initiate early feeding
      c. Observe for birth injuries (from shoulder dystocia—fractured clavicle, brachial plexus injury, facial paralysis)

F. **Hyperbilirubinemia**
   1. Physiologic Jaundice (benign)
      a. Caused by breakdown of fetal RBCs, excessive bruising, and liver immaturity.
      b. Jaundice appears after 24 hr of age.
   2. Pathologic Jaundice (underlying disease; increased RBC production or breakdown)
      a. Appears before 24 hr of age or is persistent after day 7.
      b. Usually caused by blood group incompatibility (Rh- or ABO-incompatibility) or an infection.
      c. Kernicterus (bilirubin encephalopathy) bilirubin levels at or higher than 25 mg/dL. Can lead to anemia and brain damage.
   3. Manifestations
      a. Yellowish tint to skin, sclera, and mucous membranes.
      b. Jaundice assessed best by blanching skin on the cheek or sternum.
      c. Note time of onset to distinguish between physiologic and pathologic jaundice.
      d. Assess the underlying cause by reviewing the maternal prenatal, family, and newborn history.

4. Diagnostic and Laboratory Procedures
   a. Monitor the infant's bilirubin levels every 4 hr until the level returns to normal.
   b. Assess maternal and newborn blood type to determine if there is a presence of ABO-incapability. This occurs if the newborn has blood type A, B, or AB, and the mother is type O.
   c. Review Hgb and Hct.
   d. A direct Coombs test reveals the presence of antibody-coated (sensitized) Rh-positive RBCs in the newborn.
   e. Monitor electrolyte levels for indications of dehydration during phototherapy.
   f. Transcutaneous level is a noninvasive method to measure an infant's bilirubin.

5. **Nursing Interventions**
   a. Phototherapy, sunlight, and/or exchange transfusion is administered to the newborn.
   b. Monitor vital signs.
   c. Maintain an eye mask over the newborn's eyes for protection of corneas and retinas.
   d. Keep newborn undressed. Cover male genitals to prevent possible testicular damage from heat and light waves.
   e. Avoid applying lotions or ointments to the infant because they absorb heat and can cause burns.
   f. Remove the newborn from phototherapy every 4 hr and unmask the newborn's eyes, checking for signs of inflammation or injury.
   g. Reposition the newborn every 2 hr to expose all of the body surfaces to the phototherapy lights and prevent pressure sores. Check the lamp energy with a photometer per unit protocol.
   h. Turn off the phototherapy lights before drawing blood for testing.
   i. Observe the newborn for side effects of phototherapy.
      1) Bronze discoloration: not a serious complication
      2) Maculopapular skin rash: not a serious complication
      3) Development of pressure areas
      4) Dehydration (symptoms: poor skin turgor, dry mucous membranes, decreased urinary output)
      5) Elevated temperature
   j. Monitor elimination and daily weights, watching for signs of dehydration.
   k. Monitor newborn's axillary temperature every 4 hr during phototherapy because temperature may become elevated.
   l. Feed the newborn early and frequently—every 3 to 4 hr to promote bilirubin excretion in the stools.
   m. Continue to breastfeed the newborn. Supplementing with formula may be prescribed.
   n. Maintain adequate fluid intake to prevent dehydration.
   o. Reassure the parents that most newborns experience some degree of jaundice.
   p. Explain hyperbilirubinemia, its causes, diagnostic tests, and treatment to parents.
   q. Explain that the newborn's stool contains some bile that will be loose and green.
   r. Administer an exchange transfusion for infants who are at risk for kernicterus.

Women's Health

A. **Contraception:** Methods of contraception include natural family planning, barrier, hormonal, and intrauterine methods, as well as surgical procedures.

   1. A nurse should assess a client's need/desire for contraception.

   2. A thorough discussion of benefits, risks, and alternatives of each method should be discussed.

   3. Nurses should support clients in making the decision that is best for their individualized situations.

   4. Refer to table in Unit Four: Pharmacology in Nursing – Contraceptives.

B. **Infertility:** An inability to conceive despite engaging in unprotected sexual intercourse for a period of at least 12 months

   1. Contributing Factors

      a. Structural or hormonal disorders (e.g. tubal occlusion, endometriosis, obesity)

      b. Decreased or abnormal sperm

      c. STIs (See the table on sexually transmitted infections in this unit.)

      d. Exposure to radiation or toxic substances

   2. Diagnostic Procedures

      a. Infertility Procedures

         1) Semen collection

         2) Pelvic examination

         3) Ultrasonography

         4) Hysterosalpingography

         5) Hysteroscopy

         6) Laparoscopy

   3. Collaborative Care

      a. Perform infertility assessment.

      b. **Nursing Interventions**

         1) Encourage couples to express and discuss their feelings.

         2) Monitor for adverse effects associated with medications to treat female and male infertility.

         3) Advise that the use of medications to treat female infertility may increase the risk of multiple births by more than 25%.

         4) Provide information regarding assisted reproductive therapies.

      c. Referrals to Support Groups

         1) Genetic counseling

C. **Vaginal Infections**

   1. Normal vaginal secretions are clear to cloudy, nonirritating, nonoffensive odor, with pH of 4 to 5.

   2. Most common vaginal infections: bacterial vaginosis (BV), candidiasis, and trichomoniasis.

   3. Most common causes: irritations (bath salts or bubble bath), tight-fitting clothing (especially jeans), or anything that disrupts the normal vaginal flora such as douching, sexual activity, contamination by feces.

   4. Teach preventive measures: genital hygiene, avoid douching, use condoms, void before and after intercourse, decrease dietary sugar, drink yeast-active milk, and eat yogurt with lactobacilli.

      a. If at risk for STIs, should not use IUD or diaphragm for contraception.

   5. Bacterial vaginosis: Etiology unknown. Associated with preterm labor and birth.

      a. Manifestations

         1) Increased thin vaginal discharge and fishy odor.

      b. **Collaborative Care and Nursing Interventions**

         1) Administer metronidazole.

         2) Treatment of partner is not routinely recommended.

   6. *Vulvovaginal candidiasis*, or yeast infection: Most common organism is *Candida albicans*.

      a. Contributing Factors

         1) Use of oral contraceptives, frequent use of antibiotics, and frequent douching; diabetes mellitus and immunosuppression.

         2) Ensure that both partners are treated.

      b. Manifestations

         1) Yellow or gray discharge

         2) Discomfort with urination and intercourse

         3) Irritation and itching

   7. Sexually transmitted infections (See the table on sexually transmitted infections in this unit.)

D. **Cancer**

   1. **Cervical cancer:** forms in the tissue of the cervix

      a. Contributing Factors

         1) Human papillomavirus is responsible for most cervical cancer

         2) Multiple partners with initial sex before age 18

         3) History of STIs

         4) Immunosuppression

         5) Cigarette smoking

      b. Manifestations

         1) Abnormal bleeding

         2) Pelvic pain or pain during intercourse

      c. Diagnostic Screening

         1) Pap test

         2) HPV, DNA test

      d. Collaborative Care/Treatment

         1) Conization, laser surgery, loop electrocautery excision procedure, cryosurgery, hysterectomy, radiation, and/or chemotherapy

         2) Prevention

            a) Delay initial intercourse.

            b) Avoid smoking.

            c) Practice safe sex.

            d) Gardasil (human papillomavirus quadrivalent) is a vaccine that is given as three injections over a 6-month period. Initiate as early as age 11 or up to 26 years.

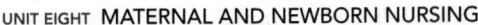

2. Endometrial cancer: Is often detected at an early stage, as it produces early vaginal bleeding between menstrual cycles or after menopause.

   a. Contributing Factors

      1) Obesity: increases risk three-fold for women who are 21 to 50 lb overweight

      2) Nulliparity

      3) Late menopause

   b. Manifestations

      1) Postmenopausal bleeding

      2) Abnormal bleeding

   c. Diagnostic Screening

      1) There is no specific screening. Endometrial biopsy performed for diagnosis.

      2) At the time of menopause, all women should be informed about the risks and symptoms of endometrial cancer.

   d. Collaborative Care

      1) Radium

      2) X-ray therapy

      3) Hysterectomy

   e. **Nursing Interventions**

      1) Assess for grieving.

      2) Provide preoperative teaching.

      3) Provide postoperative care.

      4) Assess psychosexual needs.

3. Ovarian cancer: Cancerous growth originating from different parts of the ovary.

   a. Contributing Factors

      1) Over 40 years of age

      2) Nulliparity

      3) Family history of ovarian, breast, or colon cancer

      4) History of dysmenorrhea or heavy bleeding

      5) Hormone replacement therapy

      6) Use of infertility medications

   b. Manifestations

      1) Early symptoms are not obvious.

      2) Later symptoms may include:

         a) Pressure or pain in the abdomen, pelvis, back, or legs.

         b) Swollen or bloated abdomen, nausea and indigestion, constipation or diarrhea, fatigue, shortness of breath, frequent urination, and/or vaginal bleeding.

   c. Diagnostic Screening

      1) CA 125 blood test: more than 35 u/mL is considered abnormal

      2) Intravaginal ultrasound

      3) Pelvic exam

   d. Collaborative Treatment

      1) Chemotherapy

      2) Radiation, surgery

4. **Breast Cancer:** Abnormal Growth of Breast Tissue

   a. Contributing Factors

      1) Family history (first-degree relative)

      2) Early menarche (before 12 years) and late menopause (after age 51 years)

      3) Nulligravida

      4) Early or prolonged use of oral contraceptives

      5) Long-term use of HRT

      6) Lifestyle: overweight, sedentary, excessive alcohol intake.

   b. Manifestations

      1) Lump in breast or axilla region

      2) Thickening, dimpling, redness, pain, or asymmetry in breasts

      3) Pulling, discharge, or pain in nipple area

   c. Diagnostic Screening

      1) Mammogram: Women 40 and older should get a mammogram every 1 to 2 years.

      2) Clinical breast exam: Women should receive this exam annually.

      3) Breast self-exam: Women should perform this monthly, 1 week after menses.

      4) BRCA1 and BRCA2 gene test (cannot be done within 3 months of a blood transfusion).

   d. Treatment

      1) Surgery (mastectomy) postoperative care:

         a) Head of the bed elevated 30° when awake and arm supported on pillow.

         b) Position on unaffected side.

         c) Sling on affected side while ambulating.

         d) No injections, blood pressures, or blood draws from affected side. Place sign above bed regarding these precautions.

         e) Assess incision and drainage tubes. (Drains are usually left in for 1 to 3 weeks.)

      2) Chemotherapy (combination therapy) (e.g., cyclophosphamide, doxorubicin, and fluorouracil)

      3) Radiation

      4) Hormone therapy

         a) Gonadotropin-releasing hormone (GnRH)-leuprolide (Lupron)

         b) Selective estrogen receptor modulators (SERMs)-tamoxifen and raloxifene. SERMs are used in women who are at high risk for breast cancer or who have advanced breast cancer. Tamoxifen increases risk of endometrial cancer, deep vein thrombosis, and pulmonary embolism; raloxifene does not have these side effects.

   e. Preventive Teaching

      1) Encourage screenings.

      2) Diet should include five servings of fruits and vegetables daily.

      3) Maintain healthy weight, and exercise regularly.

      4) Limit alcohol intake and avoid or cease smoking.

E. **Uterine Disorders**

1. **Myomas (uterine fibroids):** Benign fibroid tumors of the uterine muscle
   a. Contributing Factors
      1) African Americans older than age 30 who have never been pregnant
   b. Manifestations
      1) Pelvic pain or pressure
      2) Hypermenorrhea
   c. Collaborative Treatment
      1) Medication
      2) Surgery

2. **Endometriosis:** Endometrial tissue located outside of the uterus.
   a. Contributing Factors
      1) May involve retrograde menstruation
      2) Hereditary factors
      3) Impaired immune function
   b. Manifestations
      1) Severe dysmenorrhea
      2) Lower abdominal pain, pain during intercourse, back and rectal pain
      3) Abnormal bleeding
   c. Collaborative Treatment
      1) Oral contraceptives (hormone therapy), surgery, or pregnancy

F. **Menopause:** complete cessation of menstruation for 1 year

1. Manifestations
   a. Vasomotor symptoms—hot flashes
   b. Genitourinary—atrophic vaginitis, vaginal dryness, and incontinence
   c. Psychologic—mood swings, changes in sleep patterns, and decreased REM sleep
   d. Skeletal—decreased bone density
   e. Cardiovascular—decreased HDL and increased LDL
   f. Dermatologic—decreased skin elasticity and loss of hair on head and in the pubic area
   g. Reproductive—breast tissue changes, irregular menses

2. Collaborative Care and **Nursing Interventions**
   a. Assess the client's psychosocial response.
      1) Discuss menopausal hormone therapy (HT)
      2) Instruct in self-administration of HT.
      3) Advise to immediately quit smoking if applicable.
      4) Teach how to prevent and assess for development of venous thrombosis.
   b. Teach about alternate hormone therapies: dong quai and black cohosh; vitamin E. They decrease hot flashes in some women.
   c. Older adult clients may decrease risk of osteoporosis by performing regular weight bearing exercises; increasing intake of high-protein and high-calcium foods; avoiding alcohol, caffeine, and tobacco; and taking calcium with vitamin D supplements.
   d. Teach about health promotion
      1) Schedule annual exams including physical, pelvic, and mammogram.
      2) Schedule bone density test.
      3) Instruct on atypical manifestations of MI.
      4) Discuss diet, exercise, and alternative therapies.

PRENATAL AND LABOR & DELIVERY COMPLICATIONS WORKSHEET

This worksheet reviews basic knowledge of prenatal and labor & delivery complications. (Answers may be used only once; some answers may not be used.)

____ 1. Amniotic Fluid Emboli

____ 2. Abruptio Placenta

____ 3. Cardiac Disease

____ 4. Eclampsia

____ 5. Ectopic Pregnancy

____ 6. Erythroblastosis Fetalis

____ 7. Gestational Trophoblastic Disease (Hydatidiform Mole)

____ 8. HELLP Syndrome

____ 9. Hyperemesis Gravidarum

____ 10. Placenta Previa

____ 11. Prolapsed Cord

____ 12. Preterm Labor

A. Benign abnormal growth of chorionic villi. Persistent, high, hCG levels. Birth control x 1 year after D&C.

B. Low implantation of the placenta. Completely or partially covers cervical os. Usually painless, bright red bleeding.

C. Hemolytic disease of the newborn: Rh-incompatibility. Occurs when a mother who is Rh-negative has a newborn who is Rh-positive. Direct Coombs test has antibody-coated Rh-positive RBCs in the newborn.

D. Very tender, boardlike abdomen may have absent to moderate dark red bleeding.

E. Excessive pregnancy-related nausea and/or vomiting. Believed to be caused by high levels of hCG.

F. Expanding maternal plasma volume and increased cardiac output in the presence of preexisting heart condition may cause this problem.

G. Hematologic condition that coexists with severe preeclampsia involving hepatic dysfunction.

H. Most important action with this disorder is to perform a sterile vaginal exam to support the presenting part to increase blood flow to the fetus.

I. Life-threatening event where amniotic fluid, fetal cells, hair, or other debris enters the maternal circulation, resulting in respiratory distress, circulatory collapse, hemorrhage, and possible seizure activity.

J. Fertilized egg implants outside of the uterus. Cardinal sign includes sharp unilateral abdominal pain.

K. Severe preeclampsia symptoms with the onset of seizure activity.

L. Contractions with cervical change between 20 and 37 weeks gestation. Use tocolytics to stop contractions and Betamethasone to promote fetal lung maturity.

Answer Key: 1. I; 2. D; 3. F; 4. K; 5. J; 6. C; 7. A; 8. G; 9. E; 10. B; 11. H; 12. L

SEXUALLY TRANSMITTED INFECTIONS

SYMPTOMS IN WOMEN	SYMPTOMS IN MEN	COMPLICATIONS	TREATMENTS

Chlamydia
If symptoms appear, usually not until several weeks after infected.

SYMPTOMS IN WOMEN	SYMPTOMS IN MEN	COMPLICATIONS	TREATMENTS
Vaginal discharge Vaginal bleeding Painful/frequent urination Abdominal pain Fever/nausea Usually asymptomatic	Small amounts of clear or cloudy penile discharge Painful/frequent urination Swollen/tender testicles	Can pass to sexual partners and to neonate during childbirth (conjunctivitis, pneumonia) PID Can lead to infertility in women and sterility in men	Oral antibiotics, usually azithromycin or doxycycline. Preventive treatment in newborn: erythromycin (Ilotycin) ointment in eyes within 1 hr of birth.

Genital herpes
Transmission most commonly occurs from infected partner who has no visible lesion.

SYMPTOMS IN WOMEN	SYMPTOMS IN MEN	COMPLICATIONS	TREATMENTS
Most are asymptomatic Initial outbreak: painful blisters and possible systemic symptoms (fever, body aches, enlarged lymph nodes) Recurrences: mild tingling or shooting pains hours to days before herpetic eruption. Blisters last 7 to 21 days	Some have no symptoms Blisters on mouth or genital region Blisters can reoccur	No cure; symptoms are treated Can pass to sexual partners and to neonate during childbirth	Caused by a virus The antiviral medications acyclovir, famciclovir, and valacyclovir can shorten and prevent outbreaks. Cesarean birth indicated if active lesions present during the last 2 weeks before delivery. Antiviral medication (acyclovir) started at 36 weeks gestation to prevent outbreak before delivery.

Gonorrhea
Symptoms may appear 2 to 21 days after infection.

SYMPTOMS IN WOMEN	SYMPTOMS IN MEN	COMPLICATIONS	TREATMENTS
Yellow/gray vaginal discharge Vaginal bleeding between periods Symptoms mild and nonspecific Pelvic or lower abdominal pain	Yellow/green penile discharge Painful urination/bowel movement Frequent urination Swollen/tender testicles (epididymitis)	Transmitted to sexual partner and to the neonate in uterus/during childbirth (ophthalmia neonatorum) Can lead to infertility in women and sterility in men Untreated GC can cause urogenital, anorectal, conjunctival, and pharyngeal infections. Can also spread to the blood and cause disseminated gonococcal infection (DGI). DGI is usually characterized by arthritis, tenosynovitis, and/or dermatitis.	First-line treatment is single intramuscular injection of ceftriaxone, 250 mg. Ceftriaxone routinely accompanied by azithromycin or doxycycline to address the likelihood of coinfection with chlamydia Because of high reinfection rates, patients should be retested in three to six months. Preventive treatment of newborn: erythromycin ointment in eyes.

HIV
Symptoms can appear months to several years after infection.

Acute retroviral syndrome is characterized by non-specific symptoms, including fever, malaise, lymphadenopathy, and skin rash. Frequently occurs in the first few weeks after HIV infection, before antibody test results become positive.

SYMPTOMS IN WOMEN	SYMPTOMS IN MEN	COMPLICATIONS	TREATMENTS
Can be infected for several years without symptoms Weight loss/fatigue Recurring vaginal yeast infections Diarrhea/flulike symptoms Oral thrush	Can be infected for several years without symptoms Weight loss/fatigue Diarrhea/flu-like symptoms Oral thrush	There is no cure for HIV, but treatment is available. Can be passed by sex, sharing needles, during childbirth, or during breastfeeding	HIV is a virus that progressively depletes CD4 lymphocytes. Prevention counseling is key. Screening with early detection is critical. Medication includes: Antiretroviral therapy (HAART) Management for obstetrical clients includes: Antiretroviral regimens and obstetrical interventions, such as zidovudine or nevirapine and elective cesarean birth at 38 weeks of pregnancy, and education to avoid breastfeeding.

SYMPTOMS IN WOMEN	SYMPTOMS IN MEN	COMPLICATIONS	TREATMENTS

Human papillomavirus (HPV)
There are multiple strains. Some may cause genital warts and others have been linked to cervical cancer. Symptom appearance time varies.

SYMPTOMS IN WOMEN	SYMPTOMS IN MEN	COMPLICATIONS	TREATMENTS
Genital warts, also referred to as condylomas. Appear as small, flesh-colored, or gray swelling in the genital area. They can clump together and form a cauliflower shape. Itching/burning around the genitalia Abnormal pap test	Genital warts Warts can recur Itching/burning around the genitalia	Can pass to sexual partners and neonate during childbirth Warts can spread. Certain strains may lead to cancer. A rare complication includes recurrent respiratory papillomatosis (RRP).	HPV vaccines recommended for 11- or 12-year-old boys and girls. May be given to girls beginning at age 9. Medications to treat genital warts include imiquimod and podophyllin

Pelvic inflammatory disease (PID)
Several different bacteria can cause PID, and many cases have been related to chlamydia and gonorrhea.

SYMPTOMS IN WOMEN	SYMPTOMS IN MEN	COMPLICATIONS	TREATMENTS
Lower abdominal pain May have unpleasant odor Painful intercourse/urination Abnormal vaginal discharge (yellow or green) with unpleasant odor Fever, chills, and nausea and vomiting	PID does not occur in males	Can cause ectopic pregnancy Can lead to infertility May cause chronic pain in abdominal area	Depending on the severity of PID, the following may be used for treatment › Antibiotics › Hospitalization/bed rest › Outpatient intensive treatment

[handwritten notes: "semi fowler", "Fluids Mld anegisic."]

Syphilis
There are three stages of syphilis. Stage 1 symptoms can appear 1 week to 3 months after infection.

SYMPTOMS IN WOMEN	SYMPTOMS IN MEN	COMPLICATIONS	TREATMENTS
Stage 1: Primary › Sore(s) on genitalia or mouth › The sore(s) can last 2 to 6 weeks Stage 2: Secondary › Rash on body › Flu-like symptoms Tertiary (last) Stage › Neurological/ cardiovascular complications	Stage 1: Primary › Sore(s) on genitalia or mouth › The sore(s) can last 2 to 6 weeks Stage 2: Secondary › Rash on body › Flu-like symptoms Tertiary (last) Stage › Neurological/ cardiovascular complications	Can pass to sexual partners and to the neonate during pregnancy May cause miscarriage in women May cause heart disease, blindness, and/or brain damage Can lead to death	Caused by bacteria Penicillin G is drug of choice

Trichomoniasis (Trich)
Symptoms can appear 3 days to 2 weeks after infection.

SYMPTOMS IN WOMEN	SYMPTOMS IN MEN	COMPLICATIONS	TREATMENTS
May be asymptomatic Common symptom: yellowish to greenish, frothy, mucopurulent, copious, malodorous discharge. Dysuria and dyspareunia Vaginal irritation and pruritus	Often no symptoms White, watery penile discharge Painful/frequent urination	Can pass to sexual partners Can lead to prostate infection in men	Recommended treatment is metronidazole or tinidazole unless client in first trimester of pregnancy. Partner(s) should also be treated

Nursing Care of Children

Foundations of Nursing Care of Children

I Family

A. Identify legal guardian.

B. Build relationship with family and child.

C. Assess family dynamics.

D. Collaborative Care

   1. **Nursing Interventions**

      a. Respect family diversity.

      b. Assess parent-child interactions.

      c. Assist families to understand growth and development needs.

      d. Assist families to adapt to the needs of child with a health problem.

      e. Assist families to participate in care as appropriate.

      f. Use community resources for family adaptation.

Growth and Development

I Expected Growth and Development of the Infant (1st Year of Life)

A. **Physical Development**

   1. Fontanels

      a. Posterior closes by 6 to 8 weeks of age.

      b. Anterior closes by 12 to 18 months of age.

   2. Dentition

      a. First tooth appears between the ages of 6 and 10 months.

      b. Six to eight teeth by the end of first year

      c. For children under 2 years of age: Age of the child in months – 6 = Number of teeth

      d. Pain Relief for Teething

         1) Cold

            a) Refrigerated pacifier

            b) Cold teething ring

            c) Acetaminophen; ibuprofen if older than 6 months (do not use more than 3 days)

            d) Over-the-counter teething gels

      e. Tooth Care

         1) Clean teeth with cool, wet cloth.

      f. Do not give bottles to infants when they are falling asleep.

   3. Vision

      a. Infant vision is undeveloped, improves gradually

      b. At birth, can focus on objects 8 to 10 inches away

      c. Best able to discern shapes with contrast such as black/white and bright colors

      d. Red reflex should be present

   4. Measurements of Growth

      a. Height, weight, and head circumference plotted on graph

         1) Measure recumbent length (do not use tape measure).

         2) Measure weight to the nearest 10 g (0.35 oz) (Infants should be nude). Document devices (such as arm boards).

         3) Measure head circumference at widest point.

      b. Identify Issues

         1) Measurements below 5th percentile or above 95th percentile

         2) Plagiocephaly

            a) Educate parents to place infant in prone position 30 to 60 min/day.

            b) May require physical therapy or customized helmet to reshape skull.

      c. Rules of Thumb

         1) Newborns may lose up to 10% of birth weight by 3 to 4 days of age.

         2) Birth weight is reattained by 2 weeks of age.

         3) Birth weight doubles by 5 months of age.

         4) Birth weight triples by 12 months of age.

         5) Birth length increases approximately 2.5 cm (1 in) per month for the first 6 months.

         6) Birth length increases 50% by 12 months of age.

MOTOR SKILL DEVELOPMENT OF THE INFANT

AGE	GROSS MOTOR SKILLS	FINE MOTOR SKILLS
1 month	Demonstrates head lag	Strong grasp reflex
2 months	Lifts head off mattress when prone	Holds hands in an open position, grasp reflex disappearing
3 months	When in prone position, will raise head and shoulders; has slight head lag, bears weight on forearms	No longer has grasp reflex Actively holds rattle Keeps hands loosely open
4 months	Rolls from back to side	Holds object with both hands
5 months	Rolls from front to back	Able to grasp objects voluntarily Takes objects directly to mouth
6 months	Rolls from back to front	Holds bottle Picks up object if dropped
7 months	Bears full weight on feet Sits, leaning forward on both hands	Moves objects from hand to hand

MOTOR SKILL DEVELOPMENT OF THE INFANT (CONTINUED)

AGE	GROSS MOTOR SKILLS	FINE MOTOR SKILLS
8 months	Sits unsupported	Uses thumb and index finger in crude pincer grasp
9 months	Creeps on hands and knees instead of crawling Pulls to a standing position	Pincer grasp is more precise
10 months	Changes from a prone to a sitting position	Grasps rattle by its handle
11 months	Walks while holding onto something	Neat pincer grasp Deliberately drops objects for them to be picked up Places objects into a container
12 months	Sits down from a standing position without assistance Walks with one hand held	Tries to build a two-block tower without success Can turn pages in a book (many at a time)

INFANT DEVELOPMENT MILESTONES

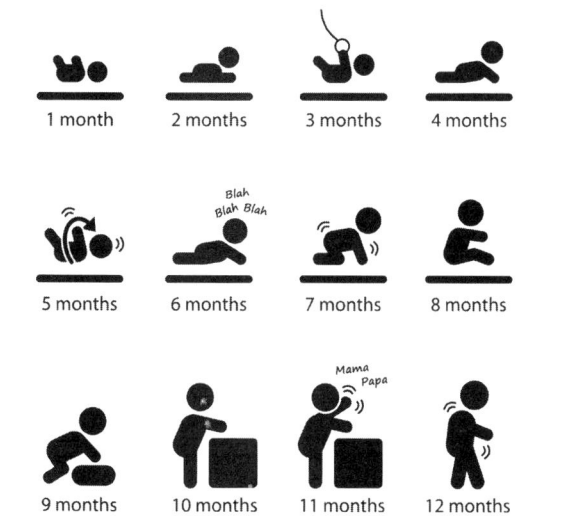

1 month 2 months 3 months 4 months

5 months 6 months 7 months 8 months

9 months 10 months 11 months 12 months

GETTY IMAGES/ISTOCKPHOTO

B. Cognitive Development

1. Piaget: Sensorimotor Phase (birth to 24 months)
   a. Separation: Learns to separate from other objects in the environment.
   b. Object permanence: Learns objects exist when hidden out of view.
      1) Occurs at approximately 9 to 10 months of age.
   c. Mental representation: Recognizes and uses symbols.
2. Language
   a. Crying is first form of verbal communication
   b. Coos and babbles; turns head to the sound of a rattle by 3 months
   c. Laughs aloud by 4 months
   d. Comprehends "no" by the age of 9 months
   e. Three to five words other than "dada" or "mama" by 12 months of age

C. Psychosocial Development

1. Erikson: Trust vs. Mistrust
   a. Trust develops as needs are met.
   b. Mistrust develops when needs are inadequately or inconsistently met, or if needs are met before vocalized by the infant.
2. Social Development
   a. Bonding
   b. Separation anxiety (4 to 8 months)
   c. Fear of strangers (6 to 8 months)
3. Body-Image Changes
   a. Discovers mouth produces pleasure.
   b. Discovers smiling causes others to react.
   c. Hands and feet are objects of play.

D. Age-Appropriate Activities

1. Solitary play
2. Shake rattles
3. Look in mirrors
4. Chew on teething toys
5. Play pat-a-cake
6. Play with blocks
7. Listen to someone read

E. Health Promotion for Infants

1. Newborn infants require medical visit with provider within 72 hr of discharge
   a. Immunizations
      1) The CDC Recommendations for Healthy Infants (less than 12 months of age)
         a) Birth: hepatitis B (Hep B)
         b) 2 months: diphtheria and tetanus toxoids and pertussis (DTaP), rotavirus vaccine (RV), inactivated poliovirus (IPV), *Haemophilus influenzae* type B (Hib), pneumococcal vaccine (PCV), and Hep B
         c) 4 months: DTaP, RV, IPV, Hib, PCV
         d) 6 months: DTaP, IPV (6 to 18 months), PCV, and Hep B (6 to 18 months); RV; Hib
         e) 6 to 12 months: seasonal influenza vaccination yearly (the trivalent inactivated influenza vaccine is available as an intramuscular injection)

NOTE: Always refer to the CDC website (www.cdc.gov) for the latest immunization requirements and schedules.

2. Nutrition
   a. Breastfeeding provides a complete diet for the first 6 months of life.
      1) Iron-fortified formula is an acceptable alternative to breast milk. Cow's milk is not recommended during the first 12 months.
      2) Vitamin D supplements within first few days of life.
      3) Iron supplements after 4 months of age for infants who are exclusively breastfed.
      4) Juice and water are not needed during the first 4 months.
      5) Do not provide fruit juice to infants younger than 1 year.
   b. Solid foods are introduced around 4 to 6 months of age.
      1) Introduce new foods one at a time and evaluate tolerance.
      2) Introduce iron-fortified cereal first.
      3) Introduce fruits and vegetables at 6 to 8 months, followed by meats.
      4) Nutritious finger foods such as cheese and raw fruit (no grapes) may be introduced at 8 to 9 months of age.
      5) Chopped, cooked, and unseasoned table foods are appropriate by 12 months of age.
      6) No citrus fruits, eggs, or meat until after 6 months; no honey during first year.
   c. Weaning
      1) Begin when infant shows signs of readiness and can drink from a cup. Usually occurs after 6 months.
      2) Stop bedtime feeding last.
3. Sleep Patterns
   a. Nocturnal sleep pattern established by 3 to 4 months of age.
   b. Sleeps through the night and takes one to two naps during the day by the age of 12 months.

II Safety for Infants

A. Aspiration
1. Provide age-appropriate toys.
2. Avoid small objects such as grapes, coins, and candy.
3. Check clothing and household objects for safety hazards such as loose buttons or drawstrings.

B. Suffocation
1. Keep plastic bags and balloons out of reach.
2. Remove pillows from crib.
3. Remove mobiles from crib by 4 to 5 months of age.
4. Firm crib mattresses with snug fit
5. Crib slats no farther apart than 6 cm (2.375 in).

C. Bodily Harm
1. Keep sharp objects out of reach.
2. Anchor furniture and heavy objects.
3. Do not leave infants unattended with animals.
4. Monitor infants for shaken baby syndrome.

D. Burns
1. Check temperature of bath water.
2. Set hot water thermostats at or below 49° C (120° F).
3. Keep working smoke detectors in the home.
4. Turn handles of pots and pans to the backs of stoves.
5. Apply sunscreen if infants will be exposed to the sun.
6. Cover electrical outlets.
7. Do not heat breast milk or formula in microwave.

E. Drowning
1. Do not leave unattended around water sources (e.g., tubs, toilets, cleaning buckets).
2. Secure fencing around swimming pools.
3. Close bathroom doors.

F. Falls
1. Keep infant seats on the ground or floor if used outside of the car.
2. Place safety gates at top and bottom of stairs.
3. Position crib mattresses in the lowest position with rails all the way up.

G. Poisoning
1. Keep poison control number readily available.
2. Avoid exposure to lead paint.
3. Keep toxins and plants out of reach. Use safety locks on cabinets.
4. Store medications in childproof containers and place out of reach.
5. Maintain working carbon monoxide detectors in home.

H. Motor Vehicle Injuries
1. Newborn infants should be placed in a federally approved car seat at a 45 degree angle; secure with safety belt.
2. Rear-facing in back seat.
3. Place shoulder harnesses in slots at or below level of infant's shoulders.
4. Place retainer clip at axillary level of infant.
5. Rear-facing until 2 years of age or the height recommended by manufacturer.
6. If air bags are near the infant (such as in a vehicle without a rear seat), the passenger seat air bag should be inactivated.

I. **Sudden Infant Death Syndrome (SIDS)**
   1. Contributing Factors
      a. Males
      b. Under 1 year of age (peak 2 to 3 months)
      c. Prematurity
      d. Low birth weight
      e. Low Apgar scores
      f. Poverty
      g. Family history of SIDS
      h. Maternal smoking or second-hand smoke
      i. Twin or multiple birth
      j. Co-sleeping
   2. Prevention
      a. Place infant on back for sleep.
      b. Encourage breastfeeding.
      c. Offer pacifier when sleeping.
      d. Prevent overheating.
      e. Remove pillows and quilts from crib; keep infant's head uncovered during sleep.
      f. Maintain up-to-date immunizations.

III Expected Growth and Development of the Toddler (Ages 1 to 3 Years)

A. **Physical Development**
   1. Anterior fontanel closes by 18 months of age.
   2. Weight: weigh four times birth weight at 30 months of age.
   3. Height: toddlers grow about 7.5 cm (3 in) per year.
   4. Head circumference: equal to chest circumference by 1 to 2 years of age.

MOTOR SKILL DEVELOPMENT OF THE TODDLER

AGE	GROSS MOTOR SKILLS	FINE MOTOR SKILLS
15 months	Walks without help Creeps up stairs	Uses a cup well Builds a tower of two blocks
18 months	Runs clumsily; falls often Throws ball overhand Jumps in place with both feet Pulls and pushes toys	Manages a spoon without rotation Turns pages in a book, two or three at a time Builds tower of three or four blocks
2 years	Walks up and down stairs by placing both feet on each step Runs with wide stance Kicks ball forward without falling	Builds a tower of six or seven blocks Turns pages in a book, one at a time
2.5 years	Jumps across the floor, off a chair or step using both feet Takes a few steps on tiptoe Stands on one foot momentarily	Draws circles and crosses Has good hand-finger coordination

TODDLER DEVELOPMENT MILESTONES

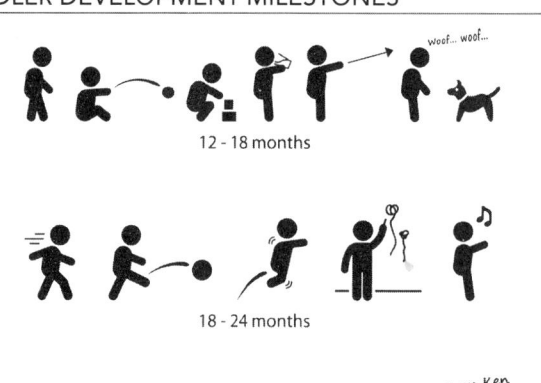

12 - 18 months

18 - 24 months

2 - 3 years

GETTY IMAGES/ISTOCKPHOTO

B. **Cognitive Development**
   1. Piaget: The sensorimotor phase transitions to the preoperational phase around 19 to 24 months of age.
      a. Object permanence is developed
      b. Memory develops
      c. Preoperational thought allows the toddler to use symbols to represent objects
   2. Language
      a. 1 year: one word sentences
      b. 2 years: two to three word sentences
      c. 3 years: simple sentences
   3. Psychosocial Development
      a. Erikson: Autonomy vs. Shame and Doubt
      b. Independence
      c. Negativism
      d. Temper tantrums
      e. Ritualism
      f. Separation anxiety peaks
   4. Moral Development
      a. Egocentric
      b. Sense good behavior is rewarded and bad is punished
   5. Self-Concept Development
      a. See themselves as separate from parents
   6. Body Image Changes
      a. Appreciates the usefulness of various body parts
      b. Develops gender identity by 3 years of age

C. **Age-Appropriate Activities**

1. Solitary Play Evolves to Parallel Play
   a. Fill and empty containers
   b. Play with blocks
   c. Look at books
   d. Push-pull toys
   e. Scribble with crayon
2. Toilet Training
   a. Begins when toddler is able to recognize the urge to urinate or defecate.
   b. Nighttime continence usually develops last.
3. Discipline
   a. Consistent with well-defined boundaries

D. **Health Promotion for Toddlers**

1. Immunizations
   a. CDC Recommendations for Toddlers (1 to 3 years of age)
      1) 12 to 15 months: inactivated poliovirus (third dose between 6 to 18 months); *Haemophilus influenzae* type B; pneumococcal conjugate vaccine; measles, mumps, and rubella; and varicella
      2) 12 to 23 months: hepatitis A (Hep A), given in two doses at least 6 months apart
      3) 15 to 18 months: diphtheria, tetanus, and acellular pertussis
      4) 12 to 36 months: yearly seasonal trivalent inactivated influenza vaccine; live, attenuated influenza vaccine by nasal spray (must be 2 years or older)
2. Nutrition
   a. Avoid snacks high in fat, sugar, and sodium.
   b. Serving size is about 1 tbsp per year of age.
   c. Should consume 24 to 28 oz of milk per day. Change from whole milk to low-fat milk after 2 years of age.
   d. Limit juice to 4 to 6 oz per day.
   e. Include 1 cup of fruit daily.
   f. No eating or drinking during play or when lying down.
   g. Prefer finger foods.
   h. Picky eaters. Physiologic anorexia occurs.
3. Sleep and Rest
   a. Average 11 to 12 hr of sleep per day and one nap.
   b. Resists going to bed.
4. Dental Care
   a. Established dental provider by 1 year of age.
   b. Adult caregiver should brush and floss teeth after meals and at bedtime.

IV **Safety for Toddler**

A. **Aspiration**
1. Avoid small objects (e.g., coins, candy) and toys with small parts.
2. Avoid common causes of choking: hot dogs, nuts, grapes, peanut butter, raw carrots, tough meat, popcorn.
3. Keep away from balloons.
4. Check clothing for drawstrings and loose buttons.
5. Teach parents emergency procedures for choking.

B. **Bodily Harm**
1. Keep sharp objects out of reach.
2. Store firearms in locked boxes or cabinets.
3. Do not leave unattended with animals.
4. Teach stranger safety.

C. **Burns**
1. Check temperature of bath water.
2. Set hot water thermostats at or below 49° C (120° F).
3. Keep working smoke detectors in the home.
4. Turn handles of pots and pans to the backs of stoves.
5. Cover electrical outlets.
6. Apply sunscreen when exposed to the sun.

D. **Drowning**
1. Do not leave unattended in bathtubs.
2. Keep toilet lids closed.
3. Supervise closely when near pools or water.
4. Teach how to swim.

E. **Falls**
1. Keep doors and windows locked.
2. Position crib mattresses in the lowest position with rails all the way up.
3. Place safety gates at top and bottom of stairs.

F. **Motor Vehicle Injuries**
1. Remain in rear-facing car seat until the age of 2 years or the height recommended by manufacturer.
2. Forward-facing car seat for toddlers over the age of 2 years, or who exceed the height recommendation.
3. Back seat is the safest area.
4. If vehicle does not have a rear seat, passenger seat air bag should be inactivated.

G. **Poisoning**
1. Keep poison control number readily available.
2. Avoid exposure to lead paint.
3. Place safety locks on cabinets that contain cleaners and other chemicals.
4. Store medications in childproof containers and place out of reach.
5. Maintain working carbon monoxide detectors in home.

H. **Suffocation**
1. Keep plastic bags out of reach.
2. Remove pillows from crib.
3. Crib mattresses should fit tightly.
4. Crib slats no farther apart than 6 cm (2.375 in).
5. Remove doors from unused appliances (such as refrigerators).

V Expected Growth and Development of the Preschooler (Ages 3 to 6 Years)

A. **Physical Development**
1. Weight: Gains 2 to 3 kg (4.4 to 6.6 lb) per year.
2. Height: Grows 6.5 to 9 cm (2.5 to 3.5 in) per year.
3. Fine and gross motor skills improve.

MOTOR SKILLS OF THE PRESCHOOLER

AGE	GROSS MOTOR SKILLS	FINE MOTOR SKILLS
3 years	Alternates feet when going up and down stairs Rides a tricycle Jumps off bottom step Stands on one foot for a few seconds	Builds a tower of nine to ten cubes Imitates cross when drawing Cannot draw a stick figure; may draw a circle with facial features
4 years	Skips and hops on one foot Throws a ball overhead Catches ball reliably	Uses scissors Laces shoes Copies square, traces cross and diamond
5 years	Jumps rope Walks backward with heel to toe Moves up and down stairs easily Throws and catches ball with ease	Ties shoelaces Uses pencil well Prints some letters Draws most of stick figure

B. **Cognitive and Language Development**
1. Piaget
   a. Preoperational phase transitions to intuitive thought.
   b. Makes judgments based on visual appearances.
2. Variations in Thinking:
   a. Magical thinking: Thoughts can cause events to happen.
   b. Animism: Inanimate objects are alive.
   c. Centration: Focuses on one aspect instead of the whole.
   d. Time: Understands sequence of daily events.
3. Language Development
   a. Enjoys talking.
   b. Speaks in three to five word sentences.

C. **Psychosocial Development**
1. Erikson: Initiative vs. Guilt
   a. Energetic learners, but lack physical abilities to be successful at everything.
   b. Guilt may occur if they misbehave or are unable to accomplish a task.
2. Self-Concept Development
   a. Feels good about mastering skills that promote independence (such as dressing self).
   b. May regress (e.g., bedwetting, sucking thumb) during times of stress, insecurity, or illness.
3. Body-Image Change
   a. Recognizes differences in appearances.
   b. Begins to compare themselves with others.
   c. Intrusive experiences (e.g., injections or cuts) are traumatic due to poor understanding of anatomy.

4. Moral Development
   a. Early preschoolers take actions based on the result of reward or punishment.
5. Social Development
   a. Older preschoolers take actions to satisfy personal needs.
   b. Begins to understand fairness.
   c. Prolonged separation (such as hospitalization) may cause anxiety.
   d. Favorite toys and appropriate play should be used.
   e. Does not exhibit stranger anxiety.
   f. Pretend play; may develop imaginary friends.

D. **Age-Appropriate Activities**
1. Associative play with some cooperation
2. Common Activities
   a. Play ball
   b. Puzzles
   c. Tricycles
   d. Pretend play and "dress-up"
   e. Painting
   f. Read books
   g. Electronic games and TV—limit screen time to 2 hr or less

E. **Health Promotion for Preschoolers**
1. Immunizations
   a. CDC Recommendations for Preschoolers (3 to 6 years of age)
      1) 4 to 6 years: diphtheria and tetanus toxoids and pertussis (DTaP); measles, mumps, and rubella (MMR); varicella; and inactivated poliovirus (IPV)
      2) 3 to 6 years: yearly seasonal influenza vaccine; trivalent inactivated influenza vaccine; or live, attenuated influenza vaccine by nasal spray
2. Nutrition
   a. Consumes half the amount of adults (1,800 kcal).
   b. May continue to be picky eaters, but more willing to try different foods at 5 years of age.
   c. Provide a diet with adequate protein, calcium, iron, folate, and vitamins A & C.
   d. Should consume five servings of fruits and vegetables per day.
   e. Should not consume sweetened beverages.
3. Dental Health
   a. Eruption of primary teeth is finalized.
   b. Parents should assist and supervise brushing and flossing.
   c. Dental trauma is common and should be immediately assessed by dentist.
4. Sleep and Rest
   a. Requires about 12 hr of sleep per day.
   b. May require daytime nap.
   c. Sleep disturbances are common.

VI Safety for Preschoolers

A. Bodily Harm

1. Place all firearms and ammunition in locked cabinets or containers.
2. Teach stranger safety.
3. Should wear protective equipment on bicycles, skateboards, and scooters (such as a helmet).

B. Burns

1. Set hot water thermostats at or below 49° C (120° F).
2. Keep working smoke detectors in the home.
3. Apply sunscreen when outside.

C. Drowning

1. Do not leave unattended in bathtubs.
2. Supervise closely when near pools or any body of water.
3. Teach water safety and how to swim.

D. Motor Vehicle Injuries

1. Use a federally approved car restraint according to the manufacturer recommendations.
2. Transition to booster seat when forward-facing car seat is outgrown.
3. An approved car restraint system is recommended until a height of 145 cm (4 feet, 9 in) is achieved or 8 to 12 years of age.
4. Safest area for children is back seat.
5. If vehicle does not have a rear seat, passenger seat air bag should be inactivated.

E. Poisoning

1. Keep poison control number readily available.
2. While this age group is more aware of dangers, poisoning is still a concern. Continue to implement precautions.

VII Expected Growth and Development of the School-Age Child (Age 6 to 12 Years)

A. Physical Development

1. Weight: Gains 2 to 3 kg (4.4 to 6.6 lb) per year.
2. Height: Grows 5 cm (2 inches) per year.
3. Prepubescence
   a. Physiological changes in females around the age of 9 years.
   b. Visible sexual maturation in males is minimal.
4. Permanent teeth erupt.
5. Bones continue to ossify.

B. Cognitive and Language Development

1. Piaget: Concrete Operations
   a. Learns to tell time.
   b. Masters concept of conservation; mass is understood first.
   c. Sees the perspective of others.
   d. Solves problems.
2. Language
   a. Defines many words and understands rules of grammar.
   b. Understands a word may have multiple meanings.

C. Psychosocial Development

1. Erikson: Industry vs. Inferiority
   a. A sense of industry is achieved through the development of personal and interpersonal skills, which allows the child to contribute to society.
   b. A sense of inferiority may occur if previous stages have not been mastered or if the child is unable or not ready to assume responsibilities.
2. Moral Development
   a. Early School-Age Years
      1) Does not understand reasoning behind rules and expectations.
      2) Believes he is wrong and others are right.
      3) Judgment guided by rewards and punishment.
      4) May interpret accidents as punishment.
   b. Later School-Age Years
      1) Can judge the intentions of an act rather than the consequences.
      2) Understands different points of view.
      3) Conceptualizes treating others as they like to be treated.
3. Self-Concept Development
   a. Develops an awareness of themselves in relation to others.
   b. Understands personal values, abilities, and physical characteristics.
   c. Gains confidence by establishing a positive self-concept.
   d. Influenced by parents, but by middle-childhood, peers and teachers are more valuable.
4. Body-Image Changes
   a. Curiosity about sexuality should be addressed with education.
   b. Knowledgeable about the body.
   c. Compares body to peers.
   d. Aware of physical disabilities in others.
   e. May be excluded if different.
   f. More modest than preschoolers and places more emphasis on privacy issues.
5. Social Development
   a. Peers are important. Peer pressure begins.
   b. Clubs and best friends are popular.
   c. Prefers same-gender companions, but develops an interest in the opposite sex by the end of the school-age years.
   d. Most relationships come from school associations.
   e. Bullying may occur in an attempt to cause harm or to control.
   f. Conformity becomes evident.

D. **Age-Appropriate Activities**
1. Play is competitive and cooperative
2. Common Activities
    a. Board games
    b. Jump rope
    c. Collecting
    d. Bicycles
    e. Organized sports
    f. Crafts
E. **Health Promotion for School-Age Children**
1. Immunizations
    a. CDC Recommendations for School-Age Children (6 to 12 years of age)
        1) If not given between 4 and 5 years of age, children should receive the following vaccines by 6 years of age: diphtheria and tetanus toxoids and pertussis (DTaP); inactivated poliovirus; measles, mumps, and rubella (MMR); and varicella
        2) Yearly seasonal influenza vaccine: trivalent inactivated influenza vaccine (TIV) or live, attenuated influenza vaccine (LAIV) by nasal spray
        3) 11 to 12 years: tetanus and diphtheria toxoids and pertussis vaccine (Tdap); human papillomavirus vaccine—HPV2 or HPV4 in three doses for females, HPV4 for males; and meningococcal (MCV4)
2. Nutrition
    a. Should eat adult portions by the end of school-age years.
    b. Obesity is a concern. Teach parents to avoid using food as a reward and emphasize physical activity.
    c. Do not skip meals.
3. Sleep and Rest
    a. Variable and depends on age, level of activity, and health status.
    b. Approximately 9 hr of sleep at the age of 11 years.
4. Health screenings
    a. Scoliosis
    b. Dental Health
        1) Obtain regular checkups; fluoride treatments if necessary.
        2) Brush after meals, snacks, and at bedtime.

VIII **Safety for School-Age Children**
A. **Bodily Harm**
1. Keep firearms locked in cabinets or boxes.
2. Identify safe play areas.
3. Teach stranger safety.
4. Teach to wear protective equipment (e.g., helmets, pads).
B. **Burns**
1. Teach fire safety and burn hazards.
2. Teach safety precautions for cooking.
3. Keep working smoke detectors in the home.
4. Use sunscreen when outside.
C. **Drowning**
1. Supervise when swimming or when near a body of water.
2. Teach water safety and how to swim.
3. Check depth of water prior to diving.
D. **Motor Vehicle Injuries**
1. Use an approved car restraint system until a height of 145 cm (4 feet, 9 inches) is achieved or 8 to 12 years of age.
2. Teach to use a seat belt when a car restraint system or booster seat is no longer required.
3. Lap belts should lay across upper thighs (not the stomach).
4. Shoulder belts should lay across chest (not the neck).
5. Do not ride in the bed of a pickup truck.
6. Teach pedestrian safety.
E. **Poisoning/Substance Abuse**
1. Keep cleaners and chemicals locked and placed out of reach.
2. Teach to say "no" to drugs and alcohol.

IX **Expected Growth and Development of the Adolescent (12 to 20 Years)**
A. **Physical Development**
1. Females
    a. Height: Grow 5 to 20 cm (2 to 8 in).
    b. Weight: Gain 7 to 25 kg (15.5 to 55 lb).
    c. Growth stops about 2 years after menarche.
2. Males
    a. Height: Grow 10 to 30 cm (4 to 12 in).
    b. Weight: Gain 7 to 30 kg (15.5 to 66 lb).
    c. Growth stops around 18 to 20 years of age.
3. Sexual maturation occurs.
B. **Cognitive and Language Development**
1. Piaget: Formal Operations
    a. Able to think of more than two categories of variables at the same time.
    b. Can evaluate own thinking.
    c. Imaginative and idealistic.
    d. More capable of using formal logic to make decisions.
    e. Understands how actions can influence others.

C. **Psychosocial Development**
1. Erikson: Identity vs. Role Confusion
   a. Develops personal identity; views themselves as unique.
   b. Peer groups greatly influence behavior
   c. See themselves as invincible
2. Sexual Identity
   a. Intimate relationships may develop
   b. Masturbation
3. Moral Development
   a. Uses internalized moral principles to solve dilemmas.
   b. Questions existing moral values to society and individuals.
4. Self-Concept Development
   a. Progresses from viewing themselves in relation to similarities with peers to recognizing unique individual characteristics.
5. Body Image Changes
   a. Normality is based on comparison with peers.
   b. Image established during adolescence is retained throughout life.
6. Social Development
   a. Peers are a support system.
   b. Friendships with best friends are stronger and last longer.
   c. Parent-child relationships change to allow independence.

D. **Age-Appropriate Activities**
1. Nonviolent video games
2. Nonviolent music
3. Sports
4. Caring for a pet
5. Career training programs
6. Reading
7. Social events (e.g., going to movies, school dances)

E. **Health Promotion for Adolescents**
1. Immunizations
   a. CDC Recommendations for Clients 13 to 18 Years of Age
      1) Include catch-up doses of any recommended immunizations not received at 11 to 12 years old.
      2) Yearly seasonal influenza vaccine: trivalent inactivated influenza vaccine or live, attenuated influenza vaccine by nasal spray.
      3) 16 to 18 years: meningococcal (MCV4) booster is recommended if first dose was received between the ages of 13 and 15 years. A booster dose is not needed if the first dose is received at age 16 or older.

2. Screenings
   a. Scoliosis
   b. Growth and development (e.g., physical health, self-image, physical activity)
   c. Social and academics (e.g., relationships, grades)
   d. Emotional well-being (e.g., mental health, sexuality)
   e. Risk reduction (e.g., tobacco, alcohol, other drugs)
   f. Violence and injury prevention
3. Nutrition
   a. Needs additional calcium, iron, protein, and zinc.
   b. Intake of folic acid, vitamin B6, vitamin A, iron, calcium, and zinc may be inadequate.
   c. Yearly Assessments of Height, Weight, and BMI to Identify Issues:
      1) Overeating—avoid using food as a reward.
      2) Undereating
4. Sleep and Rest
   a. Sleep habits change due to increased metabolism and rapid growth.
   b. Need for sleep increases.
   c. May stay up late and sleep later in the morning.
5. Dental Health
   a. Corrective appliances are common.
   b. Brush after meals, snacks, and at bedtime.
   c. Floss daily.
   d. Regular checkups.
   e. Regular fluoride treatments if necessary.
6. Sexuality
   a. Provide accurate information.
   b. Emphasize abstinence.
   c. Education: Prevent sexually transmitted infections and pregnancy.

X Safety for Adolescents
A. **Bodily Harm**
1. Keep firearms unloaded and locked in a cabinet or box.
2. Teach proper use of sporting equipment.
3. Insist on using protective equipment (e.g., helmets, pads) during activities like riding a bicycle or skiing.
4. Be aware of changes in mood. Monitor for:
   a. Poor school performance
   b. Lack of interest
   c. Social isolation
   d. Disturbances in appetite or sleep
   e. Expression of thoughts of suicide
B. **Burns**
1. Teach fire safety.
2. Apply sunscreen when outside.
3. Avoid tanning beds.

C. **Motor Vehicle Injuries**

1. Encourage driver's education courses.
2. Emphasize use of seat belts.
3. Discourage use of cell phones and driving.
4. Teach dangers of drinking and driving.
5. Role model desired behavior.

D. **Substance Abuse**

1. Monitor for signs of substance abuse.
2. Teach to say "no" to harmful substances and alcohol.

XI Child Maltreatment: Neglect and Abuse

A. Occurs across all economic and educational backgrounds and racial/ethnic/religious groups.

B. **Types**

1. Physical: causing pain or harm (e.g., shaken baby syndrome, fractures).
2. Sexual: Occurs when sexual contact takes place without consent, regardless of the victim being able to give consent. Includes any sexual behavior toward a minor and dating violence.
3. Emotional: humiliating, threatening, or intimidating behavior.
4. Neglect: failure to provide physical (e.g., food, clothes) and emotional (e.g., affection, nurturing) needs.

C. **Contributing Factors**

1. Parental
   a. Poor self-esteem
   b. Victim of abuse
   c. Lack of knowledge: parenting skills
   d. Young or single parent
   e. Social isolation
   f. Substance use disorder
2. Child
   a. 1 year old or younger
   b. Unwanted
   c. Premature
   d. Hyperactive
   e. Physically or mentally challenged
3. Environment
   a. Chronic stress
   b. Socioeconomic factors (e.g., unemployment, divorce)

D. **Manifestations of Abuse and Neglect**

1. Expected Findings
   a. Inconsistencies between the parent's and child's report.
   b. Inconsistency between nature of injury and developmental level of child.
   c. Repeated injuries requiring emergency treatment.
   d. Inappropriate responses from the parents or child.

2. Physical and Emotional Neglect
   a. Failure to thrive; lack of social smile in infant
   b. Lack of hygiene
   c. Frequent injuries; delay in seeking health care
   d. Dull affect; withdrawn
   e. School absences
   f. Enuresis
   g. Suicide attempt
   h. Self-stimulating behaviors

3. Physical Abuse
   a. Bruises in various stages of healing
   b. Burns, fractures, and/or lacerations
   c. Fear of parents
   d. Lack of emotion; withdrawn
   e. Aggression

4. Shaken Baby Syndrome
   a. Poor feeding; vomiting
   b. Bulging fontanels; retinal hemorrhages
   c. Seizures; posturing
   d. Respiratory distress

5. Sexual Abuse
   a. Bruising, lacerations, and/or bleeding of the genitals, anus, or mouth
   b. STI; frequent UTI
   c. Sudden change in behavior or personality; regressive behavior

6. Collaborative Care
   a. **Nursing Interventions**
      1) Identify abuse as soon as possible. Mandatory reporting is required of suspected or actual cases of child abuse.
      2) Do not leave child unattended. Use language the child understands.
      3) Assess for unusual bruising on abdomen, back, and/or buttocks.
      4) Document findings objectively; include diagrams and pictures.
      5) Interview child and parents separately.
   b. Diagnostic Procedures
      1) Imaging: X-Ray, CT, or MRI
      2) Laboratory: CBC, urinalysis, test for sexually transmitted infection

Adapting Nursing Care for the Child

EXPECTED VITAL SIGNS

Normal values vary by age and, in some instances, by gender.

Changes in vital signs occur with activity, medication, and illness.

At birth, heart rate and respirations are higher than adults; blood pressure is lower than adults.

As the child ages, heart rate and respirations decrease and the blood pressure increases.

The data below provides general ranges. The nurse must consider all factors when analyzing findings.

AGE	BLOOD PRESSURE	HEART RATE	RESPIRATORY RATE
0 to 30 days	65 to 75/ 40 to 50 mm Hg ·	110 to 160/min	30 to 60/min
1 month to 1 year	75 to 100/ 40 to 55 mm Hg	100 to 150/min	30 to 50/min
1 to 2 years	85 to 105/ 40 to 60 mm Hg	90 to 130/min	24 to 40/min
3 to 5 years	90 to 110/ 45 to 70 mm Hg	80 to 110/min	20 to 30/min
6 to 12 years	100 to 120/ 60 to 80 mm Hg	70 to 100/min	18 to 25/min
13 to 18 years	110 to 130/ 60 to 80 mm Hg	55 to 90/min	12 to 20/min

I Stress of Hospitalization

A. Families and children may experience major stress. The child's cognitive ability and stage of development influence their response.

B. **Stages of Separation Anxiety**

1. Protest (e.g., screaming, physical aggression)
2. Despair (e.g., withdrawal, developmental regression)
3. Detachment (e.g., interacts with strangers, appears happy)

C. **Family Responses**

1. Fear and guilt
2. Frustration
3. Alteration in family roles
4. Worry (e.g., finances, missed work, other children)

D. **Nursing Interventions**

1. Recognize stress and intervene as soon as possible.
2. Consider families of children who are ill as clients.
3. Teach the child and family what to expect.
4. Maintain a routine as much as possible.
5. Encourage parents or family members to stay with child.
6. Encourage independence and provide choices.
7. Explain treatments and procedures.
8. Provide developmentally appropriate activities.

AGE-RELATED NURSING INTERVENTIONS

AGE	INTERVENTIONS
Infant	Place infants whose parents are not in attendance close to nursing stations so that their needs may be quickly met.
	Provide consistency in assigning caregivers.
Toddler	Provide consistency in assigning caregivers.
	Encourage parents to provide routine care, such as changing diapers and feeding.
	Encourage the child's autonomy by giving appropriate choices.
Preschooler	Explain all procedures using simple, clear language. Avoid terms that can be misinterpreted by the child.
	Promote independence by encouraging the child to provide self-care.
	Encourage the child to express feelings.
	Validate fears and concerns.
	Provide toys that allow for emotional expression, such as a pounding board to release feelings of protest.
	Give choices when possible, such as "Do you want to take the pink or purple medicine first?"
	Allow younger children to handle equipment if it is safe.
School-age	Provide factual information.
	Encourage the child to express feelings.
	Maintain a normal routine for long hospitalizations, including time for school work.
	Encourage contact with peer group.
Adolescent	Provide factual information.
	Include in the planning of care to relieve feelings of powerlessness and lack of control.
	Encourage contact with peer group.

II Therapeutic Play

A. **Purpose**

1. Encourages acting out of various feelings.
2. Allows the ability to learn coping strategies.
3. Assists in gaining cooperation for medical treatment.

B. **Assessment**

1. Developmental level
2. Motor skills
3. Level of activity tolerance
4. Preferences

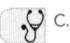 C. **Nursing Interventions**

1. Select safe toys; encourage parents to bring toys from home. (Consider isolation precautions.)
2. Select activities to enhance development.
3. Observe for clues to fears or anxieties.
4. Use dolls/stuffed animals to demonstrate procedures before they are performed.
5. Allow child to go to playroom if able.
6. Involve child life specialist in planning activities.

EFFECT OF HOSPITALIZATION ON CHILDREN

Infant

LEVEL OF UNDERSTANDING	Unable to describe illness and follow directions
	Lacks understanding of the need for therapeutic procedures
EFFECT OF HOSPITALIZATION	Displays physical behaviors as expressions of discomfort due to inability to verbalize
	Exaggerated stranger anxiety (6 to 18 months)
	May experience sleep deprivation due to strange noises, monitoring devices, and procedures

Toddler

LEVEL OF UNDERSTANDING	Limited ability to describe illness
	Poorly developed sense of body image and boundaries
	Limited understanding of the need for therapeutic procedures
	Limited ability to follow directions
EFFECT OF HOSPITALIZATION	Experiences separation anxiety
	May have regression of behavior
	May exhibit an intense reaction to any type of procedure due to the intrusion of boundaries

Preschooler

LEVEL OF UNDERSTANDING	Limited understanding of the cause of illness, but knows what illness feels like
	Limited ability to describe symptoms
	Fears related to magical thinking
EFFECT OF HOSPITALIZATION	May experience separation anxiety
	May harbor fears of bodily harm
	Might believe illness and hospitalization are a punishment

School-age child

LEVEL OF UNDERSTANDING	Beginning awareness of body functioning
	Ability to describe pain
	Increasing ability to understand cause and effect
EFFECT OF HOSPITALIZATION	Fears loss of control
	Seeks information as a way to maintain a sense of control
	May sense when not being told the truth
	May experience stress related to separation from peers and regular routine

Adolescent

LEVEL OF UNDERSTANDING	Increasing ability to understand cause and effect
	Perceptions of illness severity are based on the degree of body image changes
EFFECT OF HOSPITALIZATION	Develops body image disturbance
	Attempts to maintain composure, but is embarrassed about losing control
	Experiences feelings of isolation from peers
	Worries about outcome and impact on school/activities
	May not adhere to treatments/medication regimen due to peer influence

III Pain Management

A. Assessment of pain depends on cognitive, emotional, and physical development. Children under 4 years of age are unable to report pain accurately.

TOOLS USED IN PAIN ASSESSMENT

Faces, Legs, Activity, Cry, and Consolability (FLACC) Pain Tool *2 months to 7 years*	Pain rated on a scale of 0 to 10 Assess behaviors of child: › **F** – Face › **L** – Legs › **A** – Activity › **C** – Cry › **C** – Consolability
FACES Pain Rating Scale *3 years and older*	Rating scale uses drawings of happy and sad faces to depict levels of pain Numeric scale; 5 years and older Child rates pain on scale of 0 to 5 May substitute numbers and convert to 0 to 10 scale Child reports a number or points to level of pain on a visual scale
Oucher *3 to 13 years of age*	Pain rated on a scale of 0 to 5 using six photographs May substitute numbers and convert to a 0 to 10 scale Child organizes photographs in order of no pain to worst pain and chooses picture that best describes their feeling
Noncommunicating Children's Pain Checklist *3 years of age and older*	Observe behaviors for 10 min Score each category using 0 to 3 scale: › Vocal › Social › Facial › Activity › Body and limbs › Physiological

B. **Collaborative Care**

1. **Nursing Interventions**

   a. Use an appropriate pain tool to assess pain; reassess frequently.

   b. Include parents/provider in the assessment of pain.

   c. Administer medications in a timely manner and evaluate effectiveness.

   d. Include nonpharmacological measures.

      1) Distraction: play therapy, tell a story

      2) Relaxation: hold, rock, swaddle, reposition

      3) Imagery: guide child to use imagination

      4) Behavioral: stickers, contracts

      5) Sensory: massage, skin to skin, pacifier

   e. Use treatment room for painful procedures; allow parents to remain with child.

   f. Use appropriate terminology for developmental level.

   g. Provide choices.

2. Pharmacologic Measures
   a. Two-step approach is recommended.
      1) First step: non-opioid for mild pain in children 3 months of age or older.
         a) Nonsteroidal anti-inflammatory medications are frequently used.
      2) Second step: strong opioid for moderate or severe pain.
         a) Morphine is the medication of choice.

ANALGESIA FOR CHILDREN

ROUTE	NURSING IMPLICATIONS
Oral	Preferred route
	Takes 1 to 2 hr to reach peak analgesic effects
	Not recommended for rapid pain relief or fluctuating pain
Topical/ transdermal	Eutectic mixture of local anesthetics (EMLA) contains equal quantities of lidocaine and prilocaine in the form of a cream or disk
	› Use for any procedure in which the skin will be punctured (e.g., IV insertion, biopsy) 60 min prior to a superficial puncture and 2½ hr prior to a deep puncture
	› Place an occlusive dressing over the cream after application
	› Remove dressing and clean skin prior to procedure. Reddened or blanched skin indicates an adequate response
	› Tap skin to demonstrate to child skin is not sensitive
	› Instruct parents to apply at home prior to coming to a health care facility for a procedure
	Fentanyl
	› For children older than 12 years of age
	› Provides continuous pain control. Onset of 12 to 24 hr and a duration of 72 hr
	› May use immediate-release opioid for breakthrough pain
	› Treat respiratory depression with naloxone
Continuous Intravenous	Provide steady blood levels
Bolus	Rapid pain control in approximately 5 min
Patient-controlled analgesia (PCA)	Patient-controlled analgesia (PCA)
	Self-administration of medication
	Lockouts prevent overdosing
Family-controlled analgesia	Same concept as PCA
	Parent or caregiver manages child's pain

IV Safe Medication Administration

A. Growth and organ system maturity affect metabolism and excretion of medications in infants and children. Dosage is based on age, body weight, and body surface area (BSA).

B. **Collaborative Care**

1. **Nursing Interventions**
   a. Calculate the safe dosage. Notify provider if medication is outside of the safe dose range.
   b. Ask a second nurse to verify dosing for high risk and facility-regulated medications.
   c. Follow Rights of Medication Administration
      1) Use two client identifiers prior to administration: client name and date of birth.
      2) Use parent(s) for verification of infants or nonverbal children. Note: Two identifiers from the ID band must be confirmed (e.g., client name, date of birth, or hospital identification number).
      3) Determine parents' level of involvement with administration.
      4) Provide choices (such as left vs. right arm).
      5) Prepare child according to developmental stage and age.
   d. Routes of Medication Administration
      1) Aerosol Medications
         a) Use mask for younger children.
      2) Oral Medications
         a) Place or hold in upright position.
         b) Use smallest measuring device for liquid medication (e.g., dropper, dosing syringe, medication cup).
         c) Do not use a teaspoon or tablespoon for measuring.
         d) Allow infant to suck medication through a nipple, syringe, or dropper (do not mix in a bottle of formula or juice).
         e) Determine ability to swallow pills.
         f) Ask child to hold nose before, during, and after administration.
         g) Mix medication in small amount of sweet fluid or food (such as applesauce) or add flavoring.
      3) Optic Medications
         a) Position supine or sitting.
         b) Extend head and ask child to look up.
         c) Pull lower eyelid down and apply medication in pocket.
         d) Administer ointments before nap or bedtime.
         e) Apply light pressure to lacrimal punctum for 1 min (prevents unpleasant taste).
         f) Apply medication in nasal corner if eyes shut tight.

4) Otic Medications (should be at room temperature)

 a) Place child in prone or supine position with affected ear up.

 b) Younger than 3 years of age: Pull pinna down and back.

 c) Older than 3 years of age: Pull pinna up and back.

5) Nasal Medications

 a) Position child with head extended; hold infant in football position.

 b) Insert tip vertically, then angle prior to administration.

6) Rectal Medications

 a) Insert quickly (beyond rectal sphincters).

 b) Hold buttocks together for 5 to 10 min.

7) Injections

 a) Factors Influencing Injection Sites

  (1) Amount and viscosity

  (2) Type of medication

  (3) Muscle mass (amount and condition)

  (4) Frequency and number of medications

  (5) Access for contamination risk

8) Intradermal

 a) Administer on inside surface of forearm.

 b) TB syringe with 26- to 30-gauge needle with intradermal bevel.

 c) Insert at 15° angle.

 d) Do not aspirate.

9) Subcutaneous (SQ)

 a) Common sites: lateral aspect of upper arm, abdomen, and anterior thigh.

 b) Inject volumes less than 0.5 mL.

 c) Use 1 mL syringe with 26- to 30-gauge needle.

 d) Insert at 90° angle; 45° angle for children who are thin.

10) Intramuscular (IM)

 a) Common site: vastus lateralis (infants/small children).

 b) Apply eutectic mixture of lidocaine and prilocaine (EMLA) to the site for 60 min prior to injection.

 c) Use 22- to 25-gauge, ½- to 1-inch needle (smallest possible).

 d) Volume to be injected: 0.5 mL or less for infants; up to 2 mL for children.

 e) Assess need for assistance and secure child firmly prior to procedure.

11) Intravenous (IV)

 a) Apply EMLA to the site 60 min prior to the procedure.

 b) Use 20- to 24-gauge catheter (smallest possible).

 c) Use transilluminator.

 d) Attach extension tubing.

 e) Keep equipment out of site until ready to use.

 f) Avoid using dominant hand, or hand used for sucking.

V Nursing Care of Children: Death and Dying

A. Incorporate physical, psychological, spiritual, and emotional needs.

B. **Palliative care:** focus is on dying instead of prolonging life when a cure is not available.

 1. Nursing: Manage symptoms and provide supportive care.

C. **Hospice care:** specialized in care of a client who is dying.

 1. Nursing: Focus on pain control and comfort; allow client to die with dignity.

 2. Provide support to family who is grieving.

 3. Provide honest information regarding prognosis, disease progression, treatment options, and effects of treatments.

 4. All health care personnel must be aware of child's and family's decisions.

 5. Nurses can experience personal grief during this time.

D. **Types of Grief**

 1. Anticipatory: death is expected or a possible outcome.

 2. Complicated: extends for more than 1 year following the loss.

  a. Intense thoughts

  b. Feelings of loneliness

  c. Distressing yearning, emotions, and feelings

  d. Disturbances in personal activities

  e. Counseling may be required

 3. Parental: Intense, Long-Lasting, and Complex

  a. Secondary losses related to absence of hopes and dreams

  b. Differences in maternal and paternal grief

E. **Factors Influencing Grief, Loss, and Coping**

 1. Interpersonal relationships and social support

 2. Type and significance of loss

 3. Culture and ethnicity

 4. Spiritual and religious beliefs

 5. Prior experience with loss

 6. Socioeconomic status

CHILDREN'S RESPONSE TO DEATH/DYING

AGE	RELEVANT FACTORS
Infants/toddlers (birth to 3 years)	Little to no concept of death
	Egocentric thinking prevents toddlers from understanding death
	Mirror parental emotions (e.g., sadness, anger, depression, anxiety)
	Respond according to changes due to hospitalization (e.g., change in routine, painful procedures, immobilization, separation)
	May regress to an earlier stage of behavior
Preschool children (3 to 6 years)	Egocentric thinking
	Magical thinking allows preschoolers to believe thoughts can cause an event such as death; may feel guilt or shame
	Interpret separation from parents as punishment for bad behavior
	View death as temporary
	Lack concept of time (gone to sleep)
School-age children (6 to 12 years)	Start to respond to logical or factual explanations
	Begin to have an adult concept of death (inevitable, irreversible, universal). This generally applies to school-age children who are older (9 to 12 years)
	Experience fear of disease process, the death process, unknown, and loss of control
	Fear is often displayed through uncooperative behavior.
	May be curious about funeral services and what happens to the body after death
Adolescents (12 to 20 years)	Adult-like concept of death
	May have difficulty accepting death because they are discovering who they are, establishing an identity, and dealing with issues of puberty
	Rely more on their peers rather than the influence of their parents, which may cause the reality of a serious illness to cause adolescents to feel isolated
	May be unable to relate to peers and communicate with their parents
	May become more stressed by changes in physical appearance from the medications or illness than the prospect of death
	May experience guilt and shame

F. **Collaborative Care**

1. **Nursing Interventions**: Terminally Ill Children
   a. Allow an opportunity for anticipatory grieving.
   b. Provide consistency among nursing personnel.
   c. Encourage parents to stay with the client.
   d. Attempt to maintain a normal environment.
   e. Communicate honestly.
   f. Encourage independence.
   g. Stay with the client as much as possible.
   h. Administer analgesics to control pain.
   i. Assist with arranging religious or cultural rituals as requested.
   j. Allow for visitation of family and friends as desired.
   k. Provide opportunities for the client and family to ask questions.
   l. Remain neutral and accepting.
   m. Recognize and support differences of grieving.
   n. Give families privacy.
   o. Encourage discussion of special memories.

2. After Death
   a. Allow family to stay with the body as long as they desire.
   b. Allow family to rock or hold if desired.
   c. Offer family the option to assist with preparation of the body.
   d. Assist with preparations involving the death ritual.
   e. Encourage parents to prepare siblings for the funeral.
   f. Remain with the family and provide support.
   g. Allow family to share stories about the client's life.
   h. Refer to the client by name.
   i. Allow all family members to communicate feelings.

SECTION 4

Nursing Care of the Child who has a Congenital Anomaly

A. **Congenital Heart Disease**
   1. Contributing Factors
      a. Maternal Factors
         1) Infection in early pregnancy
         2) Alcohol and/or substance abuse during pregnancy
         3) Diabetes mellitus
      b. Genetic Factors
         1) Family history of congenital heart disease
         2) Presence of other congenital anomalies or syndromes

CONGENITAL HEART ANOMALIES

ANOMALY	HEMODYNAMICS	MANIFESTATIONS	TREATMENT
Defects with Increased Pulmonary Blood Flow			
Patent ductus arteriosus Failure of the fetal ductus arteriosus to close within minutes or a few days after birth Defect may vary in size	Blood shunts from aorta to pulmonary artery (left-to-right shunt) Oxygenated blood (aorta) mixes with deoxygenated blood (pulmonary artery)	Respiratory distress Murmur (machine hum) Bounding pulses Widened pulse pressure Poor feeding Asymptomatic or signs of heart failure	Administration of indomethacin Administration of ibuprofen (may be used for premature infants) Insertion of coils to occlude PDA during cardiac catheterization Surgical procedure: Thoracoscopic repair
Ventricular septal defect An abnormal opening in the septum between the left and right ventricle Defect may vary in size	Blood shunts from left to right ventricle and back into pulmonary artery (left-to-right shunt) Oxygenated blood (left ventricle) mixes with deoxygenated blood (right ventricle) and is pumped back into the lungs instead of the body Increased pulmonary vascular resistance Right ventricular hypertrophy Potential enlargement of right atrium	Loud, harsh murmur auscultated at left sternal border Mild cyanosis that increases with crying Heart failure	Closure during cardiac catheterization Surgical procedure: Pulmonary artery banding Complete repair with patch
Atrial septal defect An abnormal opening in the septum between the left and right atria Defect may vary in size	Blood shunts from left to right atria and flows back to the right side of the heart (left-to-right shunt) Oxygenated blood (left atria) mixes with deoxygenated blood (right atria) and increases total amount of blood that flows toward the lungs Blood is pumped back into the lungs instead of flowing to the left ventricle and to the rest of the body	May be asymptomatic May go undiagnosed until school age or adulthood Murmur Shortness of breath with activity Frequent respiratory infections Dysrhythmias Heart palpitations or skipped beats	Closure during cardiac catheterization Surgical procedure: Patch closure
Defects with Decreased Pulmonary Blood Flow			
Tetralogy of Fallot Includes four defects › Pulmonary stenosis › Ventricular septal defect (VSD) › Overriding aorta › Hypertrophy of right ventricle	Left and right ventricle pressures may be equal (because the VSD is usually large) Blood may shunt from left to right or from right to left High pulmonary vascular resistance (right-to-left shunt) High systemic vascular resistance (left-to-right shunt) Decreased blood flow to lungs and the amount of oxygenated blood returning to the left side of the heart (pulmonic stenosis) Each ventricle may distribute blood to the systemic system (depends on the position of the aorta)	Cyanosis and hypoxia ("Tet" spell) Heart sounds vary depending on defect Cardiomegaly Heart failure Systolic murmur	Palliative shunt in infant who cannot undergo primary repair Complete repair within first year

CONGENITAL HEART ANOMALIES (CONTINUED)

ANOMALY	HEMODYNAMICS	MANIFESTATIONS	TREATMENT
Defects with Mixed Blood Flow			
Transposition of great vessels (TGV) The two main arteries are reversed Aorta exits the right ventricle instead of the left Pulmonary artery originates from the left ventricle instead of the right	No exchange between systemic and pulmonary circulations Aorta exits from right ventricle and carries deoxygenated blood back to the body Pulmonary artery originates from the left ventricle and carries oxygenated blood from the lungs back to the lungs Results in inadequate oxygenated blood in the body A PDA or septal defect must be present for blood to enter the systemic or pulmonary circulation	Cyanosis Heart sounds vary depending on defect Cardiomegaly Heart failure	Intravenous prostaglandin E to keep ductus arteriosus open Balloon atrial septostomy Surgical arterial switch (within first weeks of life) Other surgical procedures depending on defect present
Defects with Obstructive Blood Flow			
Coarctation of the aorta Narrowing of the lumen of the aorta, resulting in obstruction of blood flow from the ventricle	Increased pressure proximal to defect (upper extremities) Decreased pressure distal to defect (lower extremities)	Upper extremities: elevated blood pressure, bounding pulses Lower extremities: decreased blood pressure, weak/absent pulses, cool skin Dizziness Syncope Headache Epistaxis Heart failure	Infants and children: balloon angioplasty Adolescents: placement of stents Surgical procedure: Repair of defect recommended for infants less than 6 months of age

B. **Heart failure (HF):** Impaired Myocardial Function

1. Assessment

    a. Expected Findings

        1) Impaired myocardial function

        2) Sweating

        3) Tachycardia

        4) Pallor

        5) Cool extremities

        6) Weak pulses

        7) Hypotension

        8) Gallop rhythm

        9) Cardiomegaly

    b. Pulmonary Congestion

        1) Tachypnea

        2) Dyspnea

        3) Retractions

        4) Nasal flaring

        5) Grunting

        6) Wheezing

        7) Cyanosis

        8) Cough

        9) Orthopnea

        10) Exercise intolerance

    c. Systemic Venous Congestion

        1) Hepatomegaly

        2) Peripheral edema

        3) Ascites

        4) Neck vein distention

        5) Periorbital edema

        6) Weight gain

2. Collaborative Care

    a. **Nursing Interventions**

        1) Conserve the child's energy: frequent rest periods; cluster care; provide small, frequent meals; bathing PRN; and keep crying to a minimum in cyanotic children.

        2) I&O; daily weight.

        3) Allow the child to sleep with several pillows; maintain semi-Fowler's when awake.

        4) Allow the infant to rest during feedings, taking approximately 30 min to complete the feeding.

        5) Gavage feed the infant as needed; use a high-calorie formula.

        6) Administer humidified oxygen.

        7) Monitor oxygen saturation every 2 to 4 hr.

        8) Suction airway as needed.

        9) Monitor family coping and provide support.

        10) Teach family to report signs indicating worsening of heart failure (e.g., increased sweating, decreased urinary output).

b. Medications

1) Digoxin: improves myocardial contractility

  a) Hold if apical pulse is less than 90/min for infants; less than 70/min for children.

  b) Observe for signs of toxicity: bradycardia, poor feeding, nausea, and vomiting.

  c) If given as a PO liquid, provide oral care if teeth are present to prevent tooth decay.

2) Captopril or enalapril

3) Furosemide or chlorothiazide

C. **Down Syndrome**

1. Most common chromosomal abnormality of a generalized syndrome. Affects growth and development. Cognitive and sensory impairments. Associated with many anomalies.

2. Trisomy 21 seen in 97% of cases.

3. Assessment

a. Contributing Factors

1) Exact etiology unknown

2) Maternal age greater than 35 years

3) Paternal age greater than 55 years

b. Expected Findings

1) Separated sagittal suture

2) Enlarged anterior fontanel

3) Small head

4) Flattened forehead

5) Epicanthal folds

6) Upward, outward slant to eyes

7) Small nose; depressed nasal bridge

8) Small ears

9) High-arched narrow palate

10) Protruding tongue

11) Short, broad neck

12) Shortened rib cage

13) Potential congenital heart defect

14) Protruding abdomen

15) Broad, short feet and hands with stubby toes and fingers

16) Transverse palmer crease

17) Short stature

18) Hyperflexibility, hypotonia, muscle weakness

19) Dry skin that cracks easily

c. Diagnostic Procedures

1) Prenatal: alpha-fetoprotein

2) Chromosome analysis

d. Complications

1) Cognitive impairment: Intelligence varies.

2) Social development: May be 2 to 3 years beyond mental age. Socializing has strengths.

3) Congenital anomalies: congenital heart disease (septal defects common), renal agenesis, Hirschsprung's disease, tracheoesophageal fistula, and skeletal defects.

4) Sensory: strabismus, excessive tearing, cataracts, and hearing problems.

5) Other medical conditions: upper respiratory infections, thyroid dysfunction, increased risk of leukemia

6) Growth: reduced height and weight; prone to obesity

7) Sexual development: delayed and or incomplete

NOTE: Feeding strategies for child with Down syndrome (to accommodate protruding tongue):

› Small but long, straight-handled spoon.

› Push food toward back and side of mouth.

› Refeed food, if thrust out.

4. Collaborative Care

a. **Nursing Interventions**

1) Support family at time of diagnosis.

2) Facilitate bonding; assist with holding.

  a) Wrap tightly in a blanket prior to picking up infant (hypotonicity).

3) Manage secretions (e.g., nasal aspiration, vaporizer, postural drainage).

4) Evaluate and Monitor

  a) Eyesight and hearing

  b) Thyroid functioning

  c) Height and weight

  d) Developmental milestones

5) Assess for atlantoaxial instability (neck pain, weakness, torticollis).

  a) Make appropriate referrals (e.g., social work, home health, school, genetic counseling, speech therapy, physical therapy, occupational therapy).

D. **Club Foot**

1. Also known as talipes equinovarus. Deformity of the ankle and foot involving bone deformity, malpositioning, and soft tissue contracture.

2. Assessment

a. Contributing Factors

1) Positional (intrauterine crowding)

2) Presence of other disorders (cerebral palsy)

3) Heredity

4) Idiopathic

b. Expected Findings

1) Toes are turned inward, lower than the heel.

2) Portions of the foot may turn sideways or upward.

3) Limited motion and flexibility of ankle.

4) Affected foot usually smaller and shorter.

5) If unilateral, affected extremity often shorter and atrophy of calf present.

c. Diagnostic Procedures

1) Prenatal: ultrasound

2) Visible at birth if not detected prenatally

3) Perform hip examination. Increased risk of hip dysplasia

3. Therapeutic Procedures

  a. Serial casting shortly after birth with weekly stretching of foot muscles until maximum correction is achieved.

  b. Placement of serial long-leg cast.

  c. Surgical: Percutaneous heel cord tenotomy usually performed, followed by a long-leg cast for 3 weeks.

  d. A Denis Browne bar and specialized shoes may be applied to maintain correction and prevent recurrence.

4. Collaborative Care

  a. **Nursing Interventions**

    1) Encourage parents to hold and cuddle the child.

    2) Assess and maintain the cast or corrective device.

    3) Monitor neurovascular status and skin integrity.

  b. Client Education

    1) Teach family the importance of regular cast changes.

    2) Provide information about care of cast/corrective device.

    3) Report potential complications (e.g., skin breakdown, alteration in circulation).

    4) Encourage activities to promote normal growth and development.

E. **Developmental Dysplasia of the Hip (DDH)**

1. Abnormal development of hip structures. May develop during fetal life, infancy, or childhood.

2. Acetabular dysplasia: delay in acetabular development.

3. Subluxation: incomplete dislocation of femoral head.

4. Dislocation: femoral head loses contact with acetabulum.

5. Contributing Factors

  a. Family history, gender, birth order, intrauterine position, and/or laxity of a joint

  b. Intrauterine placement, mechanical situations (e.g., size of infant, multiple births, breech presentation), and genetic factors

NOTE: Increased incidence when infants are wrapped tightly or strapped to cradle boards. Decreased incidence when mothers carry infants on their backs with legs widely abducted.

6. Expected Findings

  a. Newborn

    1) Asymmetry of gluteal and thigh folds

    2) Limited hip abduction

    3) Positive Ortolani test

    4) Positive Barlow test

  b. Child

    1) Affected leg is shorter

    2) Positive Trendelenburg sign

    3) Walks on toes on one foot

    4) Walks with a limp

7. Diagnostic Procedures

  a. Ultrasound: Should be performed at 2 weeks of age to determine the cartilaginous head of the femur.

  b. X-ray: Can diagnose DDH in infants older than 4 months.

8. Therapeutic Procedures

  a. Treatment varies with age and severity of findings. Initiate early for best outcomes.

9. Nonsurgical Interventions

  a. Pavlik harness

  b. Hip abduction braces

  c. Bryant traction (skin)

  d. Hip spica cast

10. Surgical Interventions

  a. Closed or closed reduction

  b. Osteotomy (pelvic, femur)

  c. Tenotomy

! Point to Remember

The Barlow and Ortolani maneuvers should be performed only by an experienced clinician to prevent injury to the infant's hip.

11. Collaborative Care

  a. **Nursing Interventions**

    1) Encourage holding.

    2) Promote growth and development.

    3) Pavlik Harness

      a) Maintain harness placement.

      b) Check straps every 1 to 2 weeks for adjustment.

      c) Assess neurovascular status, skin integrity.

    4) Bryant Traction (skin)

      a) Maintain alignment.

      b) Assess: neurovascular status, skin integrity, pain.

      c) Maintain traction.

    5) Hip Spica Cast

      a) Change frequently to accommodate growth.

      b) Position cast on pillows; handle with palm of hand (until dry).

      c) Assess: neurovascular status, skin integrity, pain.

      d) Turn and position; provide range of motion (of unaffected extremities).

      e) Monitor nutrition and hydration.

      f) Apply waterproof barrier around genital opening of cast (to prevent soiling).

12. Client Education and Referrals

   a. Instruct the family to keep the Pavlik harness on continuously, except during bathing, if prescribed.

   b. Instruct the family to return for follow-up visits weekly at the start of therapy and then as needed.

   c. Instruct the family to monitor and report complications.

   d. Teach and reinforce skin care (specific to procedure).

   e. Encourage parents to hold and cuddle the child.

   f. Encourage parents to meet the developmental needs of the child.

   g. Educate regarding care after discharge with emphasis on using appropriate equipment (e.g., stroller, wagon, car seat) for maintaining mobility.

F. **Spina Bifida**

   1. Failure of the osseous spine to close.

   2. Neural tube defects (NTDs) are present at birth (may not be visible).

   3. Spina bifida occulta: Protruding sac is not visible.

   4. Spina bifida cystica: Protruding sac is visible.

      a. Meningocele: Sac contains spinal fluid and meninges.

      b. Myelomeningocele: Sac includes spinal fluid, meninges, and nerves.

   5. Contributing Factors

      a. Maternal factors: medications/substances taken during pregnancy, malnutrition, insufficient intake of folic acid during pregnancy, exposure to radiation or chemicals during pregnancy

      b. Genetic

      c. Presence of other syndrome or congenital anomaly

   6. Expected Findings

      a. Spina Bifida Occulta

         1) Dimpling in lumbosacral area

         2) Port wine angioma

         3) Dark tufts of hair

         4) Subcutaneous lipoma

      b. Spina Bifida Cystica

         1) Protruding sac midline of the osseous spine

         2) Other findings vary widely depending on location of defect

         3) Flaccid, lower extremity paralysis

         4) Sensory deficits

         5) Urinary incontinence (dribbling)

         6) Bowel incontinence

         7) Prolapsed rectum

         8) Club foot, kyphosis, hip dislocation, or other skeletal defects

   7. Diagnostic Procedures

      a. Prenatal: ultrasound, amniocentesis

      b. Infant following birth: MRI, ultrasound, CT

   8. Therapeutic Procedures

      a. Surgical repair

9. Collaborative Care

   a. Interprofessional care: neurosurgery, neurology, urology, orthopedics, physical therapy, nutrition, occupational therapy, social services

   b. **Nursing Interventions**

      1) Initial Care/Preoperative

         a) Protect the sac.

            (1) Place prone in infant warmer with hips flexed, legs abducted (without clothing).

            (2) Place sterile, moist, nonadhering dressing with 0.9% sodium chloride to sac; change every 2 hr.

            (3) Avoid applying any pressure to sac.

            (4) Monitor neurological status (head circumference, fontanels, cry, suck, movement, sensory).

            (5) Inspect sac for leaks, irritation, signs of infection.

            (6) Strict I&O (intermittent catheterization may be required).

            (7) Obtain laboratory specimens as prescribed.

            (8) Administer IV antibiotics as prescribed.

            (9) Avoid rectal temperatures.

            (10) No diapering until defect is repaired and healed.

            (11) Assess and promote infant-parent bonding.

            (12) Prepare infant and family for surgical procedure.

         b) Postoperative

            (1) Maintain prone position until other positions are prescribed.

            (2) Monitor neurological status (head circumference, fontanels, cry, suck, movement, sensory).

            (3) Assess incision site & provide care (CSF leakage/ infection).

            (4) Monitor I&O.

            (5) Intermittent catheterization may be required.

            (6) Resume oral feedings.

            (7) Provide range of motion to extremities.

            (8) Administer pain medication as prescribed.

         c) Complications

            (1) Skin ulceration

            (2) Latex allergy

            (3) Increased intracranial pressure

            (4) Shunt malfunction, infection, or hydrocephalus

            (5) Bladder dysfunction

            (6) Orthopedic issues

NOTE: Think BACK—latex allergy is linked to certain foods: bananas, avocado, chestnuts, kiwi.

c. Client Education

1) Assist family with obtaining medical equipment/services needed at home.

2) Provide postoperative education (e.g., care of incision, signs of infection, medications, skin care, repositioning, range of motion exercises, findings to report to provider, activities to promote growth and development).

3) Inform parents of an increased risk for latex allergy and strategies to reduce exposure.

4) Provide list of common household items and foods that may contain latex.

5) Teach signs of an allergic reaction (e.g., urticaria, wheezing, anaphylaxis).

6) Demonstrate how to administer epinephrine and when to call 911.

7) Demonstrate how to measure head circumference and palpate fontanel.

8) Discuss signs of increased intracranial pressure and when to notify provider.

9) Inform parents of an increased risk for bladder dysfunction (spasms or flaccidity) and to monitor urine for foul odor, blood, or other signs of infection; how to perform intermittent catheterization.

10) Teach care of: shunt, cast, splint, stoma (vesicostomy).

G. **Cerebral Palsy**

1. Nonprogressive, but permanent impairment of motor function affecting muscle control, coordination, and posture (spastic, dyskinetic, ataxic). Most common permanent physical disability of childhood. May involve alterations in sensation, perception, communication, cognition, and behavior. Wide range of intelligence; 50% to 60% is within normal limits.

2. Assessment

a. Contributing Factors

1) Exact cause unknown.

2) May include prenatal, perinatal, and postnatal factors.

b. Expected Findings

1) Vary depending on type of CP

2) Delayed gross motor development; failure to meet developmental milestones

3) Abnormal Motor Performance

a) Abnormal or asymmetrical crawl

b) Stands or walks on toes; ataxia

c) Involuntary movements (e.g., facial grimacing, writhing movements of tongue)

d) Poor sucking and difficulty feeding

e) Persistent tongue thrust

f) Alterations in muscle tone

g) Increased or decreased resistance to passive movements

h) Poor head control

i) Exaggerated arching of back

j) Abnormal posture

k) Persistence of primitive reflexes (e.g., Moro, plantar, palmar grasp reflex, hyperreflexia, ankle clonus)

3. Diagnostic Procedures

a. Complete neurological assessment

b. Metabolic and genetic testing

c. General movements assessment (children greater than 2 years and younger than 5 years of age)

4. MRI

5. Collaborative Care

a. **Nursing Interventions**

1) Adapt interventions/communication according to child's developmental level.

2) Communicate with the child directly; include parents as needed.

3) Keep head of bed elevated (especially for increased amount of oral secretions).

4) Ensure suction is available; suction oral secretions as needed.

5) Identify risk for aspiration; implement precautions.

6) Implement safety precautions (pad side rails and arms of wheelchair).

7) Provide pulmonary hygiene.

8) Ensure adequate nutrition; administer gastrostomy feedings if applicable.

9) Position correctly for feeding (head positioning/manual jaw control methods as needed).

10) Provide high-calorie milk products (for children 1 year of age or older).

11) Provide diet high in fruit and fiber (prevents constipation).

12) Assess for pain/muscle spasms and administer medications as prescribed.

13) Provide skin care (asses skin; turn frequently; keep skin dry).

14) Monitor growth and development.

15) Evaluate need for speech and hearing evaluation or other referrals.

16) Incorporate family in plan of care.

17) Determine family coping and support and evaluate need for respite care.

b. Medications

1) Baclofen: Skeletal muscle relaxant

2) Diazepam

3) Botulinum toxin A: used primarily for spasticity in lower extremities

4) Antiepileptics: control seizure activity

c. Therapeutic Measures

1) Physical therapy (braces, splints, wheelchair)

2) Occupational therapy (utensils for eating and writing)

3) Speech-language therapy (oral-motor skills, adaptive communication techniques)

4) Special education (early intervention programs)

5) Behavioral therapy

6) May include gastrostomy, tenotomy, procedures to correct orthopedic and or dental problems

d. Client Education and Referrals

1) Emphasize the need for frequent rest periods.

2) Review feeding schedule and feeding techniques if changes were made during hospitalization.

3) Provide information regarding expected responses, side effects, and adverse reactions to medications.

4) Teach pulmonary hygiene techniques.

5) Discuss measures to prevent skin breakdown.

6) Encourage to adhere to immunization schedule.

7) Encourage parents to provide a stimulating environment and incorporate therapeutic measures into daily activities (adapt environment for safety).

e. Complications

1) Visual and hearing impairment

2) Behavioral problems

3) Difficulty with speech and communication

4) Cognitive impairment

5) Orthopedic (scoliosis, hip dislocation)

6) Nystagmus/amblyopia

7) Otitis media

8) Seizures

H. **Congenital Gastrointestinal Disorders**

1. **Hypertrophic pyloric stenosis**

a. Description and Contributing Factors

1) Thickening of the pyloric sphincter, which causes an obstruction. Most common within first 5 weeks of life.

b. Manifestations

1) Projectile vomiting after feeding or intermittently

2) Constant hunger

3) Palpable olive shaped mass in right upper abdominal quadrant

4) No evidence of pain

5) Possible peristaltic wave moving left to right when lying supine

6) Signs of dehydration (sunken fontanel, no tears, decreased wet diapers, dry mouth)

7) Failure to gain weight

c. Diagnostic Procedures

1) Abdominal ultrasound shows elongated mass surrounding pyloric area.

d. **Nursing Interventions**

1) Preoperative

a) Monitor vital signs.

b) Assess for signs of dehydration.

c) Administer IV fluids (corrects electrolyte imbalances).

d) Insert NG tube (decompression).

e) NPO

f) Strict I&O

2) Postoperative

a) Monitor vital signs.

b) Administer IV fluids.

c) Strict I&O

d) Daily weights

e) Assess for signs of infection.

f) Clear liquid diet 4 to 6 hr after surgery; advance to breast milk or formula as tolerated.

g) Document tolerance to feedings (may have some vomiting during the first 24 to 48 hr after surgery).

e. Medications

1) Analgesics

f. Therapeutic Measures

1) Surgical removal of aganglionic section of bowel

2) Temporary colostomy may be required

g. Client Education and Referrals

1) Report any signs of infection or intolerance of feedings.

2. **Hirschsprung's Disease (congenital aganglionic megacolon)**

a. Description and Contributing Factors

1) Occurs when a section of the colon is aganglionic, resulting in decreased motility and obstruction.

b. Manifestations

1) **Newborn:** failure to pass meconium within 24 to 48 hr, refusal to eat, episodes of vomiting bile, and abdominal distention

2) **Infant:** failure to thrive, constipation, abdominal distention, episodes of vomiting and diarrhea

3) **Older child:** constipation, abdominal distention, visible peristalsis, ribbon-like stool, palpable fecal mass, and a malnourished appearance

c. Diagnostic Procedures

1) Rectal biopsy to confirm absence of ganglionic cells

d. **Nursing Interventions**

1) Preoperative

a) If malnourished, provide high-protein, high-calorie, low-fiber diet; TPN may be required.

b) Monitor for signs and symptoms of enterocolitis and/or bowel perforation.

c) Administer IV fluids.

d) Bowel prep with saline enemas.

2) Postoperative

a) Assess surgical site.

b) Assess bowel sounds and bowel function.

c) Monitor for irregular passage of stool (i.e., constipation or incontinence).

e. Medications

　1) Analgesics

　2) Antibiotics

f. Therapeutic Measures

　1) Surgical removal of aganglionic section of bowel

　2) Temporary colostomy may be required

g. Client Education and Referrals

　1) Teach wound care; colostomy care if applicable.

　2) Teach to monitor for signs of infection.

　3) Teach parents to monitor for complications after discharge (e.g., enterocolitis, fecal incontinence, obstruction).

　4) Teach parents how to perform daily anal dilations (if required).

　5) Teach to monitor for signs and symptoms of dehydration.

3. **Intussusception**

a. Description and Contributing Factors

　1) The telescoping of the intestine upon itself, may progress to ischemia

　2) Common in infants and children between 3 months and 6 years of age

b. Manifestations

　1) Intervals of sudden abdominal pain, appears normal between episodes

　2) Empty lower right quadrant (Dance sign)

　3) Palpable, sausage-shaped mass in the right upper quadrant of the abdomen and/or a tender, distended abdomen

　4) Stools that are mixed with blood and mucus that resemble the consistency of red currant jelly

c. Diagnostic Procedures

　1) Ultrasonography

　2) Rectal examination reveals mucus and blood

d. **Nursing Interventions**

　1) Preoperative

　　a) NPO

　　b) Administer IV fluids (correct and prevent dehydration).

　　c) Insert NG tube (decompression).

　　d) Monitor stools.

　2) Postoperative

　　a) Observe for passage of water-soluble contrast (if used).

　　b) Monitor incision if surgery is required.

　　c) Monitor stool patterns (intussusception may recur).

! Point to Remember

Passage of normal brown stool usually indicates intussusception has resolved itself. Report immediately; diagnostic and therapeutic procedures may be altered.

e. Medications

　1) Antibiotics per prescription

f. Therapeutic Measures

　1) Air enema (with or without contrast) performed by radiologist

　2) Ultrasound-guided hydrostatic (saline) enema

　3) Surgery, if enema is unsuccessful

g. Client Education and Referrals

　1) Teach parents to monitor stools and for signs and symptoms of intussusception

4. **Cleft Lip (CL) and Cleft Palate (CP)**

a. Description and Contributing Factors

　1) Cleft lip results from incomplete fusion of the oral cavity during intrauterine life.

　2) Cleft palate results from incomplete fusion of the palatine plates during intrauterine life.

　3) Contributing factors: family history, exposure of alcohol, cigarette smoke, anticonvulsants, or steroids during pregnancy. Deficiency of folate during pregnancy.

b. Manifestations

　1) Cleft lip is visible at birth.

　2) Cleft palate may be detected by visual inspection of oral cavity or by palpating the hard and soft palate with a gloved finger.

c. Diagnostic Procedures

　1) Cleft lip and cleft palate may be diagnosed prior to birth by routine ultrasound.

d. **Nursing Interventions**

　1) Preoperative

　　a) Evaluate and promote bonding.

　　b) Inspect lip; palpate palate using gloved finger.

　　c) Assess ability to suck.

　　d) Refer to lactation consultant/social services.

　　e) Inform parents noisy feeding is common and not a sign of choking.

　　f) Instruct parents to observe for "facial sign" indicating feeding should be stopped briefly (e.g., raised eyebrows, wrinkled forehead, watery eyes).

　　g) Cleft Lip

　　　(1) Encourage breastfeeding.

　　　(2) Use wide base nipple for bottle feeding and squeeze cheeks together to decrease width of cleft.

　　h) Cleft Palate or Cleft Lip and Palate

　　　(1) Position upright while cradling head during feeding.

　　　(2) Use modified bottles/feeders (one-way flow valve, squeezable bottles).

　　　(3) Use wide or long nipples with a cut slit.

　　　(4) Burp after every ounce.

　　　(5) Transition to cup feeding prior to CP repair.

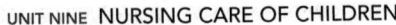

2) Postoperative—Cleft Lip

  a) Maintain airway.

  b) Obtain vital signs.

  c) Major goal: Protect the site.

  d) Avoid prone position; position upright in infant seat.

  e) Apply elbow restraints immediately after surgery (varies by surgeon).

  f) Monitor and supervise closely to prevent damage to sutures (fingers in mouth).

  g) Administer pain medication.

  h) Clean suture line using cotton tip applicator. Saline, water, or diluted hydrogen peroxide may be used.

  i) Apply thin layer of antibiotic ointment to suture line.

3) Postoperative Cleft Palate

  a) Administer oxygen (usually by face mask).

  b) Position to prevent airway obstruction; may be placed on abdomen in the immediate postoperative period.

  c) Observe closely for signs of airway obstruction, hemorrhage, and laryngeal spasm.

  d) Report croup, stridor, difficulty breathing, or frequent swallowing.

  e) Assess pain; administer medications.

  f) Clear liquids for 24 hr; liquid diet for 2 weeks.

  g) Use open cup for liquids.

  h) Avoid placing suction catheters, pacifiers, tongue depressors, rigid spoons, straws, or hard-tipped sippy cups in mouth.

  i) Apply elbow restraints.

  j) Remove restraints to allow movement (supervise closely).

e. Medications

  1) Analgesics

  2) Antibiotics

f. Therapeutic Measures

  1) Cleft lip repair typically performed between 2 to 3 months

  2) Cleft palate repair typically performed between 6 to 12 months

g. Client Education and Referrals

  1) Discuss proper feeding techniques.

  2) Teach parents how to clean incision.

  3) Monitor operative site for infection/bleeding/crusting.

  4) Discuss proper positioning for sleep.

  5) Discuss the proper use of restraints.

Nursing Care of the Child who has an Acute Condition

A. **Gastrointestinal Disorders**

  1. **Acute Gastrointestinal Infections**

    a. Contributing Factors

      1) Age: the younger the child, the more susceptible and serious

      2) Underlying poor health (e.g., malnutrition, immunocompromised)

      3) Environment: crowding, poor sanitation, lack of access to clean water

      4) Lack of knowledge: poor food preparation and storage, inadequate handwashing

      5) Antibiotic and other medication therapies can exacerbate

    b. Expected Findings

      1) Diarrhea

      2) Vomiting

      3) Malaise

      4) Fever

      5) Poor appetite

      6) Dehydration

      7) Weight loss

      8) Stool examination, culture positive for ova, parasites, or bacteria

      9) Enzyme-linked immunosorbent assay (ELISA) positive for rotavirus or giardia

    c. Laboratory Tests and Diagnostic Procedures

      1) Stool examination for blood, ova, parasites

      2) Stool culture for bacteria

      3) ELISA for rotavirus, giardia

      4) CBC

      5) Electrolytes

    d. Therapeutic Procedures and Medications

      1) Antimicrobials (e.g., antibiotic, antiparasitic)

      2) Antipyretics

      3) Antiemetics if unable to tolerate anything orally

> **NOTE:** Older antiemetics (e.g., promethazine, metoclopramide) should not be routinely administered to children due to the potential for adverse effects (e.g., somnolence, nervousness, irritability, and dystonic reactions).

      4) Intravenous fluids only if unable to tolerate oral fluids

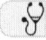

e. **Nursing Interventions**

1) Provide oral rehydration therapy. Administer 5 to 10 mL every 1 to 5 min. Vomiting is not a contraindication unless severe.

2) After rehydration, alternate with water, breast milk, lactose-free formula.

3) Reintroduce a normal diet as soon as possible; lessens severity of illness and improves weight gain.

4) Weigh daily; weight is the best indicator of fluid gains and losses.

5) Monitor electrolytes, blood glucose, and acid-base status.

6) Carefully monitor intake and output.

7) No rectal temperature.

8) If hospitalization is required, give nothing by mouth and prepare to administer parenteral fluids.

f. Client Education

1) Teach to observe for signs of dehydration by counting diapers, voiding; seek medical attention if dehydration is suspected, especially for infants, due to the risk for hypovolemia shock.

2) Teach the importance of handwashing, proper food storage, and clean water.

GASTROINTESTINAL INFECTIONS OF CHILDREN

MANIFESTATIONS	TRANSMISSION
Escherichia coli (E. coli)	*bacterial*
Watery, then bloody diarrhea, abdominal cramping; may develop hemolytic uremic syndrome	Contaminated food (beef, milk, fresh produce), water; person to person
Clostridium difficile (C. diff)	*bacterial*
Mild, watery diarrhea; may develop pseudomembranous colitis	Associated with alteration in normal intestinal flora by antibiotics
Salmonella	*bacterial*
Mild to severe N&V, abdominal cramping, bloody diarrhea	Undercooked meat, eggs, poultry; person to person
Enterobius vermicularis (pinworm)	*helminthic*
Perianal itching, enuresis	Fecal-oral
Giardia lamblia	*parasitic*
Diarrhea, greasy stools, abdominal cramping, vomiting, anorexia	Contaminated food, water, animals; person to person
Rotavirus	*viral*
Most common cause of diarrhea in children younger than 5 years	
Mild-moderate fever; vomiting followed by watery diarrhea	Often nosocomial; Fecal-oral

KEY POINT: Fruit juice, carbonated drinks, gelatin, caffeine, broth, and sports drinks do not help diarrhea and vomiting. A BRAT (bananas, rice, applesauce, and toast) diet is also contraindicated. All have low nutritional value and may disrupt electrolyte balance.

2. **Hyperbilirubinemia**

a. Bilirubin is a byproduct of the breakdown of red blood cells. When the immature liver is unable to process bilirubin for excretion, excessive amounts accumulate, primarily in sclera, nails, and skin, manifesting as jaundice.

b. Contributing Factors

1) Prematurity

2) Breastfeeding

3) Liver compromise

4) Diabetic mother

5) Native American or Asian

6) Birth injury that causes bruising or hematoma

7) Decreased intake

8) Hereditary hemolytic disease

9) Sibling with history of hyperbilirubinemia

10) Exclusive breastfeeding with excessive weight loss

11) Rh-negative mother

c. Expected Findings

1) Jaundice seen in sclera, nails, or skin, occurring when unconjugated bilirubin levels exceed 5 mg/dL

d. Laboratory Tests and Diagnostic Procedures

1) Serum bilirubin

2) Coombs (direct, indirect)

3) Transcutaneous bilirubinometry

e. Therapeutic Procedures and Medications

1) Phototherapy

2) Exchange transfusion for dangerously high bilirubin levels

3) Immunoglobulin if caused by blood incompatibility

4) Tin-mesoporphyrin (prevents bilirubin formation)

f. **Nursing Interventions**

1) Regularly observe for jaundice by blanching skin over bony prominences and observing sclera, mucous membranes, and nails.

2) Assess color in natural daylight.

3) Obtain transcutaneous bilirubinometry readings (not accurate if neonate is under phototherapy).

4) Weigh daily.

5) Assess voiding and stooling.

6) Assess feeding patterns and hydration.

7) Initiate breastfeeding within first hour of birth.

8) Encourage rooming in.

9) For Infants Under Phototherapy

a) Expose as much skin as possible to light.

b) Ensure that opaque mask is in place over infant's eyes; remove when taken out from under lights.

c) Monitor for temperature instability.

g. Client Education

   1) Teach the importance of adequate intake.

   2) Instruct to leave under the lights as much as possible, with mask in place.

   3) Explain how to monitor for jaundice and to notify health care provider if it worsens.

   4) Explain the importance of monitoring urinary and stool output.

TYPES OF HYPERBILIRUBINEMIA OF THE NEWBORN

Physiologic Jaundice

CAUSE	Immature liver function Increased bilirubin load from increased number of RBCs in newborn
ONSET	After first 24 hr
DURATION	Decreases 5th to 7th day
THERAPY	Increase feeding frequency Monitor stool, use phototherapy for significant increase in bilirubin

Breastfeeding Jaundice

CAUSE	Decreased intake before mother's breast milk comes in; infrequent stooling
ONSET	3rd to 5th day
DURATION	Varies
THERAPY	Frequent breastfeeding, NO supplements (can decrease breast milk production); phototherapy for significant increase in bilirubin

Hemolytic Disease

CAUSE	ABO or Rh blood incompatibility
ONSET	1st 24 hr; bilirubin levels increase greater than 5mg/dL/day
DURATION	Depends on severity
THERAPY	Immunoglobulin, tin-mesoporphyrin, exchange transfusion; encourage mother to pump and store breast milk for future feeding RhoGAM to prevent Rh incompatibility

3. **Acute Appendicitis**

  a. Inflammation of the vermiform appendix caused by obstruction due to fecalith (hardened stool is most common), inflamed lymphoid tissue following a viral infection, or a parasite

  b. Contributing Factors

   1) Age: peak incidence is ten years

   2) Recent viral infection

   3) Intestinal helminth infection

  c. Expected Findings

   1) Focal abdominal tenderness in the periumbilical area, progressing to right lower quadrant

    a) McBurney's point, located two-thirds the distance between the umbilicus and anterosuperior iliac spine

    b) Rovsing's sign: tenderness in the right lower quadrant that occurs during palpation or percussion of other abdominal quadrants

   2) Nausea, vomiting, anorexia, poor feeding

   3) Diarrhea or constipation

   4) Lethargy

   5) Pain in right hip when walking

   6) Low-grade fever (38° C [100.4° F])

   7) Decreased or absent bowel sounds

   8) Tachypnea, tachycardia

   9) Rigid abdomen

   10) If perforation occurs:

    a) Sudden relief from pain, followed by an increase

    b) Temperature elevations of 38.8° to 39.4° C (102° to 103° F), chills

    c) Progressive abdominal distention

    d) Tachycardia, tachypnea

    e) Pallor

  d. Laboratory Tests and Diagnostic Procedures

   1) Complete blood count (white cell count greater than 10,000 mm³ and elevated C-reactive protein are common, but not specific)

   2) Urinalysis

   3) Computerized tomography

   4) Ultrasound

  e. **Unruptured Appendix**

   1) Therapeutic Procedures and Medications

    a) IV fluids

    b) IV antibiotics

    c) Electrolyte replacement

    d) Laparoscopic incisions to surgically remove the appendix

    e) Analgesics

   2) **Nursing Interventions**

    a) Perform thorough pain assessment and continue to monitor; instruct the child to point to the area of pain; note change in activity.

    b) Prepare child for surgery; ensure consents have been signed.

    c) Monitor vital signs.

    d) Maintain NPO.

    e) Maintain bed rest until surgery; allow child to assume position of comfort.

    f) Avoid applying heat to abdomen.

    g) Monitor bowel sounds; palpation should be very gentle.

    h) After surgery, monitor oxygen status, vital signs, level of consciousness; administer oxygen as needed.

    i) Monitor, provide incision care, as prescribed.

    j) Assess abdomen for distention; monitor for passage of flatus, stool.

    k) Administer analgesics as needed.

    l) Encourage early ambulation.

    m) Provide a small pillow or stuffed animal for abdominal support.

3) Client Education

    a) Teach incision care.

    b) Teach to monitor for signs of infection.

f. **Ruptured Appendix**

1) Therapeutic Procedures

    a) IV fluids, antibiotics, electrolytes

    b) NG suction

    c) Surgery (wound may be left open or closed)

    d) Analgesics

2) **Nursing interventions** are the same as for unruptured, plus:

    a) After surgery, provide wound care, irrigation as prescribed; note quantity and character of drainage.

    b) Maintain NG to low, intermittent suction.

    c) Administer analgesics on a routine schedule for the first few days after surgery.

    d) Ambulate in room; sit in a chair at least three times per day.

    e) Due to emergent nature of surgery, encourage child and parents to express feelings and ask questions.

4. **Necrotizing Enterocolitis**

a. Acute inflammatory disease related to ischemia of the bowel, immature GI defenses, and bacterial proliferation; causes devastating damage to the bowel wall, which results in tissue death. Onset is usually between four and ten days after feedings are initiated.

b. Contributing Factors

1) Prematurity

2) Neonate with complications: respiratory distress, birth asphyxia, shock, polycythemia, infection

3) Intrauterine growth restriction

4) Neonate who has received an exchange transfusion and/or enteral feedings

c. Expected Findings

1) Abdominal distension

2) Lethargy

3) High gastric residuals

4) Apnea that worsens

5) Hypotension

6) Anemia

7) Metabolic acidosis

8) Leukopenia, leukocytosis

9) Electrolyte imbalance

10) Sausage-shaped dilation of the intestine

11) Pneumatosis (bubbly appearance of thickened bowel wall)

12) Bloody stools

13) Bile-stained emesis

14) Hypothermia

15) Decreased urinary output

d. Laboratory Tests and Diagnostic Procedures

1) Abdominal radiography

2) CBC

3) Arterial blood gases

4) Blood culture

5) Electrolyte panel

e. Therapeutic Procedures and Medications

1) Prevent by withholding feedings for 24 to 48 hr for any neonate who has experienced complications; minimize enteral feedings; encourage breastfeeding.

2) NPO

3) NG to low, intermittent suction

4) IV fluids and antibiotics

5) Correction of hypovolemia, electrolyte imbalances

6) Oxygen (intubation likely)

7) Serial abdominal x-rays, every 4 to 6 hr

8) Surgical intervention to remove necrotized bowel; possible temporary colostomy

f. **Nursing Interventions**

1) Monitor bowel sounds, gastric residuals, and stool.

2) Monitor vital signs, including blood pressure; oxygen saturation.

3) Monitor arterial blood gases.

4) Avoid rectal temperatures.

5) Leave undiapered to prevent pressure on abdomen.

6) Position supine or on side.

7) Measure abdominal girth.

8) Institute strict handwashing; isolate infants with confirmed cases.

9) Maintain on oxygen, respiratory support, as needed.

10) Monitor for septicemia, disseminated intravascular coagulation, hypoglycemia.

11) If surgery is performed, provide routine postoperative care, including analgesia.

12) Perform colostomy care, if indicated.

13) Provide emotional support to parents; encourage them to share feelings and ask questions.

g. Client Education

1) Teach the protective quality of breast milk (confers passive immunity, macrophages, lysozymes).

2) Prepare parents for surgical intervention, as needed, and for possible long-term complications, including short bowel syndrome, colonic stricture, fat malabsorption, failure to thrive.

B. **Urinary Disorders**

1. **Minimal Change Nephrotic Syndrome**

   a. Glomeruli become permeable to protein, primarily albumin, which reduces the serum albumin level and lowers the serum osmotic pressure; cause is unknown.

   b. Contributing Factors

      1) Occurs primarily in preschool children; peak incidence is between 2 and 3 years of age

      2) Often preceded by viral upper respiratory infection

   c. Expected Findings

      1) Facial puffiness, especially around the eyes, seen upon rising in the morning; dissipates through the day

      2) Swelling of abdomen, genitalia, lower extremities; more prominent during the day

      3) Gradual or rapid onset of anasarca (generalized edema)

      4) Ascites

      5) Diarrhea, anorexia

      6) Dark, frothy urine; decreased output

      7) Extreme pallor

      8) Fatigue, irritability

      9) Muehrcke (white) lines in nails

      10) Increased susceptibility to infection

      11) Hypoalbuminemia

      12) Hypercholesterolemia

      13) Massive proteinuria, high specific gravity, hyaline casts

      14) Increased platelets (500,000 to 1,000,000/mm³)

      15) Hyponatremia (around 130 to 135 mEq/L)

      16) Hypocalcemia

   d. Laboratory Tests and Diagnostic Procedures

      1) Serum protein, serum albumin

      2) Electrolyte panel

      3) CBC

      4) Lipid panel

      5) Urinalysis

      6) Specific gravity

      7) Renal biopsy

      8) Blood urea nitrogen and creatinine

   e. Therapeutic Procedures and Medications

      1) Corticosteroids

      2) Immunosuppressants

      3) Diuretics

      4) Antibiotics

      5) Usual vaccines (no live vaccines), plus pneumococcal conjugate and pneumococcal polysaccharide vaccines

      6) Sodium-restricted diet during periods of massive edema

   f. Nursing Interventions

      1) Engage in quiet activity.

      2) Strictly monitor intake and output; monitor urine for protein.

      3) Monitor edema: daily weight, daily measurement of abdominal girth.

      4) Monitor skin integrity.

      5) Monitor vital signs.

      6) Protect from contact with anyone who has an infection.

      7) Elevate edematous parts; clean skin and separate with clothing, cotton, or antiseptic powder.

      8) Maintain on low-sodium diet; consult with dietitian to provide palatable foods.

      9) After edema subsides, allow to resume normal activities.

   g. Client Education

      1) Teach parents how to check urine for protein.

      2) Review requirements for low-sodium diet.

      3) Discuss medication administration, possible side effects.

      4) Reassure parents that symptoms will dissipate as recovery continues.

      5) Discuss ways to address social isolation, boredom.

2. **Acute Glomerulonephritis**

   a. Most commonly, a postinfectious disorder associated with pneumococcal, streptococcal, and viral infections; thought to be a response to the deposition of immune complexes in the glomeruli

   b. Contributing Factors

      1) Recent pneumococcal, streptococcal, or viral infection

      2) Most prevalent in summer and early fall

      3) Family history of the disease

   c. Expected Findings

      1) Edema of the face, worse in the morning; spreads to gonads, abdomen, lower extremities throughout the day

      2) Anorexia

      3) Severely decreased urinary output

      4) Cloudy, smoky brown urine (often described as tea or cola-colored); proteinuria, hematuria; decreased glomerular filtration rate

      5) Headache, abdominal discomfort, dysuria

      6) Lethargy, irritability, pallor

      7) Mild to moderate increase in blood pressure

      8) Azotemia

      9) May have elevated streptococcal antibody titers

      10) Decreased glomerular filtration rate

      11) Decreased serum complement (C3) level; returns to normal eight to ten weeks after the disease

      12) Hyperkalemia, acidosis, hypocalcemia, and hyperphosphatemia

      13) Generalized cardiac enlargement, pulmonary congestion, and pleural effusion during edematous phase

d. Laboratory Tests Diagnostic Procedures

   1) Urinalysis

   2) Blood urea nitrogen, creatinine, glomerular filtration rate

   3) Antistreptolysin O (ASO) titer

   4) Serum complement level

   5) Electrolyte panel

   6) Chest x-ray

e. Therapeutic Procedures and Medications

   1) Sodium and water restriction if output is significantly reduced

   2) Diuretics, unless renal failure is severe

   3) Antihypertensives

   4) Antibiotics for persistent streptococcal infection

   5) Fluid restriction if glomerular filtration rate is significantly decreased

f. **Nursing Interventions**

   1) Encourage activity as desired.

   2) Daily weight.

   3) Monitor vital signs, level of consciousness, changes in behavior.

   4) Limit sodium in diet; limit potassium if oliguric; limit protein with severe azotemia.

   5) Note volume and character of urine.

   6) Monitor intake.

   7) If fluids are restricted, evenly divide fluids while the child is awake; serve in small cups.

   8) Monitor skin; elevate edematous parts; encourage frequent movement and repositioning.

   9) Refer for a dietary consult.

g. Client Education

   1) Discuss dietary restrictions with child and parents; have the child identify palatable foods that are allowed.

   2) Teach the importance of adhering to follow-up appointments.

   3) Teach how to provide fluids, if the child is on a fluid restriction.

   4) Discuss ways to prevent infection transmission.

   5) Encourage plans for activity that allow for frequent rest.

3. **Urinary Tract Infection**

a. An infection of the lower urinary tract (urethra and bladder), upper urinary tract (ureters, kidneys), or both. Diagnostic factors are pyuria and at least 50,000 colonies per mL of a single pathogenic organism in a clean catch or sterile urine specimen. Escherichia coli is responsible for 85% of cases.

b. Contributing Factors

   1) Female

   2) Caucasian

   3) Uncircumcised male

   4) Vesicoureteral reflux

   5) Sexual activity, masturbation

   6) Incomplete emptying of the bladder resulting in urinary stasis, dysfunctional voiding

   7) Inadequate fluid intake

   8) Urinary tract abnormalities

   9) Constrictive clothing or diapers, synthetic underwear, prolonged wearing of wet clothing

   10) Constipation

   11) Catheters

   12) Pinworms

   13) Bubble baths, hot tubs, whirlpool baths

   14) Beginning of toilet training

c. Expected Findings

   1) Thick, cloudy urine with mucous strands

   2) Pyuria (at least 10 white blood cells/mL of uncentrifuged urine)

   3) Bacterial growth in urine culture

   4) Infants

      a) Irritability, lethargy

      b) Screaming with urination

      c) Poor feeding, vomiting, diarrhea

      d) Fever

      e) Newborns may exhibit fever or hypothermia, jaundice, cyanosis, tachypnea

      f) Hematuria

   5) Children

      a) Abdominal, flank, back pain

      b) Dysuria, malodorous urine

      c) Hematuria

      d) Incontinence in previously toilet-trained child

      e) Enuresis

      f) Boys may dribble urine

      g) Straining to urinate

      h) High fever, severe flank and abdominal pain, and leukocytosis are symptoms of pyelonephritis

      i) May be asymptomatic or display symptoms inconsistent with urinary tract infection (respiratory, gastrointestinal)

d. Laboratory Tests and Diagnostic Procedures

   1) Urinalysis

   2) Urine culture

   3) Ureteral catheterization

   4) Bladder washout

   5) Renography

   6) Ultrasound

   7) Voiding cystourethrogram

   8) Intravenous pyelography

   9) Dimercaptosuccinic acid scan

e. Therapeutic Procedures and Medications

   1) Antibiotics, intravenously for pyelonephritis

   2) Analgesics

   3) Treatment of contributing anatomic defects

f. **Nursing Interventions**
   1) Ensure that clean-catch urine specimens are collected properly.
   2) Collect first morning urine for analysis.
   3) Assist with suprapubic aspiration or collect catheterized specimen for culture.
   4) Encourage adequate fluid intake.
   5) Encourage frequent urination and complete emptying of bladder.
   6) Monitor urine output, character.
   7) Administer mild analgesia as needed.
   8) Encourage high-fiber diet.

g. Client Education
   1) Teach females to wipe from front to back.
   2) Teach "double voiding" to ensure adequate emptying: urinate, stop, and attempt to urinate again.
   3) Teach importance of wearing cotton underwear, nonrestrictive clothing.
   4) Demonstrate how to retract and clean foreskin, if uncircumcised.
   5) Discuss need to promptly change out of wet clothing.
   6) Instruct to avoid bubble baths, whirlpool tubs, hot tubs.
   7) Emphasize importance of adequate fluid intake.
   8) Encourage sexually active adolescents to void immediately after intercourse.
   9) Emphasize importance of completing antibiotic regimen.

C. **Respiratory Disorders**
1. **Tonsillitis**
   a. Tonsillitis refers to inflamed tonsils, usually accompanied by pharyngitis, and is often caused by a virus or bacterium.
   b. Contributing Factors
      1) Exposure to pathogenic organism
      2) Increased susceptibility in younger children, due to immature immune system
   c. Expected Findings
      1) Halitosis
      2) Snoring
      3) Nasal-sounding voice
      4) Difficulty swallowing, breathing
      5) Mouth-breathing
      6) Edema, inflammation, erythema
      7) Difficulty hearing due to blocked Eustachian tubes
      8) Throat pain that worsens with swallowing
      9) Fever
      10) Persistent cough
      11) Possible positive throat culture for Group A beta-hemolytic streptococcus
   d. Laboratory Tests
      1) Throat culture
      2) CBC
      3) Clotting times

CROUP SYNDROMES

	Acute Epiglottitis	Acute Laryngotracheal Bronchitis	Acute Spasmodic Laryngitis
ETIOLOGY	Bacterial, usually *H. influenzae*	Viral (RSV, influenza A, B), *mycoplasma pneumonia*, measles, parainfluenza types 1, 2, 3	Viral; possibly allergy-related
AGE MOST AFFECTED	2 to 5 years	Infant, child younger than 2 years	1 to 3 years
ONSET	Progresses rapidly	Gradual onset of symptoms	Child goes to bed well; "midnight" or "twilight" croup awakens child
EXPECTED FINDINGS	Stridor, drooling, tripod position (chin pointing out, mouth opened, tongue protruding), high fever, dysphagia, dyspnea, muffled, frog-like voice, tachypnea, tachycardia	Inspiratory stridor, barking, brassy cough, hoarseness, restlessness, irritability, substernal retractions, low-grade fever Symptoms are usually worse at night	Wakes suddenly with dyspnea, barking, metallic cough, stridor, hoarseness, restlessness Symptoms disappear during the day; recurrent
THERAPEUTIC PROCEDURES AND MEDICATIONS	MEDICAL EMERGENCY Possible intubation, tracheostomy, lateral neck radiograph, antibiotics (droplet precautions for first 24 hr after IV antibiotics initiated), corticosteroids, humidified O_2, IV fluids, child is very frightened	Cool air (take outside)/cool mist for mild croup; steroids, oral/IV fluids, nebulized racemic epinephrine as prescribed; nebulized budesonide	Cool mist, steroids, racemic epinephrine, supportive care
NURSING INTERVENTIONS	Encourage position of comfort; droplet isolation; provide calm reassurance to child and caregiver, monitor O_2 status; ensure intubation equipment is at bedside; DO NOT put anything in the mouth (e.g., tongue depressor, culture swab)	Frequently monitor VS including pulse oximetry, be alert to s/s of impending respiratory obstruction: tachypnea, tachycardia, retractions, nasal flaring, restlessness; encourage caregiver to stay with, hold child to calm; provide reassurance	Usually managed at home; cool mist vaporizer; encourage quiet activity

e. Therapeutic Procedures and Medications

 1) Antibiotics, if positive for Group A beta-hemolytic streptococcus

 2) Antipyretics

 3) Analgesics

 4) Topical anesthetics

 5) Antiemetics

 6) Tonsillectomy

f. **Nursing Interventions**

 1) Tonsillitis

 a) Soft or liquid diet

 b) Cool-mist vaporizer

 c) Cool liquids

 d) Warm saline gargles

 2) Tonsillectomy

 a) Prepare child and parents for surgery; ensure consents are signed.

 b) Note bleeding tendencies; note clotting times.

 c) Obtain baseline vital signs.

 d) Report any symptoms of an upper respiratory infection.

 e) Report loose teeth.

 3) Postoperatively

 a) Discourage coughing, clearing throat, blowing nose.

 b) Monitor for signs of hemorrhage: frequent swallowing, repeated throat clearing, hematemesis.

 c) Monitor for airway obstruction, stridor, drooling, restlessness, agitation, tachypnea, cyanosis.

 d) Position to facilitate drainage; elevate head of bed.

 e) Restrict food and fluid until swallowing with no signs of hemorrhage are observed.

 f) Offer ice chips, sips of water, cool liquids, ice pops.

 g) Refrain from offering red or brown foods that may be mistaken for blood.

 h) Apply ice collar.

 i) Advance to soft foods.

 j) Administer narcotic analgesics on a regular schedule.

g. Client Education

 1) Provide information about what to expect on admission and after surgery.

 2) Teach to avoid irritating or spicy foods.

 3) Teach to avoid gargles, vigorous tooth-brushing.

 4) Discuss strategies for continued pain management

 5) Identify the signs of hemorrhage, respiratory obstruction; instruct to seek emergency care if present.

 6) Instruct to notify health care provider if child develops persistent cough, severe ear pain, or fever.

D. **Bronchitis (Tracheobronchitis)**

 1. Inflammation of the trachea and bronchi. It is usually associated with an upper respiratory section and typically caused by a virus or *M. pneumoniae* (common in children 6 years of age or older). It begins with a dry, hacking cough that becomes productive in two to three days. Symptoms intensify at night. It is treated symptomatically with analgesics, antipyretics, cough suppressants, and humidity. Cough suppressants can interfere with clearing of secretions. It usually resolves in five to ten days. Adolescents with chronic bronchitis should be screened for marijuana and tobacco use.

 2. **Bronchiolitis**

 a. Most commonly caused by respiratory syncytial virus, which is the most common lower respiratory infection in children and is the most frequent cause of hospitalization of infants. Parainfluenza viruses and adenoviruses are also causes.

 b. Contributing Factors

 1) Male

 2) Under 2 years; peaks between 2 and 7 months

 3) Crowded living conditions

 4) Chronic disease

 5) Daycare

 6) Exposure to second-hand smoke

 7) Prematurity

 c. Expected Findings

 1) Rhinorrhea, pharyngitis

 2) Fever

 3) Coughing, sneezing

 4) Possible eye or ear infection

 5) Irritability, lethargy

 6) Poor feeding or refusal to feed

 7) Wheezing, crackles, diminished breath sounds

 8) Retractions, nasal flaring

 9) Dyspnea

 10) Tachypnea, apneic episodes

 11) Copious secretions

 12) Cyanosis

 13) Tests on nasopharyngeal secretions are positive for RSV antigen

 d. Laboratory Tests and Diagnostic Procedures

 1) Rapid immunofluorescent antibody-direct fluorescent antibody staining

 2) Enzyme-linked immunosorbent assay

 3) Testing for coexisting infection: urinalysis, lumbar puncture

 4) Arterial blood gases

 5) Electrolytes

 e. Therapeutic Procedures and Medications

 1) Bronchodilators are not recommended.

 2) Oxygen, mechanical ventilation

 3) Ribavirin (only medication approved for treatment for children hospitalized with RSV; controversial due to high cost)

4) Corticosteroids (controversial but may be used)

5) IV fluids

6) Palivizumab for prevention in at-risk children

f. **Nursing Interventions**

1) Droplet and contact precautions.

2) Administer oxygen if oxygen saturation is not consistently maintained at or above 90%, after suctioning and repositioning.

3) Monitor airway and breath sounds.

4) Limit visitors and number of hospital personnel.

5) Assign only to nurse with no other at-risk patients.

6) Suction with normal saline before feeding and PRN.

7) Encourage fluids; offer small amounts (5 to 10 mL) of fluid frequently.

8) Monitor vital signs and oxygenation status.

9) Encourage breastfeeding.

10) Do not administer chest physiotherapy.

g. Client Education

1) Teach scrupulous handwashing.

2) Discourage smoking in the home.

3) Teach how to instill saline drops and suction with bulb syringe.

3. **Respiratory Distress Syndrome (RDS)**

a. A condition of surfactant deficiency and immature thorax, often referred to as hyaline membrane disease, that results in hypoxia. It is most common in premature infants. It is rare in drug-exposed infants or neonates who were exposed to intrauterine stress (e.g., preeclampsia, hypertension).

b. Contributing Factors

1) Prematurity

2) Diabetic mother, hypoglycemia

3) Multifetal pregnancy

4) Cesarean section

5) Cold stress

6) Birth asphyxia

7) Family history of RDS

8) Sepsis

9) Cardiac or respiratory abnormality

10) Premature rupture of membranes

11) Maternal use of depressants close to delivery

c. Expected Findings

1) Tachypnea (respiratory rate is greater than 60 breaths/minute)

2) Peristernal, pericostal retractions

3) Nasal flaring

4) Labored breathing with prolonged expiration

5) Inspiratory crackles

6) Expiratory grunt

7) Mottling

8) Low oxygen saturation

9) Respiratory or mixed acidosis, hypercapnia

10) Atelectasis

11) As condition worsens: flaccidity, nonresponsiveness, apnea, decreased breath sounds, central cyanosis

d. Laboratory Tests and Diagnostic Procedures

1) Arterial blood gases

2) Chest x-ray

3) Cultures of blood, urine, and cerebrospinal fluid

4) Blood glucose

e. Therapeutic Procedures and Medications

1) Mechanical ventilation, CPAP

2) Oxygen

3) IV fluids

4) NPO in acute phase

5) Total parenteral nutrition

6) Exogenous surfactant

7) Prophylactic antibiotics

8) Caffeine

9) Inotropes

10) Electrolytes

11) Sodium bicarbonate

f. **Nursing Interventions**

1) Monitor response to therapy: respiratory effort, arterial blood gases.

2) Monitor vital signs, oximetry, color, pulses.

3) Place in prone position initially, to increase chest expansion.

4) Suction only when necessary.

5) Place under radiant warmer or other controlled environment to eliminate heat loss and prevent cold stress.

6) Encourage parents to hold, touch, talk to baby, as status allows.

7) Encourage parental participation in care (e.g., pump and store breast milk, assist with repositioning).

g. Client Education

1) Orient to the neonatal intensive care unit.

2) Explain all procedures.

3) Encourage kangaroo (skin-to-skin) hold, as condition allows.

4) Instruct how to pump and store breast milk

Point to Remember

Do not give anything by mouth to infants with a respiratory rate greater than 60 breaths/minute or to children with severe respiratory distress.

E. **Neurosensory Disorders**

1. **Meningitis**

   a. Inflammation of meninges, the covering of the spinal cord and brain, caused by bacterial or viral (also called aseptic) infection. The mortality rate is higher for bacterial meningitis and can result in permanent neurological disability.

   b. Contributing Factors

      1) Premature rupture of fetal membranes
      2) Head trauma
      3) Head, neck, back surgery
      4) Cochlear implant
      5) More common in late winter, early spring
      6) Crowded living conditions, daycare
      7) Recent viral illness

   c. Expected Findings

      1) Positive cerebrospinal fluid, blood culture (bacterial)
      2) Cerebral spinal fluid if bacterial: cloudy, elevated white blood cell count, elevated protein, decreased glucose, positive Gram stain; if viral: clear, slightly increased white blood cell count, normal or slightly increased protein, normal glucose, negative Gram stain
      3) Neonates and Infants

         a) Poor suck
         b) Poor feeding
         c) Temperature instability
         d) High-pitched cry
         e) Nuchal rigidity (older infants)
         f) Vomiting, diarrhea
         g) Bulging fontanels (late)
         h) Irritability
         i) Seizures

      4) Children and adolescents

         a) Headache
         b) Seizures
         c) Nuchal rigidity
         d) Photophobia
         e) Decreased level of consciousness
         f) Vomiting
         g) Sensory alterations (e.g., seeing spots, halos)
         h) Positive Kernig's, Brudzinski's signs (not reliable under age 2 years)
         i) Irritability, agitation, delirium, stupor, coma
         j) Hyperactivity with variable reflex response
         k) Fever and chills

   d. Laboratory Tests and Diagnostic Procedures

      1) Lumbar puncture with culture of cerebral spinal fluid
      2) Blood culture
      3) Nose, throat cultures
      4) Computerized tomography (CT)
      5) Magnetic resonance imaging (MRI)

   e. Therapeutic Procedures and Medications

      1) IV fluids
      2) Isolation
      3) Oxygen, mechanical ventilation
      4) Antibiotics, primarily cephalosporins (if bacterial)
      5) Antipyretics
      6) Corticosteroids
      7) Analgesics
      8) Antiepileptics

   f. **Nursing Interventions**

      1) Droplet precautions, as soon as meningitis is suspected.
      2) Quiet, low-light, low-stimulus environment.
      3) Position with head of bed slightly elevated or side-lying; no pillow.
      4) Monitor vital signs, urine output, and neurological status.
      5) Maintain NPO until neurological status has improved; advance to clear liquids, diet as tolerated.
      6) Monitor pain level; provide comfort measures.
      7) If fontanels are bulging, measure head circumference.
      8) Monitor hydration, fluid volume, intake and output; restrict fluids if exhibiting signs of increased intracranial pressure.
      9) Implement seizure precautions.
      10) Provide information and reassurance to child and parents.

   g. Client Education

      1) Encourage parents to ensure vaccines are given at the appropriate times. Children should receive the Hib and PCV vaccines at 2, 4, and 6 months of age, then again between 12 and 15 months of age.
      2) Explain isolation procedures.
      3) Emphasize the importance of adhering to the medication regimen.

! Point to Remember

Development of a puerperal or petechial rash in an ill child could indicate meningococcemia and requires immediate medical attention.

2. **Reye Syndrome**
   a. Metabolic encephalopathy characterized by significantly decreased level of consciousness, hepatic dysfunction, and fever. The cause is unknown. An association between use of aspirin in children and Reye syndrome has been identified.
   b. Contributing Factors
      1) Recent viral illness (usually influenza or varicella)
      2) Use of aspirin and other salicylates
      3) Winter months
   c. Expected Findings
      1) Cerebral edema
      2) Fatty liver, clotting abnormalities
      3) Seizures
      4) Personality changes, delirium, combativeness
      5) Profuse vomiting
      6) Lethargy, irritability, coma
      7) Elevated liver enzymes
      8) Elevated serum ammonia
      9) Prolonged clotting times
   d. Laboratory Tests and Diagnostic Procedures
      1) Liver enzymes (alanine aminotransferase [ALT], aspartate aminotransferase [AST])
      2) Electrolytes
      3) Serum ammonia
      4) Clotting times
      5) Liver biopsy
      6) Cerebral spinal fluid analysis (to rule out meningitis)
   e. Therapeutic Procedures and Medications
      1) Oxygen, respiratory support
      2) Occupational and physical therapy for resulting neurological deficits
      3) Dietary consultation
      4) Osmotic diuretic (mannitol)
      5) Vitamin K
   f. **Nursing Interventions**
      1) Position with head of bed elevated 30°; head in neutral position.
      2) Seizure precautions
      3) Monitor vital signs, oxygen saturation, level of consciousness.
      4) Bleeding precautions.
      5) Strict intake and output.
      6) Monitor pain response; provide comfort measures.
      7) Provide information and reassurance to child and parents.

   g. Client Education
      1) Instruct to avoid administering aspirin or other salicylates to children.
      2) Assist to identify lesser known sources of salicylates (bismuth subsalicylate, methyl salicylate).
      3) Provide a list of acceptable over-the-counter medications for children.

3. **Neonatal Seizure**
   a. The most common cause is hypoxic-ischemic encephalopathy secondary to asphyxia; intracranial hemorrhage is second most common cause; others include infection, kernicterus, hypoglycemia, birth injury, and electrolyte imbalance
   b. Contributing Factors
      1) Prematurity
      2) Diabetic mother, hypoglycemia, hyperglycemia
      3) Rh-negative mother
      4) Delivery complications (e.g., dystocia, prolonged labor, malpresentation, hemorrhage)
      5) Congenital anomaly
      6) Narcotic withdrawal, secondary to maternal use
      7) PKU
      8) Perinatal infection
      9) Intracranial hemorrhage
      10) Uremia, kernicterus
   c. Expected Findings
      1) Clonic
         a) Unilateral
         b) Slow, jerking movements
         c) May migrate from one part of body to another
         d) Last 1 to 3 seconds
         e) May be focal or multifocal
      2) Tonic
         a) Extension, stiffening of extremities or stiffened, flexed arms
         b) Sustained posturing of limbs, neck
         c) May be focal or generalized
      3) Subtle
         a) More common in preterm infants
         b) Repeated blinking
         c) Sucking
         d) Fluttering of eyelids
         e) Pedaling, swimming movements of extremities
         f) Apnea
      4) Myoclonic
         a) Rapid jerking of extremities
         b) Asynchronous twitching
         c) Bilateral jerks of extremities
         d) May be focal, multifocal, or generalized

d. Laboratory Tests and Diagnostic Procedures
1) Blood glucose
2) Serum electrolytes
3) Cerebrospinal fluid analysis
4) Electroencephalogram
5) Computerized tomography (CT) scan
6) Ultrasound
7) Electroencephalography

e. Therapeutic Procedures and Medications
1) Correct underlying problem.
2) Oxygen, respiratory support
3) Antiepileptics
4) Benzodiazepines

f. **Nursing Interventions**
1) Carefully monitor at-risk neonate for seizure activity.
2) Implement seizure precautions; implement seizure-response regimen as prescribed.
3) Monitor vital signs, oxygen status, level of consciousness.
4) Keep parents informed of neonate's condition; interpret behaviors.
5) Encourage parents to participate in care, hold, talk to, touch infant.

g. Client Education
1) Ensure parents understand how to respond if infant has a seizure.
2) Discuss medication regimen and expected response.
3) Stress the importance of maintaining follow-up appointments.

4. Substance-Exposed Infant
a. A substance-exposed neonate will begin to display signs of drug withdrawal 12 to 24 hr after birth, depending on the type of drug, amount, route, and length of exposure; symptoms may last several weeks.
b. Contributing Factors
1) Maternal use of drugs, prior to knowledge of pregnancy
2) Maternal substance use and addiction
c. Expected Findings
1) Perspiration (highly unusual in the normal neonate)
2) Hypertonicity, hyperactive reflexes
3) Tachypnea, tachycardia, apnea, nasal flaring
4) Cyanosis, mottling
5) Jitteriness, tremors, frantic movement
6) Poor feeding, projectile vomiting, diarrhea
7) Excessive but ineffective sucking
8) Poor, restless sleep; increased wakefulness
9) Sneezing, yawning
10) Intractable, high-pitched cry
11) Fever

12) Stuffy nose
13) Seizures
14) Excoriated areas on face and knees
15) Positive drug screen

d. Laboratory Tests and Diagnostic Procedures
1) Blood glucose
2) CBC
3) Electrolytes
4) Drug screen of meconium, urine, hair
5) Chest x-ray

e. Therapeutic Procedures and Medications
1) Prenatal drug screening
2) IV fluids, electrolytes
3) Phenobarbital
4) Morphine
5) Tincture of opium
6) Methadone
7) Buprenorphine
8) Clonidine

f. **Nursing Interventions**
1) Provide quiet, low-light environment.
2) Feed on demand; monitor amount ingested, response to feedings.
3) Monitor hydration and electrolyte status.
4) Swaddle, but maintain hands close to mouth for sucking.
5) Implement the Neonatal Abstinence Scoring System to evaluate.
6) Monitor reflexes, behavior, activity in relation to feeding and other stimulation.
7) Involve mother in care; remain nonjudgmental.
8) Ensure supervisory care is in place prior to discharge.

g. Client Education
1) Demonstrate bonding behaviors.
2) Discuss options for drug rehabilitation.
3) Identify purpose of referral to Child Protective Services.

F. **Neoplastic Disorders**
1. Cancer in children is rare. Acute lymphoblastic leukemia, lymphoma, and central nervous system tumors are the most common types, all of which occur more frequently in males.
2. Contributing Factors
a. Family history of cancer
b. Exposure to cigarette smoke
c. Excessive sun exposure
d. Immunosuppressive drugs
e. Radiation exposure
f. Epstein-Barr infection
g. Male
h. Caucasian
i. Down syndrome

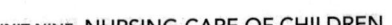

COMMON CHILDHOOD CANCERS

	DESCRIPTION	EXPECTED FINDINGS	TREATMENT
Acute Lymphocytic Leukemia	Most common form of childhood cancer Malignancy of bone marrow and lymphatic system; causes overproduction of immature WBCs, deficiency in platelets, RBCs Occurs primarily between age 2 to 5 years More common in Caucasian males; greater risk in children with Down syndrome Relapse most commonly occurs in the testes	Low-grade, unresolving fever Pallor, bruising, petechiae, lethargy, joint pain, headache, N&V, weakness, anorexia	IV, intrathecal chemotherapy Corticosteroids Bone marrow transplant Hematopoietic stem cell transplant
Hodgkin Disease	Malignancy of the lymph system, primarily lymph nodes Primarily occurs between age 15 to 19 years	Painless, enlarged subclavicular or cervical nodes Nonproductive cough, abdominal pain, low-grade fever, anorexia, pruritus, night sweats, weight loss	Chemotherapy Radiation
Brain Tumor	Most common solid tumor in children; about 25% of childhood cancers Most occur in brainstem or cerebellum Can originate from any cranial cell; glial tumors are most common, followed by astrocytomas	Depends on location and size Headache upon awakening, vomiting unrelated to food, ataxia, dysmetria, dysarthria, nystagmus, behavioral changes	Radiotherapy prior to surgery Proton radiation Chemotherapy
Neuroblastoma	Most common cancer of infancy; median age is 22 months Solid, extracranial tumor that arises from fetal cells that form the adrenal medulla and sympathetic nervous system Primary site is the abdomen 70% of all cases have metastasized prior to diagnosis	Firm, painless abdominal mass that crosses midline Urinary frequency or retention (due to bladder compression) S/S of metastasis: periorbital edema, supraorbital ecchymosis, exophthalmos, hepatomegaly, respiratory dysfunction, fatigue, anorexia, weight loss	Surgery followed by radiation Chemotherapy One of the few tumors that may spontaneously regress
Osteosarcoma	Most common bone cancer in children Occurs most frequently after age 10 years, after a growth spurt More than half occur in the femur	Localized pain, often relieved with flexion Limping, other gait change	Surgery: limb salvage, amputation Chemotherapy
Wilms Tumor (nephroblastoma)	Most common childhood cancer of the kidney 75% occur under age 5 years 5% are familial	Painless abdominal mass that does not cross the midline Weight loss, enlarged liver, spleen, anemia,	Surgery Chemotherapy Note: NEVER palpate the abdomen; doing so may cause tumor cells to disseminate

3. Expected Findings
    a. Unusual swelling or mass
    b. Unexplained fatigue
    c. Unexplained pallor
    d. Headaches, vomiting with headaches
    e. Sudden vision changes
    f. Prolonged fever or illness
    g. Limp, other change in gait
    h. Localized pain
    i. Unexplained bruising tendency
    j. Sudden unexplained weight loss
    k. Anemia
    l. Hematuria
    m. Thrombocytopenia
    n. Neutropenia, leukemic blasts
    o. Mass visible on imaging

4. Laboratory Tests and Diagnostic Procedures
    a. Complete blood count
    b. Urinalysis
    c. Blood urea nitrogen, creatinine
    d. Bone marrow, organ biopsy
    e. Computerized tomography (CT) scan
    f. Magnetic resonance imaging (MRI)
    g. Positron emission tomography (PET) scan
    h. Lumbar puncture
    i. Serum chemistry
    j. Liver function tests

5. Therapeutic Procedures and Medications
    a. Chemotherapy
    b. Surgery
    c. Radiation
    d. Bone marrow transplant
    e. Analgesics

f. Antiemetics

g. Corticosteroids

h. Cell-stimulating medications (e.g., epoetin alfa, filgrastim, oprelvekin)

i. Topical anesthetics (e.g., viscous lidocaine, EMLA cream)

j. Antihistamines

k. Antibiotics

6. **Nursing Interventions**

a. Encourage frequent intake of small amounts of fluids.

b. Monitor for anaphylaxis for 20 min after chemotherapy infusion.

c. Maintain strict asepsis.

d. Monitor VS.

e. Screen visitors and prohibit those with signs of infection.

f. Provide favorite foods, but do not pressure to eat; engage child in menu selection.

g. Institute bleeding and neutropenic precautions.

h. Monitor weight.

i. Premedicate and prepare for painful procedures.

j. Provide pharmacological and nonpharmacological pain relief.

k. Use medical play to demonstrate procedures; allow child to safely manipulate equipment.

l. Prepare for hair loss; let child decide how to manage.

m. Ensure sun protection when outside.

n. Promote cleanliness and regular hygiene practices.

o. Encourage peer visits, contact.

p. Maintain as normal a routine as possible, including continuation of schooling.

q. Encourage child to dress in own clothing.

r. Encourage oral hygiene, use of soft toothbrush.

s. Encourage discussion of fears, feelings.

t. Provide uninterrupted time for family.

7. Client Education

a. Carefully explain all procedures to caregiver and child; adapt to child's developmental level.

b. Explain what to expect as treatment progresses, including common side effects.

c. Teach ways to handle side effects.

d. Ensure parents understand explanations of medical care and prognostic statistics.

e. Discuss participation in support groups, other support organizations.

G. **Infectious Disorders**

1. **Otitis Media**

a. An infection and inflammation of the middle ear; if there is fluid, it is referred to as otitis media with effusion. It is among the most common childhood illnesses.

b. Contributing Factors

1) Less than 24 months of age

2) Cleft lip/palate

3) Daycare; entering school for the first time

4) Passive cigarette smoke exposure

5) Bottle feeding

6) Propping the bottle

7) Recent upper respiratory infection

8) Winter and spring months

9) Allergies

10) Enlarged adenoids

11) Nonadherence to vaccine schedule

12) Down syndrome

c. Expected Findings

1) Ear pain, rubbing, tugging at ear, rocking head from side to side

2) Pain worsens with sucking or chewing

3) Fever

4) Enlarged, painful postauricular and cervical lymph glands

5) Bulging tympanic membrane

6) Inconsolable crying

7) Anorexia, nausea, vomiting

8) Irritability, restlessness, poor sleeping

9) Purulent drainage from ear

10) Transient hearing loss, balance problems

11) Feeling of fullness in the ear

12) Nonspecific symptoms including rhinitis, cough, and diarrhea

13) Drainage from ear accompanied by immediate pain relief, indicates tympanic rupture

14) Decreased or no tympanic movement with pneumatic otoscopy

d. Diagnostic Procedures

1) Pneumatic otoscopy

2) Acoustic reflectometry

3) Tympanometry

e. Therapeutic Procedures and Medications

1) Antibiotics

2) Antipyretics

3) Analgesics

4) Topical anesthetics

5) Myringotomy with tympanostomy tube placement

f. **Nursing Interventions**
   1) Apply heat over ear and lie on affected side.
   2) Clean drainage from external ear.
   3) Ear wicks should be loose and kept dry.
   4) Monitor for hearing loss.
   5) Provide comfort measures.
   6) Position upright.

g. Client Education
   1) Stress the importance of adherence to vaccine schedule.
   2) Discourage propping the bottle.
   3) Encourage breastfeeding.
   4) Discourage exposure to passive smoking.
   5) Instruct to notify health care provider when symptoms initially occur.
   6) If the child has tympanostomy tubes, instruct to keep water out of the ears and to notify provider when tubes come out.

2. *Enterobiasis vermicularis* (pinworms)

a. The most common helminthic infection in the United States. Eggs float through the air and may be ingested or inhaled. They hatch in the upper intestine and mature, migrate out of the intestine, and lay eggs, which are viable for 2 to 3 weeks on indoor surfaces.

b. Contributing Factors
   1) Close proximity to others (e.g., classrooms and daycare)
   2) Hand-to-mouth behavior in children
   3) Temperate climate

c. Expected Findings
   1) Intense anal itching
   2) Enuresis
   3) Poor sleep, nighttime restlessness
   4) Irritability

d. Diagnostic Procedure
   1) Tape test: Parents are instructed to wrap a tongue depressor with tape, sticky side out, and firmly press the tape against the perianal area. This is done when the child awakens for three consecutive mornings. They are placed in a jar or plastic bag and brought in for microscopic examination.

e. Medications
   1) Antihelminthics (e.g., pyrantel pamoate, pyrvinium pamoate, albendazole—available over-the-counter)

f. **Nursing Interventions**
   1) Trim fingernails short.
   2) Dress child in one piece pajamas.
   3) Encourage showering rather than bathing.

g. Client Education
   1) Advise that pyrantel pamoate will turn GI contents red and will stain clothing.
   2) Discuss the need for treatment of all family members: initial dose, then repeat 2 weeks later.
   3) Teach the importance of good handwashing.

3. *Pediculosis capitis* (head lice)

a. Infestation of the scalp and hair with lice. The female lays eggs (nits) at night, on the hair shaft, close to scalp, which hatch in 7 to 10 days. The louse sucks blood of the host. With a host, the life span of the female is around one month.

b. Contributing Factors
   1) Close proximity to others, such as in classrooms or daycare
   2) School age
   3) Common sharing of objects that touch the head such as hats or combs

c. Expected Findings
   1) Intense itching of scalp
   2) Small red bumps on scalp
   3) Small white specks attached to hair shaft, usually close to the scalp

d. Medications
   1) Permethrin cream rinse (available over-the-counter)
   2) Pyrethrin with piperonyl butoxide (available over-the-counter, contraindicated for those with chrysanthemum or ragweed allergy)
   3) Malathion
   4) Benzyl alcohol (for children over 2 years)
   5) Spinosad (for children over 4 years)
   6) Ivermectin lotion (if child is over 6 months)

e. **Nursing Interventions**
   1) Assure child and caregiver that anyone can get head lice; it is not due to lack of cleanliness.
   2) Carefully inspect the head and hair to identify.
   3) Use "nit" comb on hair after shampooing with pediculicide.

f. Client Education
   1) Caution against sharing objects that touch the head (e.g., hats, combs, barrettes, scarves, coats).
   2) Instruct to repeat the treatment in 7 to 10 days.
   3) Teach caregiver to use nit comb; run in sections from scalp to ends.
   4) Suggest that the caregiver play "beauty parlor" with child when treating.
   5) Advise to cover child's eyes while treating.
   6) Instruct to treat all members of the household.
   7) Advise to wash linens, towels, clothing in hot water and dry in hot dryer; seal nonwashable objects in a plastic bag for two weeks.
   8) Thoroughly vacuum carpets, car seats, pillows, stuffed animals.
   9) Soak combs, brushes, hair accessories in lice-killing agent for 1 hr.

COMMUNICABLE DISEASES OF CHILDHOOD

	TRANSMISSION, INCUBATION, COMMUNICABILITY	EXPECTED FINDINGS	THERAPEUTIC PROCEDURES	NURSING INTERVENTIONS (STANDARD PRECAUTIONS APPLY TO ALL)
Chickenpox (varicella-zoster)	Contact, airborne Incubation 2 to 3 weeks Communicable 1 day before macule eruption to when all lesions have crusted	Fever, malaise, loss of appetite for first 24 hr; then macules, papules, vesicles, crusts; pruritus, irritability Complications: encephalitis, secondary infection	Meds: Acyclovir, diphenhydramine, or other antihistamine Prevention: Varicella vaccine	Airborne and contact precautions until all lesions are crusted; skin care, tepid oatmeal baths; trim fingernails and keep clean; lightweight clothing; distract from itching; NO aspirin (possible Reye syndrome)
Diphtheria (*Corynebacterium diphtheria*)	Direct contact, droplet; spread via nasal discharge and lesions Incubation 2 to 5 days Communicable 2 to 4 weeks after disease onset	Malaise, cold-type symptoms, sore throat, epistaxis, thick, white, or gray membrane covering throat, fever, hoarseness, lymphadenopathy (bull's neck) Complications: septic shock, myocarditis, neuropathy	Equine antitoxin, penicillin G, strict bed rest, O₂, tracheostomy PRN Prevention: diphtheria vaccine; series given in infancy and childhood as part of combination vaccine with periodic boosters	Droplet precautions; contact precautions with skin lesions; provide complete care, conserve client's energy; monitor VS, especially for respiratory obstruction; suction PRN
Fifth Disease (erythema infectiosum; caused by human parvovirus B19)	Contact with respiratory secretions, blood, and blood products Incubation 4 to 21 days Communicability period not certain	3 Stages › Stage I: "Slapped face" erythema on cheeks (days 1 to 4) › Stage II: Appears 1 day after onset of Stage I; maculopapular rash › Stage III: Rash subsides but reappears if skin is irritated Complications: aplastic crisis (rash usually absent), acute arthritis	Antipyretics, anti-inflammatory medications, analgesics, blood transfusion for aplastic crisis	Usually isolation is unnecessary Droplet precautions if hospitalized; not likely to be contagious after rash appears; may return to school or daycare
Mononucleosis (Epstein-Barr virus)	Direct contact with oral secretions, blood, and blood products Incubation 30 to 50 days Communicability period is unknown Seen primarily in adolescents and young adults	Malaise, sore throat, fever, lymphadenopathy, unusual fatigue, headache, rash (sometimes), epistaxis Complications: splenic rupture, respiratory failure, neurological events (e.g., seizure, meningitis), pancytopenia	IV hydration, rest, analgesics, antipyretics	Monitor airway status; monitor for hemorrhage (secondary to splenic rupture); encourage saltwater gargles, anesthetic throat spray or lozenges; counsel re: importance of rest
Mumps (paramyxovirus)	Direct contact with saliva, droplet Incubation 14 to 21 days Communicable immediately before and after swelling of parotid glands	Fever, headache, earache aggravated by chewing Parotitis beginning third day, pain tenderness Complications: deafness, myocarditis, arthritis, hepatitis, pancreatitis, meningitis, orchitis, oophoritis	Analgesics, antipyretics, IV hydration PRN Prevention: mumps vaccine (included in MMR)	Droplet and contact precautions Encourage rest, fluids; provide soft foods; apply warm or cool compresses to inflamed areas (per client preference)
Pertussis (whooping cough; caused by *Bordetella pertussis*)	Direct contact with droplets; indirect contact with contaminated objects Incubation 6 to 20 days Communicable during phase with upper respiratory symptoms, before cough	Coryza, sneezing, watery eyes, low-grade fever Paroxysmal "whooping" cough, worse at night, causing bulging eyes, cyanosis, protruding tongue that may last until mucus plug is dislodged—lasts 4-6 weeks; vomiting of mucus Complications: pneumonia, rib fractures, hemorrhage, seizures, otitis media, atelectasis, hernia, prolapsed rectum	Prophylactic antibiotics, oxygen, IV fluids, mechanical ventilation if needed	Droplet precautions Offer small amounts of fluid, frequently; monitor for airway obstruction

	TRANSMISSION, INCUBATION, COMMUNICABILITY	EXPECTED FINDINGS	THERAPEUTIC PROCEDURES	NURSING INTERVENTIONS (STANDARD PRECAUTIONS APPLY TO ALL)
Poliomyelitis (three types; caused by enteroviruses)	Direct contact with oropharyngeal secretions or oral-fecal route; less common through sneeze or cough Incubation 7 to 14 days Period of communicability is unknown	It appears in three different forms: abortive, nonparalytic, and paralytic Fever, headache, vomiting, loss of appetite, nausea, abdominal pain; fatigue; pain in neck, back, legs in more severe form Paralytic: onset has same symptoms as nonparalytic followed by recovery, then CNS paralysis Complications: permanent paralysis, respiratory failure, hypertension	Bed rest, mechanical ventilation PRN, physical therapy, sedatives for anxiety, analgesics Prevention: immunization administered in series in infancy and childhood	Position in alignment, use footboard, pressure-relieving mattress; apply moist warm packs, assist with ROM exercises; encourage participation in ADLs; assist with ambulation; encourage high-protein, high-fiber diet, encourage fluids
Roseola (exanthem subitum caused by human herpes virus type 6)	Occurs in children younger than 3 years; transmission is unknown—thought to be from saliva of adults, who do not have symptoms Incubation 5 to 15 days Communicability is unknown	High fever for 3 to 7 days in otherwise healthy child; temperature suddenly drops to normal with appearance of rosy-pink maculopapular rash that begins on trunk and lasts 1 to 2 days; disappears when blanched; bulging fontanels Complications: febrile seizures, encephalitis	Antipyretics; otherwise supportive Only standard precautions	Teach caregiver to monitor temperature and to administer antipyretics
Rubella Virus (German measles)	Contact with nasopharyngeal secretions, blood, stool, urine Incubation 14 to 21 days Communicable 7 days before and 5 days after appearance of rash	Prodrome doesn't occur in children; in adolescents, consists of low-grade fever, malaise, coryza, cough, and lasts 1 to 5 days Rash: maculopapular, begins on face and spreads downward; lasts 3 days Complications: rare; greatest risk is teratogenic effect; supportive: analgesics, antipyretics	Prevention: childhood vaccine (part of MMR)	Droplet precautions Provide comfort measures; instruct caregiver to keep child away from pregnant women
Rubeola (measles, virus)	Direct contact; more prevalent in winter Incubation 10 to 20 days Communicable 4 days before and 5 days after rash	Fever, malaise, cough, allergy-type nasal irritation, watery eyes, Koplik spots on buccal mucosa Maculopapular rash appears on face third or fourth day and moves down body; anorexia, abdominal pain, lymphadenopathy, photophobia Complications: otitis media, pneumonia, obstructive laryngitis, encephalitis	Rest, antipyretics, antibiotics in high-risk children, vitamin A Prevention: rubeola vaccine (included in MMR)	Airborne precautions Encourage rest, quiet activity; maintain low-light environment; cool-mist vaporizer, encourage soft, bland diet, tepid baths
Scarlet Fever (group A beta-hemolytic streptococci)	Direct contact with nasopharyngeal secretions Incubation 2 to 5 days, with range of 1 to 7 Communicable during incubation and throughout illness, around 10 days; after that may persist for months	Begins with abrupt high fever, generalized punctate rash appears, except on face; abdominal pain, halitosis; tonsils are swollen, very red, and covered in white patches of exudate; white strawberry tongue, turns red; generalized rash appears, except on face, about 12 hr after onset; face is flushed; circumoral pallor; sandpaper-like rash on torso; sloughing on palms and soles Complications: peritonsillar abscess, sinusitis, otitis media, acute glomerulonephritis, acute rheumatic fever (arthralgia), rheumatic heart disease (valve damage)	Penicillin, or erythromycin, if allergic; rest, analgesics, antipyretics, local anesthetics for throat pain	Droplet precautions until child has been on antibiotic for 24 hr; rest, quiet activity; emphasize importance of full course of antibiotics to caregiver; gargles, cool mist vaporizer; encourage fluids and soft foods; teach family how to prevent spread (discard toothbrush)

SECTION 6

Nursing Care of the Child who has a Chronic Condition

A. **Gastrointestinal Disorders**

1. **Celiac Disease (gluten-sensitive enteropathy)**

   a. An immune-mediated disease that causes damage to the small intestine and villi when exposed to foods containing gluten.

   b. Contributing Factors

      1) Type I diabetes mellitus or other autoimmune disorder (such as rheumatoid arthritis)

      2) Caucasian

      3) Introduction of solid foods

   c. Expected Findings

      1) Failure to thrive

      2) Chronic diarrhea; steatorrhea

      3) Aphthous ulcers (canker sores)

      4) Fatigue

      5) Abdominal pain and distention

      6) Anemia

      7) Irritability

      8) Muscle wasting

      9) Celiac crisis: copious watery diarrhea and vomiting

      10) Positive serologic markers

      11) Mucosal inflammation, crypt hyperplasia, and villous atrophy seen with endoscopy

   d. Laboratory Tests and Diagnostic Procedures

      1) Serologic blood test for tissue transglutaminase and antiendomysial antibodies in children 18 months of age or older (positive result indicates disease)

      2) Gastrointestinal endoscopy and biopsy

   e. Medications

      1) Nutritional supplements

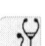

   f. **Nursing Interventions**

      1) Restrict gluten from diet

      2) Maintain a high-calorie, high-protein diet

      3) Restrict lactose during periods with acute symptoms

      4) Consult with dietitian

      5) Encourage child and parents to express concerns

   g. Client Education

      1) Instruct to read food labels, look for hidden sources of gluten.

      2) Use the BROWS acronym to teach major sources of gluten: barley, rye, oats, wheat, spelt.

      3) Assist to identify nongluten sources of grains: rice, corn, millet.

      4) Discuss support organizations (such as Celiac Sprue Association).

B. **Respiratory Disorders**

1. **Cystic Fibrosis**

   a. Genetic disorder that affects exocrine (mucus) glands so that secretions are thick and viscous, obstructing organs. It affects multiple systems but manifests primarily in lungs, GI tract, skin, and pancreas.

   b. Contributing Factors

      1) Caucasian

      2) Family history

   c. Expected Findings

      1) Chronic, dry cough

      2) Cyanosis, clubbing

      3) Dyspnea, wheezing

      4) Repeated respiratory infections

      5) Meconium ileus in newborn

      6) Abdominal distention, intestinal obstruction

      7) Steatorrhea

      8) Failure to thrive, gain weight

      9) Hypoalbuminemia

      10) Rectal prolapse

      11) Skin tastes salty; tears, saliva have excessive sodium and chloride

      12) Hyponatremia, hypochloremia

      13) High sweat chloride

      14) Atelectasis

      15) Hemoptysis

      16) Voracious appetite

      17) Barrel chest, thin arms and legs

      18) Anemia

      19) Fat-soluble vitamin deficiency

      20) Viscous cervical mucus; decreased or absent sperm

   d. Laboratory Tests and Diagnostic Procedures

      1) Nutritional panel to detect a deficiency of fat-soluble vitamins (A, D, E, and K)

      2) Sputum culture

      3) DNA testing

      4) Chest x-ray

      5) Pulmonary function tests

      6) Abdominal x-ray

      7) Stool analysis

      8) Sweat chloride test

   e. Therapeutic Procedures and Medications

      1) Oxygen

      2) IV fluids

      3) Feeding tube (for intractable weight loss)

      4) Chest physiotherapy

      5) High-calorie diet

      6) Vaccines

      7) Palivizumab for RSV prevention

266

8) Pancreatic enzymes (must be administered within 30 min of eating)

9) Multivitamin, vitamins A, D, E, K

10) Dornase alfa (decreases mucus viscosity)

11) Antibiotics (including nebulized)

12) Antifungals

13) Bronchodilators

14) Anticholinergics

15) H_2 blockers, proton pump inhibitors, stool softeners

16) Surgery for meconium ileus, if indicated

17) Lung, heart, pancreas, liver transplant for advanced disease

f. **Nursing Interventions**

1) Monitor respiratory effort, breath sounds.

2) Monitor for fatigue.

3) Monitor for weight loss, muscle wasting.

4) Involve the child and caregiver in scheduling care activities.

5) Encourage to view care activities as part of a normal daily routine.

6) Provide airway clearance therapy (ACT) twice daily; more frequently, as indicated.

7) Perform chest physiotherapy (CPT) as need determines; avoid doing so right before or after meals (shaker vest, manual cupping).

8) Encourage a high-protein, high-calorie diet, snacks in between meals.

9) Monitor blood glucose.

10) Encourage moderate aerobic exercise.

11) Refer for dietary consult.

12) Provide support and reassurance for child and parents.

g. Client Education

1) Provide information about access to medical equipment and medications.

2) Teach caregiver how to perform airway clearance techniques, chest physiotherapy.

3) Discuss medication schedule, administration, therapeutic and side effects.

4) Instruct to monitor for deteriorating respiratory status and to notify provider or seek emergency care.

5) Teach to monitor nutritional status, growth, weight.

6) Demonstrate use of nebulizer.

7) Teach nasal lavage (used for chronic sinusitis).

8) Emphasize importance of adherence to vaccine schedule.

9) Teach about diet and ways to increase caloric intake.

10) Provide information about support groups and organizations.

11) Instruct to maintain normalcy in daily routine, relationship with child.

C. **Hematologic Disorders**

1. **Sickle Cell Anemia**

a. A genetic disease in which abnormal sickle hemoglobin (HgS) replaces normal hemoglobin.

b. Contributing Factors

1) Both parents carry the sickle cell trait.

2) African American or of Middle Eastern, Mediterranean, or Indian descent

3) Family history of the disease

c. Expected Findings

1) Organ dysfunction, enlargement (spleen, liver, kidneys), cirrhosis

2) Osteoporosis

3) Chronic anemia (hemoglobin is less than 10 g/dL)

4) Hands and feet are cool to touch

5) Increased susceptibility to infection, sepsis

6) Pallor, pale mucous membranes

7) Jaundice

8) Shortness of breath, fatigue

9) Pain

10) Retinal detachment

11) Delayed growth, puberty

12) Systolic murmur

13) Enuresis, renal failure

14) Skeletal deformities; shoulder hip avascular necrosis

15) Vaso-Occlusive Crisis

a) Extreme pain in joints, hands, feet

b) Swelling of joints and extremities

c) Severe abdominal pain

d) Priapism

e) Hematuria

f) Symptoms of stroke

g) Dyspnea; acute chest syndrome

h) Visual disturbances

i) Shock

j) Elevated white blood cells, bilirubin and reticulocytes; decreased hemoglobin

k) Peripheral blood smear reveals sickled cells

16) Sequestration

a) Blood pools excessively in spleen, liver

b) Reduced blood volume can cause hypovolemia and shock (tachycardia, tachypnea, thready pulse, hypotension)

d. Laboratory Tests and Diagnostic Procedures

1) Sickle cell screening of newborn

2) CBC (for anemia)

3) Sickle-turbidity: detects presence of HbS; does not differentiate trait from disease

4) Hemoglobin electrophoresis—for definitive diagnosis

5) DNA sequencing

6) Transcranial Doppler test: detects risk for CVA (performed annually for children 10 to 16 years of age with disease)

7) Sickle Cell Crisis

a) CBC

b) Bilirubin and reticulocyte levels

c) Peripheral blood smear

e. Therapeutic Measures and Medications

1) Hydroxyurea

2) Penicillin prophylaxis

3) Exchange transfusion (erythrocytapheresis)

4) Chelation with deferoxamine, if multiple transfusions required

5) Splenectomy

6) Crisis Management

a) IV fluids

b) Oxygen, if hypoxic (of little value until circulation is improved)

c) Electrolyte replacement, correction of metabolic acidosis

d) Opioid analgesia

e) Blood transfusion

f) Antibiotics

g) Bed rest

Point to Remember

Meperidine is not used for treatment of pain in sickle cell anemia. It produces a metabolite that can cause tremors, anxiety, myoclonus, and generalized seizures, as levels rise with repeated doses. Children with sickle cell disease are particularly at risk for seizures.

f. **Nursing Interventions**

1) Use the acronym HOP when planning care for vaso-occlusive crisis: hydration, oxygen, pain management.

2) Monitor oxygenation status.

3) Monitor hydration; calculate fluid requirements and ensure intake exceeds minimum.

4) Provide fluids in a special cup to encourage fluid intake.

5) Exclude anyone with an infection from visiting.

6) Strict intake and output.

7) Apply warm compresses to painful joints; avoid cold compresses.

8) Monitor for signs of reaction, associated with blood transfusion.

9) Monitor and measure the size of the spleen.

10) Bed rest; conserve energy.

11) Passive range of motion, as is tolerated.

12) Weigh daily.

13) Monitor potassium and other electrolyte levels.

14) Monitor for complications of stroke and chest syndrome (e.g., severe thoracic pain, fever, cough, dyspnea, tachycardia, hypoxia).

15) Refer for genetic testing and counseling.

16) Provide support and information to parents, siblings, and other close family members.

g. Client Education

1) Encourage frequent rest breaks during physical activities.

2) Discourage from contact sports if spleen is enlarged.

3) Instruct to avoid low-oxygen environments (e.g., nonpressurized airplane, high altitudes).

4) Emphasize the importance of hydration.

5) Teach about fluid sources other than water (e.g., ice pops, sherbet, soup).

6) Teach parents to recognize signs of dehydration.

7) Encourage clothing that prevents sweating.

8) Discourage long periods of sun exposure.

9) Discourage limiting fluids if enuresis occurs.

10) Emphasize the importance of avoiding communicable illnesses; importance of scrupulous hand hygiene; promote adherence to vaccine schedule.

11) Teach the signs of crisis and infection; instruct to seek medical help immediately.

12) Teach parents how to palpate the spleen to detect sequestration early.

13) Emphasize the importance of good nutrition.

14) Advise wearing of medical alert tag.

15) Discuss support groups and organizations.

2. **Hemophilia**

a. Group of bleeding disorders; the result of a deficiency of a clotting factor, which causes difficulty controlling bleeding, most often as the result of the inheritance of the associated X-linked recessive trait that is passed from a carrier mother to her son.

b. Contributing Factors

1) Family history of the disease

2) Affected father; trait-carrying mother

c. Expected Findings

1) Prolonged bleeding (may be first noticed following newborn procedures such as injections, heel sticks, circumcision)

2) Epistaxis, bleeding gums, prolonged bleeding after tooth loss

3) Hematuria, tarry stools

4) Bruising, hematoma out of proportion to injury

5) Hemarthrosis, joint pain

6) Anemia

d. Laboratory Tests and Diagnostic Procedures

1) DNA testing

2) aPTT (PT is normal)

3) Factor-specific assay

4) CBC (platelets are normal)

e. Therapeutic Procedures and Medications

1) IV infusion of deficient factor. (Cryoprecipitate is no longer recommended since recombinant factor VIII concentrate became available. It is considered to be a medication and does not carry the risks of blood product administration.) Factor VIII should be administered immediately if an injury occurs. It may also be administered prophylactically.

   a) Administer missing factor.
      (1) Hemophilia A: factor VIII
      (2) Hemophilia B: factor IX

2) Blood transfusion

3) Corticosteroids

4) 1-deamino-8-d-arginine vasopressin (DDAVP—used for mild cases; can be administered intranasally or parenterally)

5) Epsilon-aminocaproic acid (EACA) prevents clot destruction and is used with mouth trauma surgery; the child swishes the medication around in the mouth and then swallows it.

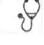

f. **Nursing Interventions**

1) Avoid unnecessary punctures; venipunctures are preferred over finger or heel sticks; administer parenteral medications subcutaneously instead of intramuscularly when possible.

2) Monitor urine and stool for blood.

3) Do not administer aspirin or other salicylates; use of NSAIDS is discouraged; acetaminophen is acceptable.

4) Provide a soft toothbrush, water irrigation device for oral care.

5) Monitor for signs of bleeding such as headache, slurred speech, change in level of consciousness.

6) Respond immediately to an injury.

   a) Administer replacement clotting factor immediately.

   b) Immobilize, elevate, and apply ice to affected joints.

   c) Monitor for adverse response: headache, tachycardia, hypotension, change in level of consciousness.

g. Client Education

1) Encourage regular exercise and physical therapy (passive range of motion exercises should not be performed after any acute incident).

2) Teach parents to create a safe environment that allows for normal development.

3) Encourage participation in noncontact sports like swimming, golf, walking, jogging, fishing, bowling.

4) Teach parents how to administer clotting factor intravenously (beginning when child is 2 to 3 years of age); teach the child to self-administer at 8 to 12 years of age.

5) Emphasize need to administer clotting factor without delay, if injury occurs.

6) Encourage use of soft toothbrush and, when appropriate, electric razor.

7) Work with the school nurse and teach to prepare the child for entering school.

8) Emphasize importance of adhering to vaccine schedule.

9) Instruct how to identify signs of bleeding.

10) Discuss how to respond to injuries using the RICE acronym (rest, ice, compression, elevation).

11) Inform the family about community resources and support groups.

D. **Musculoskeletal Disorders**

1. **Idiopathic Scoliosis**

a. A spinal deformity characterized by lateral curvature and spinal rotation, which causes rib asymmetry. It usually becomes evident at age ten or older and is the most common spinal deformity.

b. Contributing Factors

1) Etiology is unknown, but there appears to be a genetic aspect.

2) Preadolescent growth spurt

3) Female

4) Age between 8 to 15 years of age

c. Expected Findings

1) Ill-fitting clothes

2) Asymmetry in scapula, ribs, flanks, shoulders, and hips

3) One leg shorter than the other

4) Head and hips not aligned (uncompensated) or head aligns with gluteal cleft (compensated)

5) Spinal curvature

d. Diagnostic Procedures

1) Screening: observe from behind; the child wears clothing that provides a clear view of the spine (shorts, briefs) and bends forward from the waist; trunk is parallel to the floor and arms hang freely (Adam's position), making asymmetry apparent. Screen before and during growth spurts.

2) Radiography

   a) Cobb technique: determines degree of curvature

   b) Risser scale: determines skeletal maturity

3) Scoliometry

e. Therapeutic Procedures and Medications

1) Bracing and exercise for moderate curvatures of 25° to 45°

2) Spinal fusion with rod placement if curvature is 45° or more

3) Postoperative opioid analgesics

f. **Nursing Interventions**

1) Bracing and Exercise

   a) Assist with fitting brace.

   b) Monitor skin integrity.

   c) Reinforce a positive self-image.

2) Spinal Fusion with Rod Placement

  a) Preoperative

    (1) Refer for preoperative testing, including type and cross-match for blood, pulmonary function testing.

    (2) Orient the adolescent and family to the hospital, including the intensive care unit.

  b) Postoperative

    (1) Monitor neurologic status of extremities and promptly report any impairment.

    (2) Carefully monitor for pain, using age-appropriate tool.

    (3) Use log-rolling technique to turn frequently.

    (4) Encourage pulmonary hygiene.

    (5) Monitor skin for pressure areas.

    (6) Keep skin clean and dry.

    (7) Monitor surgical sites and drains; provide wound care as prescribed.

    (8) Assess bowel function; monitor for ileus.

    (9) Monitor hematocrit and hemoglobin; observe for bleeding.

    (10) Monitor for infection.

    (11) Perform range of motion on unaffected extremities; encourage mobility when able to tolerate.

    (12) Provide diversionary activities; encourage visits with family and friends.

g. Client Education

  1) Bracing and Exercise

    a) Explain the process thoroughly and ensure understanding.

    b) Provide guidance when selecting clothing and activities.

    c) Encourage independence and socialization.

  2) Spinal fusion with Rod Placement

    a) Preoperative

      (1) Discuss options for autologous blood donation.

      (2) Discuss postoperative expectations. Inform about monitors, NG tube, chest tubes, urinary catheter, and patient-controlled analgesia.

      (3) Teach pulmonary hygiene techniques: turn, cough, deep breath, incentive spirometry; discuss respiratory therapy techniques.

      (4) Instruct about the log-rolling technique.

      (5) Allow time for questions and clarification of medical terms.

    b) Postoperative

      (1) Reinforce expected course of recovery.

      (2) Encourage the family to arrange the environment to encourage independence.

      (3) Emphasize the importance of follow-up care.

CPR Guidelines for Infants and Children

A. **Cardiac Arrest**

Refer to the American Heart Association "CPR and ECC Guidelines"

1. C–A–B sequence

2. Begin compressions and rescue breathing, using a ratio of 15:2 (1 or 2 rescuers).

3. Compression rate should be approximately 100/min.

4. Chest should be compressed to the anteroposterior diameter: 1.5 inches in infants; 2 inches in children up to puberty.

5. If available, use AED.

6. Compression-only CPR generally is not effective for children; however, it is preferable to no CPR.

B. **Choking**

1. Infant

  a. Pick up and hold face down along forearm with infant's head away from the body, angled down.

  b. Administer five back blows.

  c. Turn face up and administer five chest thrusts.

  d. Repeat until obstruction is cleared.

  e. Open the mouth; remove obstruction if it is visible and can safely be cleared.

  f. Prepare to administer CPR.

2. Child Over 1 Year

  a. Observe for signs of choking: hands to throat, inability to talk, dyspnea, ineffective cough, noisy or absent breathing, cyanosis.

  b. Deliver five abdominal thrusts (Heimlich maneuver).

  c. Assess for breathing.

  d. Repeat sequence.

  e. If unsuccessful, prepare to perform CPR.

! Point to Remember

Never perform a blind finger sweep. The object may be pushed further into the airway.

Activities

Answers for all activities are at the end of the activities section.

PRIORITIZING NURSING CARE OF THE CHILD

Match each clinical situation to the priority nursing action, listed below. Each will be used once.

CLINICAL SITUATION

1. A 3-year-old toddler who has diarrhea and has been febrile for 2 days

2. A 4-week-old infant who has hypertrophic pyloric stenosis and is vomiting.

3. A neonate born with a myelomeningocele in the lumbar region

4. A 5-year-old child who is receiving chemotherapy for acute lymphocytic leukemia

5. A 10-year-old child who has sickle cell anemia and is having a vaso-occlusive crisis

1. _____

2. _____

3. _____

4. _____

5. _____

PRIORITY ACTIONS

a. Monitor for hypotension, wheezing, nausea, vomiting, and urticaria.

b. Place on bed rest and minimize activity.

c. Administer oral rehydration fluids.

d. Administer replacement electrolytes intravenously.

e. Monitor respirations and level of consciousness.

INFANT VOCALIZATION

Match the developmental task for vocalization to the age. Select from the list below.

CLINICAL SITUATION

1. 2 months

2. 4 months

3. 6 months

4. 8 months

5. 10 months

6. 12 months

1. _____

2. _____

3. _____

4. _____

5. _____

6. _____

PRIORITY ACTIONS

a. Comprehends "bye-bye"

b. Begins to imitate sounds

c. Coos

d. Imitates animal sounds

e. Laughs out loud

f. Combines syllables ("dada") but doesn't understand meaning

NURSING CARE OF THE CHILD WITH A COMMUNICABLE DISEASE

Fill in the blanks with the information that pertains to the identified communicable disease. There are several options for symptoms and interventions.

VARICELLA (CHICKENPOX)

Transmitted via _____ particles

and _____ _____

with open vesicles or lesions.

List three symptoms:

a. _____

b. _____

c. _____

Describe rash: _____ that progresses

to _____

List three nursing interventions:

a. _____

b. _____

c. _____

Report to the Center for Disease Control: ☐ Yes ☐ No

PERTUSSIS

Transmitted via _____

List three symptoms:

a. _____

b. _____

c. _____

List three nursing interventions:

a. _____

b. _____

c. _____

Report to the Center for Disease Control: ☐ Yes ☐ No

MEASLES (RUBEOLA)

Transmitted via _____

List three symptoms:

a. _____

b. _____

c. _____

List three nursing interventions:

a. _____

b. _____

c. _____

Report to the Center for Disease Control: ☐ Yes ☐ No

RESPIRATORY SYNCYTIAL VIRUS (RSV)

Transmitted via _____

List three symptoms:

a. _____

b. _____

c. _____

List three nursing interventions:

a. _____

b. _____

c. _____

Report to the Center for Disease Control: ☐ Yes ☐ No

ROTAVIRUS

Transmitted via _____

List three symptoms:

a. _____

b. _____

c. _____

List three nursing interventions:

a. _____

b. _____

c. _____

Report to the Center for Disease Control: ☐ Yes ☐ No

IMMUNIZATIONS

Identify the immunization(s) to be given, based on the developmental stages. Select from the list below. Several will be used more than once.

NEWBORN	INFANT	TODDLER	PRESCHOOLER	SCHOOL-AGE	ADOLESCENT

WORD LIST

Diphtheria, tetanus, and pertussis (DTaP)

Tetanus, diphtheria, and pertussis (Tdap)

Rotavirus (RV)

Influenza

Measles, mumps, rubella (MMR)

Meningococcal (Men)

Human papillomavirus (HPV)

Pneumococcal conjugate (PCV13)

Hepatitis B (Hep B)

Human papillomavirus (HPV)

Hepatitis A (Hep A)

Varicella (VAR)

Inactivated polio virus (IPV)

Haemophilus influenzae type b (Hib)

Answers to Activities

PRIORITIZING NURSING CARE OF THE CHILD ANSWERS

CLINICAL SITUATION	PRIORITY ACTION	RATIONALE
1. A 3-year-old toddler who has diarrhea and has been febrile for 2 days	c. Administer oral rehydration fluids.	Fluid volume deficit, which could lead to hypovolemic shock, is the primary concern. Oral rehydration replaces fluid loss from diarrhea and is preferred over intravenous therapy.
2. A 4-week-old infant who has hypertrophic pyloric stenosis and is vomiting	d. Administer replacement electrolytes intravenously.	Children who have this condition are especially prone to depletion of potassium, sodium, and chloride. All of these electrolytes are contained within gastric secretions. A serious imbalance could be life-threatening.
3. A neonate born with a myelomeningocele in the lumbar region	e. Monitor respirations and level of consciousness.	80% to 85% of children who are born with a myelomeningocele develop hydrocephalus, which can affect respiration and neurological function. Feeding difficulties, irritability, lethargy, seizures, and episodes of apnea should be reported immediately.
4. A 5-year-old child who is receiving chemotherapy for acute lymphocytic leukemia	a. Monitor for hypotension, wheezing, nausea, vomiting, and urticaria.	Many chemotherapeutic agents have anaphylactic potential. Children should be monitored carefully while the medication is infusing and for one hour afterwards for signs of anaphylaxis. Emergency equipment and medications must be immediately available.
5. A 10-year-old child who has sickle cell anemia and is having a vaso-occlusive crisis	b. Place on bed rest and minimize activity.	The primary objective in treatment of a vaso-occlusive crisis is to minimize oxygen expenditure and improve oxygen utilization, which occurs by limiting physical activity.

INFANT VOCALIZATION ANSWERS

CLINICAL SITUATION	VOCALIZATION
1. 2 months	c. Coos
2. 4 months	e. Laughs out loud
3. 6 months	b. Begins to imitate sounds
4. 8 months	f. Combines syllables ("dada") but doesn't understand meaning
5. 10 months	a. Comprehends "bye-bye"
6. 12 months	d. Imitates animal sounds

NURSING CARE OF THE CHILD WITH A COMMUNICABLE DISEASE ANSWERS

VARICELLA (CHICKENPOX)

Transmitted via <u>airborne</u> particles and <u>direct</u> <u>contact</u> with open vesicles or lesions.

List three symptoms:

› Fever

› Lymphadenopathy

› Intense pruritus

Describe rash: <u>Maculopapular rash</u> that progresses to <u>vesicles</u>

List three nursing interventions:

› Place airborne and contact precautions until all vesicles are dried and crusted over.

› Bathe and change sheets and clothes daily.

› Apply calamine lotion.

› Keep fingernails short; apply mittens.

› Maintain a cool environment.

› Provide diversionary activities to distract from scratching.

› Teach child to apply pressure instead of scratching.

› Remove loose crusts.

› Avoid use of aspirin.

Report to the Center for Disease Control: <u>Yes</u>

PERTUSSIS

Transmitted via <u>droplet</u>

List three symptoms:

› Coryza

› Sneezing

› Watery eyes

› Low-grade fever

› Dry hacking cough that becomes paroxysmal

› Cough is followed by a sudden inspiration which produces a "whooping" sound

› Flushed cheeks or cyanosis during cough

› Mucus plug dislodged by cough

› Vomiting after coughing

List three nursing interventions:

› Place on droplet precautions.

› Offer small amounts of fluids frequently.

› Position on side.

› Provide humidified oxygen.

› Monitor for airway obstruction, hypoxia.

› Emphasize need for child to finish entire course of antibiotics.

Report to the Center for Disease Control: <u>Yes</u>

MEASLES (RUBEOLA)

Transmitted via <u>airborne particles</u>

List three symptoms:

› Fever and malaise

› Coryza, cough, conjunctivitis

› Koplik spots on buccal mucosa before rash

› Maculopapular rash that starts on the face and spreads down

› Anorexia, abdominal pain

› Lymphadenopathy

› Photophobia

List three nursing interventions:

› Place on airborne precautions.

› Encourage rest.

› Provide antipyretics.

› Maintain low-light environment.

› Clean eyes with warm saline.

› Provide a cool mist vaporizer.

› Encourage fluids and soft foods.

› Bathe in tepid water.

Report to the Center for Disease Control: <u>Yes</u>

RESPIRATORY SYNCYTIAL VIRUS (RSV)

Transmitted via <u>droplet, direct or indirect contact</u>

List three symptoms:

› Rhinorrhea

› Low-grade fever

› Cough

› Respiratory symptoms: wheezing, retractions, crackles, dyspnea, tachypnea, crackles, diminished breath sounds

› Lethargy

› Poor feeding

› Apneic episodes

List three nursing interventions:

› Place on droplet and contact precautions.

› Screen visitors for illness.

› Encourage breastfeeding mothers to pump and store milk.

› Provide small of amounts of fluid frequently.

› Monitor oxygenation.

› Suction PRN.

› Teach parents to suction nares using saline drops and a bulb syringe.

› Administer antipyretics.

Report to the Center for Disease Control: <u>No</u>

ROTAVIRUS

Transmitted via <u>fecal-oral, contact</u>

List three symptoms:

› Watery diarrhea

› Vomiting

› Fever

› Abdominal pain

› Anorexia, poor feeding

› Irritability

› Signs of dehydration: absence of tears, dry mucous membranes, decreased output, weight loss, warm, dry skin, sunken fontanel

List three nursing interventions:

› Place on contact precautions.

› Administer oral rehydration in small amounts (1-2 tsp) frequently (every 5-10 min while awake).

› Administer and monitor IV fluids if unable to tolerate oral fluids.

› Weigh daily.

› Monitor intake and output.

› Monitor for signs of hypovolemic shock: lethargy, pallor, tachycardia, tachypnea.

› Monitor specific gravity.

› For infants, instruct parents to alternate oral rehydration solution with breast milk or formula.

› Progress to diet as tolerated.

Report to the Center for Disease Control: <u>No</u>

IMMUNIZATIONS ANSWERS

NEWBORN	INFANT	TODDLER	PRESCHOOLER	SCHOOL-AGE	ADOLESCENT
Hepatitis B (Hep B)	Hepatitis B (Hep B)	Hepatitis B (Hep B)	Diphtheria, tetanus, and pertussis (DTaP)	Influenza	Influenza
	Rotavirus (RV)	Diphtheria, tetanus, and pertussis (DTaP)	Inactivated polio virus (IPV)	Meningococcal	Meningococcal
	Diphtheria, tetanus, and pertussis (DTaP)	*Haemophilus influenzae* type b (Hib)	Influenza	Tetanus, diphtheria, and pertussis (Tdap)	
	Haemophilus influenzae type b (Hib)	Pneumococcal conjugate (PCV13)	Measles, mumps, rubella (MMR)	Human papillomavirus (HPV)	
	Pneumococcal conjugate (PCV13)	Inactivated polio virus (IPV)			
	Inactivated polio virus (IPV)	Influenza			
	Influenza	Measles, mumps, rubella (MMR)			
		Varicella (VAR)			
		Hepatitis A (Hep A)			

Source: http://www.cdc.gov/vaccines/schedules/hcp/imz/child-adolescent.html

Index

Autism spectrum disorders (ASDs), 179
Automobile safety. *See* Motor vehicle safety
Autonomy, defined, 16
Avoidant personality disorder, 181

Love and belonging needs, 5, 172, 173
LPN (licensed practical nurse), 13
Lumbar puncture, 148
Lumen occlusion, 30
Lung cancer, 89
Lupus, 161–162
LVN (licensed vocational nurse), 13
Lymphomas, 158

M

Macular degeneration, 155
Magico-religious beliefs, 24
Magnesium imbalances, 82–83
Magnesium toxicity, 198
Magnetic resonance imaging (MRI), 110, 149
Major depressive disorder. *See* Depression
Malpractice, defined, 17
Management and leadership process, 10–12
Mandatory reporting requirements, 17
Mania, 180
Mantoux test, 85
MAOIs (monoamine oxidase inhibitors), 54, 180
Maslow's Hierarchy of Needs, 5, 172, 173
Mass casualty disaster triage, 22
Mastitis, 213
Maternal nursing, 189–224. *See also* Newborn nursing; Women's health
  labor and delivery, 201–210
  postpartum care, 61, 210–213
  pregnancy, 190–200
  reproductive system, 190
  standards of care for, 210
Maternal serum alpha-fetoprotein screening (MSAFP), 194
Maternal substance abuse, 217–218, 260
McDonald's rule of due date calculation, 191
Measles (Rubeola virus), 72, 265
Mechanical soft diets, 167
Mechanical ventilation, 92
Medical asepsis (clean technique), 70

Medical-surgical nursing, 77–169
  acid-base imbalances in, 84–85
  burns, assessment and management of, 162–164
  cardiovascular system disorders, 94, 128–137, 196–198, 242–243
  diet and nutrition in, 165–168
  endocrine system functions and disorders, 95, 116–125, 198–199
  end-of-life care, 165
  fluids and electrolytes, 79–85, 169
  gastrointestinal system disorders, 95–109, 219, 247–252, 266
  genitourinary system disorders, 94, 95, 141–147, 253–255
  hematologic system disorders, 125–128, 267–269
  immune system disorders, 160–162
  musculoskeletal system disorders, 110–116, 269–270
  neurosensory disorders, 57–58, 66–67, 147–157, 198, 258–260
  ocular disorders, 58, 155–156
  oncology nursing, 158–160
  perioperative care, 93–95
  respiratory system disorders, 30, 72–73, 85–92, 218, 255–257, 266–267
Medications. *See also* Pharmacology; Routes of administration; *specific names and types of medications*
  actions, interactions, and reactions, 29, 31
  for cardiovascular system, 32–36
  in children, 29, 238–239
  in complementary and alternative therapies, 62–64
  in elderly populations, 29
  for endocrine system, 39–42
  for gastrointestinal system, 46–47
  for genitourinary system, 48–49
  half-life of, 29
  for hematologic system, 42–46
  for immune system, 50–52
  in labor and delivery, 204–206
  for musculoskeletal system, 52–53
  for nervous system, 54–58
  for pain and inflammation, 58–59, 206, 238
  pregnancy and breastfeeding considerations, 29
  for reproductive system, 59–61
  for respiratory system, 36–39
  safety in administration of, 29, 30, 238–239

Meglitinides, 39
Melatonin, 64
Ménière's disease, 157
Meningitis, 258
Meningocele, 245
Meningococcal disease, 72
Meningococcemia, 258
Menopause, 222
Mental health, defined, 172
Mental health nursing, 171–187
  anger/violence, abuse, and assault, 185–186
  anxiety and anxiety disorders, 54, 176–177
  assessment in, 174
  for children and adolescents, 178–179
  cognitive disorders, 183–184
  communication skills in, 175–176
  crisis intervention in, 22
  defined, 172
  depressive/bipolar disorders, 179–180, 212
  eating disorders, 184
  group therapy in, 176
  legal aspects of, 187
  nurse-client relationship in, 175
  personality disorders, 181–182
  schizophrenia, 178
  substance abuse and dependence, 182, 217–218, 233, 235, 260
  theoretical models, 172–174
  trauma- and stressor-related disorders, 22, 23, 186
Mental illness, defined, 172
Mental status examinations (MSEs), 174
Meperidine, 268
Metabolic acidosis, 84
Metabolic alkalosis, 84
Metabolic syndrome, 122
Methicillin-resistant *Staphylococcus aureus* (MRSA), 72
Methylergonovine, 61
Methylxanthines, 37
MI (myocardial infarction), 131
Minimal change nephrotic syndrome, 253
Misdemeanors, 17
Molar pregnancy, 200
Monoamine oxidase inhibitors (MAOIs), 54, 180
Mononucleosis, 264
Mormons, 26

Morphine, 103, 238

Morse Fall Scale, 75–76

Motor disorders, 178–179

Motor skill development, 226–227, 229, 231

Motor vehicle safety, 228, 230–233, 235

Movement disorders, 178

MRI (magnetic resonance imaging), 110, 149

MRSA (methicillin-resistant *Staphylococcus aureus*), 72

MS (multiple sclerosis), 153

MSAFP (maternal serum alpha-fetoprotein screening), 194

MSEs (mental status examinations), 174

Mucolytics, 38

Mucosal protectants, 46

Multigeneration antibiotics, 50–51

Multimedia test questions, 3

Multiple choice test questions, 3

Multiple myeloma, 158

Multiple response test questions, 3

Multiple sclerosis (MS), 153

Mumps, 264

Musculoskeletal system disorders, 110–116
  amputations, 115–116
  arthritis, 110–112
  arthroplasty, 115
  in children and adolescents, 269–270
  diagnostic tests for, 110
  fractures, 112–113
  gouty arthritis, 112
  medications for, 52–53
  osteoarthritis, 110–111
  osteomyelitis, 114
  osteoporosis, 114
  rheumatoid arthritis, 111

Muslims, 25

Myasthenia gravis, 154–155

Myelomeningocele, 245

Myocardial infarction (MI), 131

Myomas, 222

Myopia, 155

Myxedema coma, 120

N

Nägele's rule of due date calculation, 191

Narcissistic personality disorder, 181

Nasal route of administration, 239

Nasogastric feeding tubes, 97

Nasointestinal feeding tubes, 97, 98

Natural disasters, 20, 21

Naturalistic beliefs, 24

Nausea, 94

NCLEX-RN®
  assessment and remediation prior to, 3
  day of exam procedures, 7
  general information regarding, 2
  question types, 2–4, 28
  test-taking strategies for, 4–6

NDRIs (norepinephrine dopamine reuptake inhibitors), 180

Nearsightedness, 155

Necrotizing enterocolitis, 252

Negative symptoms of schizophrenia, 178

Neglect, 185, 235

Negligence, defined, 17

Neonatal period, 213–216. *See also* Newborn nursing

Nephroblastoma, 261

Nephrosis, 143

Nephrotic syndrome, 253

Nerve conduction studies, 110

Neuroblastoma, 261

Neurogenic shock, 135

Neurological disorder medications, 57–58

Neurosensory disorders, 147–157
  ALS (Lou Gehrig's disease), 154
  assessment of, 147–148, 155–157
  auditory, 156–157
  cerebrovascular accidents, 151–152
  in children and adolescents, 258–260
  diagnostic procedures for, 148–149
  Guillain-Barré syndrome, 155
  head injuries, 149
  hyperthermia, 150
  intracranial pressure elevations, 149–150
  medications for, 54–58
  meningitis, 258
  multiple sclerosis, 153
  myasthenia gravis, 154–155
  ocular, 155–156
  Parkinson's disease, 57, 153
  Reye syndrome, 259
  seizure disorders, 57–58, 66–67, 150–151, 198, 259–260
  spinal cord injuries, 152–153
  status epilepticus, 151
  surgical procedures for, 155
  transient ischemic attacks, 151

New Ballard Score for newborns, 215

Newborn nursing, 213–219
  Apgar scoring, 213
  assessment of newborns, 213–215
  breastfeeding guidelines, 29, 210, 215–216
  circumcision care, 216
  complications of, 217–219, 222
  formula-feeding guidelines, 216
  gestational age assessment, 215
  hyperbilirubinemia and, 219, 250–251
  hypoglycemia and, 218
  maternal substance abuse and, 217–218, 260
  neonatal period, 213–216
  physical and reflexes assessment, 214–215
  posterm infants, 219
  preterm births and, 195, 208–209, 218–219
  reactivity periods and, 215
  respiratory distress syndrome and, 218, 257
  seizures and, 259–260
  vital sign assessment, 213–214

Nicotine use, 217

Nitrates, organic, 35

Nitroglycerin, 130

Noncommunicating Children's Pain Checklist, 237

Nonmaleficence, defined, 16

Non-mass-casualty situations, 22

Non-stress tests (NSTs), 192–193

Nontherapeutic communication, 175–176

Nonurgent injuries, 22

Nonviral hepatitis, 107

Norepinephrine dopamine reuptake inhibitors (NDRIs), 180

NSAIDs (nonsteroidal anti-inflammatory drugs), 53, 58

Nurse-client relationship, 175

Thyroidectomy, 121

Thyroid gland, 120–121

Thyroid hormone antagonists, 41

Thyroid hormones, 40

Thyroid storm, 120

TIAs (transient ischemic attacks), 151

Time orientation, cultural differences in, 24

Tissue donation, 16

TMS (transcranial magnetic stimulation), 180

Tobacco use, 217

Tocolytics, 61

Toddlers, 229–230, 236, 237, 240. *See also* Child and adolescent nursing

Tonsillitis, 255–256

Topical route of administration, 238

Tort law, 17

Total joint arthroplasty, 115

Total parenteral nutrition (TPN), 30, 98

Tourette disorder, 178

Toxic drug levels, 29, 31

Tracheobronchitis, 256–257

Tracheostomy care, 91

Traction devices, 113

Transcranial magnetic stimulation (TMS), 180

Transdermal route of administration, 238

Transesophageal echocardiogram (TEE), 129

Transference, 172, 173

Transferring and lifting clients, 67

Transient hyperglycemia, 123

Transient ischemic attacks (TIAs), 151

Transmission-based precautions, in infection control, 71–73

Transplants, 145

Transurethral resection of prostate (TURP), 146

Trauma-related disorders, 22, 23, 186

Triage, 22

Trichomoniasis, 220, 224

Tricyclic antidepressants (TCAs), 54, 177, 180

Trough levels, 29

T-SPOT.TB test, 85

Tuberculosis (TB), 73, 85, 88

TURP (transurethral resection of prostate), 146

2-amino-2-deoxyglucose (glucosamine), 63

Type 1 and type 2 diabetes, 122

U

Ulcerative colitis, 102–103

Ulcers, 100–101

Ultrasounds, 192

Umbilical cord, 190, 194, 209, 213

Unintentional torts, 17

Universal Protocol (Joint Commission), 93

Unlicensed assistive personnel (UAP), 13

Unruptured appendix, 251–252

Unstable (preinfarction) angina, 130

Urea breath tests, 96

Urgent injuries, 22

Urinalysis, 137, 169, 199

Urinary catheterization, 142

Urinary diversion, 146

Urinary retention/hesitancy, 94, 147

Urinary system disorders. *See* Genitourinary system disorders

Urinary tract infections, 95, 254–255

Urolithiasis, 143

Uterine contractions, 201

Uterine disorders, 222

Uterine fibroids, 222

V

Vaccines. *See* Immunizations

Vacuum assisted delivery, 207

Vaginal exams, 199, 201, 210

Vaginal infections, 220

Valerian root, 62

Valvular disorders, 132

Vancomycin-resistant enterococci (VRE), 73

Variance reports, 12

Variant (Prinzmetal's) angina, 130

Varicella zoster (chickenpox), 71, 264

Varicose veins, 134

Vascular disease, 133

Vasodilators, 34

Vasospasms, 197

Vehicular safety. *See* Motor vehicle safety

Venous thromboembolism (VTE), 134

Ventilation, mechanical, 92

Veracity, defined, 16

Video test questions, 3

Violence, 185–186. *See also* Abuse

Virtual colonoscopy, 96

Vision problems, 155–156

Vital signs in children, 213–214, 236

Vitamins, 62–64

Voluntary admissions, 187

Vomiting, 250

VRE (vancomycin-resistant enterococci), 73

VTE (venous thromboembolism), 134

Vulnerable groups, community health nursing for, 20

W

Walkers, 69

Wharton's jelly, 190

Whipple procedure, 109

WHO (World Health Organization), 161

Whooping cough, 264

Wills, 16

Wilms tumor, 261

Women's health, 220–224. *See also* Maternal nursing

cancer, 220–221

contraception, 59–60, 220

infertility, 220

menopause, 222

sexually transmitted infections, 223–224

uterine disorders, 222

vaginal infections, 220

Working phase in nurse-client relationship, 175

Worksheets

acid-base imbalances, 85

addictive disorders, 182

anger/violence, abuse, and assault, 186

anxiety disorders, 177

child and adolescent nursing, 179, 271–276

cognitive disorders, 184

communication, 175

delegation, 13

depressive/bipolar disorders, 180

eating disorders, 184

endocrine system disorders, 125

herbal therapies, 64

labor and delivery medications, 206

leadership style, 10

mass casualty disaster triage, 22

medication categories, 32

Morse Fall Scale, 75–76

neurosensory system disorders, 157

personality disorders, 182

prenatal, labor, and delivery complications, 222

prioritization, 15, 271, 274

respiratory system disorders, 92

schizophrenia, 178

side effects and adverse reactions, 31

theory review, 174

World Health Organization (WHO), 161

Wounds, postoperative complications and, 94, 95

Y

Yeast infections, 220

References

Berman, A., Snyder, S., & Frandsen, G. (2016). Kozier & Erb's fundamentals of nursing: Concepts, process, and practice (10th ed.). Upper Saddle River, NJ: Prentice-Hall.

Burchum, J. R., & Rosenthal, L.D. (2019). Lehne's pharmacology for nursing care (10th ed.). St. Louis, MO.

Cherry, B., & Jacob, S. R. (2019). Contemporary nursing: Issues, trends, & management. (8th ed.). St. Louis, MO: Elsevier.

U.S. Food and Drug Administration. (2019). Drugs@ FDA: FDA approved drug products. Retrieved from https://www.accessdata.fda.gov/scripts/cder/daf/

Halter, M. J. (2018). Varcarolis' foundations of psychiatric mental health nursing: A clinical approach (8th ed.). St. Louis, MO: Elsevier.

Hinkle, J. L., & Cheever, K. H. (2018). Brunner and Suddarth's textbook of medical-surgical nursing (14th ed.). Philadelphia: Wolters Kluwer.

Hockenberry, M.J., & Wilson, D. (2018). Wong's Nursing Care of Infants and Children (11th ed).St. Louis, MO: Mosby.

Ignatiavicius, D. D., & Workman, M. L. (2018). Medical-surgical nursing (9th ed.). St. Louis, MO: Elsevier.

Lilley, L. L., Rainforth-Collins, S., & Snyder, J. S. (2017). Pharmacology and the nursing process (8th ed.). St. Louis, MO: Elsevier.

Lowdermilk, D. L., Perry, S. E., Cashion, M.C., & Aldean, K.R. (2016). Maternity & women's health care (11th ed.). St. Louis, MO: Elsevier.

Marquis, B.L., & Huston, C. J. (2017). Leadership roles and management functions in nursing: Theory and application. (9th ed.). Philadelphia: Wolters Kluwer.

Potter, P. A., Perry, A. G., Stockert, P., & Hall, A. (2017). Fundamentals of nursing (9th ed.). St. Louis, MO: Elsevier.

Silbert-Flagg, J., & Pillitteri, A. (2018). Maternal & child health nursing: Care of the childbearing and childrearing family (8th ed.). Philadelphia: Wolters Kluwer.

Vallerand, A. H., Sanoski, C. A. & Deglin, J. H. (2019). Davis's drug guide for nurses (16 ed.). Philadelphia.

Practice Questions

Nursing Leadership and Management

1. During a home health assessment, the nurse witnesses a school-age child fall from a second story window. Which of the following is the priority action?

   A. Tell the child not to move.

   B. Provide support to the parents.

   C. Apply pressure to bleeding.

   D. Place the child on a rigid board.

2. A unit manager observes several nurses working throughout the day. Which of the following actions represents a breach in client confidentiality?

   A. Shredding a client's printed laboratory results

   B. Giving report to the oncoming nurse at the bedside

   C. Logging off the computer prior to leaving workstation area

   D. Posting positive information about a client on a social media website

3. A client who is newly admitted requests information about advance directives. The nurse should include which of the following statements in the discussion?

   A. "An advance directive may not be changed."

   B. "Advance directives are only discussed with terminally ill clients."

   C. "You will need to designate a relative to act as your health care proxy."

   D. "I will give you a pamphlet with written information about advance directives."

4. A nurse completes a home health assessment on an older adult who has a broken arm and burn marks to the chest. The caregiver states injuries were sustained from a fall. Which of the following actions is needed at this time?

   A. Administer ibuprofen PRN.

   B. Implement seizure precautions.

   C. Contact adult protective services.

   D. Provide teaching to promote safety.

5. A client arrives to the emergency department and reports a headache, neck stiffness, and sensitivity to light. Which of the following is the priority nursing action?

   A. Notify recent contacts.

   B. Administer acetaminophen.

   C. Implement droplet precautions.

   D. Decrease environmental stimuli.

6. A bladder irrigation is prescribed for a client who has an occluded indwelling urinary catheter. Which of the following actions should the nurse take when unsure of how to perform this procedure?

   A. Refuse to perform and notify provider.

   B. Refer to the policy and procedure manual.

   C. Instill solution slowly and observe for signs of pain.

   D. Delay irrigation and inform next nurse assigned.

7. A charge nurse reviews abbreviations used in client documentation. Which of the following is an approved entry?

   A. Enoxaparin 30 mg SC BID

   B. Zolpidem 5.0 mg PO qhs

   C. Digoxin .125 mg IV q 24 h

   D. Furosemide 60 mg PO daily

8. A nurse participates in quality improvement to decrease hospital readmissions for clients who have heart failure. Which of the following actions should the nurse expect to perform?

   A. Discuss staff performance appraisals with team.

   B. Compare performance to current practice standard.

   C. Reinforce evidence-based practice guidelines to staff.

   D. Interview all nurses caring for clients who are readmitted.

9. A nurse assigns care for a client who has diabetes mellitus to the licensed practical nurse (LPN) and assistive personnel (AP). Which of the following tasks should be delegated to the LPN?

   A. Measure urinary output.

   B. Apply antiembolic stockings.

   C. Assist with bedside commode.

   D. Obtain capillary blood glucose.

10. A client who has stage IV pancreatic cancer decides to discontinue all treatment. Which of the following actions should the nurse take?

    A. Offer alternative medications.

    B. Encourage the client to reconsider.

    C. Ask the client to discuss the decision.

    D. Request a mental health consultation.

11. A nurse receives a client's medication prescription over the telephone from the provider. Which of the following actions should the nurse take?

    A. Repeat the prescription back to the provider.

    B. Ensure the provider signs the prescription immediately.

    C. Instruct the provider to submit the prescription electronically.

    D. Request another nurse to witness the provider's prescription.

12. A nurse receives an end-of-shift report. Which of the following client assessment findings should the nurse address first?

    A. Blood pressure of 105/70 mm Hg in a client who is dehydrated

    B. New onset of confusion in a client who has a left femur fracture

    C. Blood glucose of 140 mg/dL in a client who has diabetes mellitus

    D. Decreased bowel sounds in a client who is 2 days postoperative

13. A nurse should prepare to notify public health officials about which of the following client infections? (Select all that apply.)

    A. Gonorrhea

    B. Hepatitis C

    C. *Clostridium difficile*

    D. *Chlamydia trachomatis*

    E. Meningococcal disease

14. A client has a new diagnosis of stage IV lung cancer. When the partner requests the diagnosis be withheld from the client, which of the following actions should the nurse take?

    A. Withhold the diagnosis from the client.

    B. Contact the institution's ethics committee.

    C Document the request in the medical record.

    D. Request additional information from the partner.

15. A nurse reviews the plan of care for a client who has myasthenia gravis. Which of the following interventions requires a revision?

    A. Monitor for sudden increases in weakness.

    B. Perform pulmonary percussion and postural drainage.

    C. Refer to speech and occupational therapy for evaluation.

    D. Assist with daily activities prior to medication administration.

Pharmacology in Nursing

1. A client who has COPD is prescribed ipratropium bromide. The nurse should instruct the client to report which of the following symptoms immediately?

    A. Nausea

    B. Eye pain

    C. Dry mouth

    D. Constipation

2. An older adult who is receiving a blood transfusion develops an increase in blood pressure and crackles bilaterally. Which of the following medications should the nurse administer?

    A. Lisinopril

    B. Ampicillin

    C. Furosemide

    D. Diphenhydramine

3. A nurse provides teaching to a client who is prescribed spironolactone. The nurse should limit the intake of which of the following foods? (Select all that apply.)

    A. Bananas

    B. White rice

    C. Tomatoes

    D. Avocados

    E. Sweet potatoes

4. A client is prescribed acetaminophen 650 mg PO every 4 hr PRN pain. Which of the following findings should alert the nurse to question this prescription?

    A. Manual BP 145/86 mm Hg

    B. Reports drinking six beers daily

    C. Oral temperature of 37° C (98.6° F)

    D. Smokes two packs of cigarettes weekly

5. A school-age child who has ADHD is observed having an increased ability to focus and complete tasks. The nurse recognizes which of the following medications may have been a contributing factor?

    A. Disulfiram

    B. Alprazolam

    C. Chlorpromazine

    D. Methylphenidate

6. An unresponsive client who has a respiratory rate of 8/min and pinpoint pupils is brought to the emergency department. The nurse should administer which of the following medications?

    A. Naloxone

    B. Disulfiram

    C. Methadone

    D. Succinylcholine

7. A nurse provides discharge instructions to a client who is newly prescribed lisinopril. Which of the following statements indicates teaching was effective? (Select all that apply.)

    A. "I can continue using a salt substitute on food."

    B. "It is an emergency if my mouth starts to swell."

    C. "If I develop a cough, my doctor will be notified."

    D. "My potassium level will need to be monitored."

    E. "Getting up quickly may cause me to feel dizzy."

8. A nurse provides care to a client who is receiving chemotherapy IV. After reviewing the policy, which of the following is an appropriate action if chemotherapy drips on the floor?

    A. Use a spill kit

    B. Dry the liquid

    C. Document waste

    D. Call housekeeping

9. A client has a documented allergy to sulfamethoxazole-trimethoprim. The nurse should question the prescription for which of the following medications?

    A. Glipizide

    B. Sertraline

    C. Amoxicillin

    D. Loratadine

10. A nurse prepares to administer morphine 2 mg IV to a client. The vial available contains morphine 4 mg per 2 mL. Which of the following actions should be taken?

    A. Administer 2 mL of morphine.

    B. Call pharmacy for the exact medication dose.

    C. Waste morphine 1 mL with another nurse as witness.

    D. Notify the charge nurse of an inaccurate narcotic count.

11. The electronic medication list from the referring clinic is different from the client's medication. Which of the following actions should the home health nurse perform?

    A. Clarify prescriptions with provider.

    B. Document the recent prescriptions.

    C. Disregard the missing prescriptions.

    D. Call pharmacy to order prescriptions.

12. An older adult who is receiving TPN states, "I am having trouble breathing." The nurse should perform which of the following actions?

    A. Check serum blood glucose.

    B. Evaluate fluid volume status.

    C. Replace filter on IV infusion set.

    D. Administer furosemide by mouth.

13. A client who has cellulitis reports a pain level as two on a zero to 10 scale. The nurse should plan to administer which of the following medications?

    A. Morphine IV

    B. Ibuprofen PO

    C. Fentanyl patch

    D. Hydromorphone IM

14. A client is prescribed sucralfate for treatment of a duodenal ulcer. The nurse recognizes which of the following statements indicates effective teaching? (Select all that apply.)

    A. "Treatment will be completed in 2 weeks."

    B. "I should drink 2000 mL of water each day."

    C. "Exercise should be limited during treatment."

    D. "This will turn into a paste and cover the ulcer."

    E. "My diet will include more fruits and vegetables."

    F. "The medication will be taken 1 hr before meals."

15. A client who has a deep vein thrombosis is receiving a heparin infusion. Current lab values include an aPTT of 40 seconds. Which of the following actions should the nurse implement?

    A. Stop the infusion.

    B. Increase the infusion.

    C. Decrease the infusion.

    D. No change in the infusion.

16. A nurse prepares to administer ketamine IM to a preschooler who weighs 40 lb. The dose prescribed is 2.5 mg/kg and the vial contains 50 mg/mL. How many mL should the nurse administer? _____ mL

17. A young adult is newly prescribed levetiracetam for a seizure disorder. Which of the following information should the nurse discuss?

    A. Take medication with food to reduce nausea.

    B. Massage gums daily to prevent gingival hyperplasia.

    C. Regular blood tests will be required to monitor levels.

    D. Mild periods of drowsiness may occur during the day.

18. A client is prescribed clozapine. The nurse should monitor for which of the following complications?

    A. Dyslipidemia

    B. Osteoporosis

    C. Hypertension

    D. Thrombocytopenia

19. A client is prescribed alendronate tablets. Which of the following information should the nurse include in the teaching?

    A. Take at mealtime with 60 mL of water.

    B. Sit upright for 30 min after administration.

    C. Increase the amount of vitamin D in your diet.

    D. Wear sunglasses when exposed to outside sunlight.

20. A client who is prescribed phenelzine asks the nurse, "Why must I stop adding Parmesan cheese to pasta?" The nurse understands which of the following complications may occur?

    A. Sedation

    B. Agranulocytosis

    C. Hypertensive crisis

    D. Extrapyramidal syndrome

21. Which of the following actions should the nurse implement prior to administering levothyroxine to a client who has continuous enteral feeding?

    A. Place in high Fowler's position.

    B. Flush the tube with 60 mL of water.

    C. Pause the infusion pump for 30 min.

    D. Inject air into tube to verify correct placement.

22. A nurse cares for a client who has an implanted venous port. Which of the following actions should be implemented prior to administering medications?

    A. Withdraw and discard 10 mL of blood.

    B. Access port using a non-coring needle.

    C. Flush port with 5 mL heparin 1000 units/mL.

    D. Auscultate and document presence of bruit.

23. Prior to administering a client's scheduled dose of enoxaparin sodium, which laboratory finding should the nurse evaluate?

    A. PT

    B. INR

    C. aPTT

    D. Platelets

24. A client is to receive morphine 4 mg IV bolus through an existing continuous infusion. Identify the sequence of actions the nurse should follow when administering the medication. (Place the steps in selected order of performance. All steps must be used.)

    A. Inject medication.

    B. Withdraw syringe.

    C. Aspirate for blood return.

    D. Connect syringe to IV line.

    E. Clean port with antiseptic swab.

    F. Pinch tubing above injection port.

25. A client who has acute pulmonary edema is to receive furosemide 40 mg IV. Which of the following is an appropriate action by the nurse?

    A. Administer over 2 min.

    B. Dilute with 0.9% sodium chloride.

    C. Monitor the client for hyperkalemia.

    D. Determine if the client has peripheral edema.

Fundamentals for Nursing

1. A nurse prepares to perform a dressing change. Which of the following identifiers should the nurse use to ensure client safety? (Select all that apply.)

    A. Name

    B. Birthdate

    C. Phone number

    D. Facility armband

    E. Photo identification

    F. Hospital room number

2. Identify the sequence a nurse should follow when moving clients who can partially bear weight from a bed to a chair. (Place the steps in selected order of performance. All steps must be used.)

    A. Apply the transfer belt to the client.

    B. Rock the client to a standing position.

    C. Grasp the transfer belt along the client's sides.

    D. Assist the client to a sitting position on the side of bed.

    E. Request the client pivot on the foot farther from the chair.

3. A nurse provides care to a client who has a sealed radiation implant. Which of the following actions should be implemented? (Select all that apply.)

    A. Limit each visitor to 1 hr per day.

    B. Wear a lead apron when providing care.

    C. Instruct visitors to stand 6 ft from client.

    D. Double glove to dispose of the radiation source.

    E. Place "Caution: Radioactive Material" sign on the door.

4. A school nurse teaches a course about health and safety for 11-year-old students. Which of the following topics would be appropriate for this class? (Select all that apply.)

    A. Activity and exercise

    B. STIs and pregnancy

    C. Alcohol and drug use

    D. Memory and cognition

    E. Peer pressure and violence

    F. Eating disorders and nutrition

5. A nurse provides care to a client who is admitted for sepsis. Which of the following circumstances requires an occurrence report? (Select all that apply.)

    A. Eye glasses are lost.

    B. Visitor falls in hallway.

    C. Syncopal episode occurs.

    D. Oxygen therapy is refused.

    E. Blood cultures are positive.

6. A nurse provides teaching to a client regarding the use of a hearing aid. Which of the following information is needed? (Select all that apply.)

    A. "Avoid hairspray while wearing the aid."

    B. "A whistling sound indicates proper fit."

    C. "The hearing aid can be worn continuously."

    D. "Batteries should be removed when not in use."

    E. "Follow-up with an audiologist is recommended."

7. A nurse provides end-of-life care to a client of Chinese heritage. Which of the following rituals may be practiced by the family following death?

    A. The bed will be placed facing east.

    B. The oldest child will bathe the body.

    C. A window will be opened by the partner.

    D. A priest will place an amulet on the pillow.

8. A client states "I have not been sleeping well." The nurse should recommend which of the following activities prior to bedtime?

    A. Walk briskly.

    B. Watch television.

    C. Take a warm bath.

    D. Drink a glass of wine.

9. A nurse provides discharge education to a client who has a methicillin-resistant Staphylococcus aureus skin infection. Which of the following statements should be included?

    A. "Discontinue antibiotics after a scab forms."

    B. "Do not share athletic equipment with others."

    C. "Discard soiled bandages in a sealed plastic bag."

    D. "Keep the infected area covered with a dry bandage."

    E. "Showering is recommended rather than taking a bath."

    F. "Wash all uninfected skin areas prior to infected areas."

10. A nurse reviews client room assignments. Which of the following infectious diseases requires droplet precautions? Select all that apply.

    A. Mumps

    B. Measles

    C. Varicella

    D. Pertussis

    E. Pneumonia

11. A nurse provides teaching to a client about the use of a cane. Which of the following instructions should the nurse include?

    A. Move the stronger leg forward with the cane.

    B. Hold the cane on the stronger side of the body.

    C. Keep the cane handle within 5 cm (2 in) of waist level.

    D. Place the cane approximately 30 cm (12 in) in front of foot.

12. A nurse teaches an older adult about measures to prevent constipation. Which of the following information should be included?

    A. Drink at least 4 cups of fluid daily.

    B. Eat one cup of yogurt with breakfast.

    C. Consume 10 grams of fiber each day.

    D. Take docusate sodium as prescribed.

13. A nurse observes a stage I pressure ulcer on a client's heel. Which of the following treatments should the nurse initiate?

    A. Wet-to-dry dressing

    B. Oral antibiotic therapy

    C. Pressure-relieving device

    D. Intermittent wound irrigation

14. A nurse provides teaching to a client who has a newly applied short-arm fiberglass cast. Which of the following instructions should the nurse discuss? (Select all that apply.)

    A. Expect injured area to be warm and painful.

    B. Report numbness or tingling to your provider.

    C. Keep arm elevated above the heart during rest.

    D. Blow cool air from a hair dryer to relieve itching.

    E. Wrap cast with plastic covering prior to showering.

15. A nurse provides care for a client who has dementia and is recovering from knee arthroplasty. Which of the following findings requires intervention?

    A. Hgb 14 g/dL

    B. Facial grimacing

    C. Respirations 23/min

    D. Serous drainage on dressing

16. A client requires vital sign assessments every 30 min. Which of the following actions should the nurse implement when using an electronic blood pressure device?

    A. Elevate the extremity prior to inflating the cuff.

    B. Ensure three fingers fit between the cuff and skin.

    C. Compare the initial reading with auscultation results.

    D. Remove the device and assess the skin every 2 hours.

17. A nurse provides care to a client who is on a clear-liquid diet. Which of the following food choices may be included? (Select all that apply.)

    A. Hard candy

    B. Chicken broth

    C. Orange sherbet

    D. Vanilla milkshake

    E. Chocolate pudding

    F. Fruit-flavored gelatin

18. A client requires an enteral feeding tube. Which of the following actions should the nurse perform immediately following insertion?

    A. Flush tube with 30 mL of sterile water.

    B. Inject 60 mL of air to verify placement.

    C. Aspirate gastric contents to measure pH.

    D. Apply low intermittent suction as prescribed.

19. A nurse provides care for a client who is agitated. Which of the following actions would be appropriate to implement? (Select all that apply.)

    A. Restrain the client.

    B. Reduce room noise.

    C. Play soothing music.

    D. Assess for urinary retention.

    E. Administer a benzodiazepine.

20. A nurse observes a staff member's behavior when a client becomes angry. Which of the following reactions requires an immediate intervention?

    A. Maintains eye contact.

    B. Walks away from the client.

    C. Speaks in short sentences.

    D. Provides the client personal space.

Adult Medical Surgical Nursing

1. After obtaining a blood specimen from a client's peripherally inserted central catheter (PICC), which of the following actions should the nurse take next?

    A. Resume continuous IV infusion.

    B. Perform sterile dressing change.

    C. Instill heparin solution 10 units/mL.

    D. Flush with 20 mL 0.9% sodium chloride.

2. A client is admitted to the telemetry unit for sustained paroxysmal supraventricular tachycardia. Which of the following medications should the nurse prepare to administer?

    A. Atropine

    B. Adenosine

    C. Nitroprusside

    D. Norepinephrine

3. A nurse provides care for a client who was just admitted to the emergency department reporting chest pain. Which of the following diagnostic tests should the nurse prioritize?

    A. Echocardiogram

    B. Chest radiograph

    C. Electrocardiogram

    D. Cardiac angiography

4. A nurse provides care for a client who is diagnosed with syndrome of inappropriate antidiuretic hormone (SIADH). Which of the following laboratory values would be expected? (Select all that apply.)

    A. Sodium 128 mEq/L

    B. Potassium 5.0 mEq/L

    C. Magnesium 1.5 mEq/L

    D. Urine specific gravity 1.035

    E. Serum specific gravity 290 mOsm/kg

5. A nurse provides care for a client who has a Jackson-Pratt (JP) drain. Which of the following actions will ensure proper function?

    A. Coil tubing of drain.

    B. Empty bulb every day.

    C. Keep bulb compressed.

    D. Place drain to wall suction.

6. A nurse provides education to a preoperative client regarding use of an incentive spirometer (IS). Identify the sequence the client should follow. (Place the steps in selected order of performance. All steps must be used.)

    A. Sit up.

    B. Inhale slowly.

    C. Exhale slowly.

    D. Hold breath for 3 to 5 seconds.

    E. Create a tight seal around mouthpiece.

    F. Perform 10 (IS) breaths per hour while awake.

7. A nurse plans care for a client who requires continuous ambulatory peritoneal dialysis. Which of the following actions is appropriate? (Select all that apply.)

    A. Notify provider of cloudy or opaque effluent.

    B. Prepare client for exchange two or three times weekly.

    C. Apply mask to client during system connect and disconnect.

    D. Require client to remain in reclining position during exchange.

    E. Warm dialysate bag by applying heating pad prior to installation.

8. A nurse plans care for a client who has a serum potassium of 7 mEq/L. Which of the following actions should be implemented? (Select all that apply.)

    A. Place on a cardiac monitor.

    B. Obtain a serum creatinine level.

    C. Infuse 100 mL of 10% glucose IV.

    D. Begin IV infusion of regular insulin.

    E. Administer sodium polystyrene sulfonate.

    F. Initiate 0.33% sodium chloride IV fluid bolus.

9. A nurse provides care to a client who is on continuous ECG monitoring and observes the rhythm below. Which of the following activities should be implemented?

    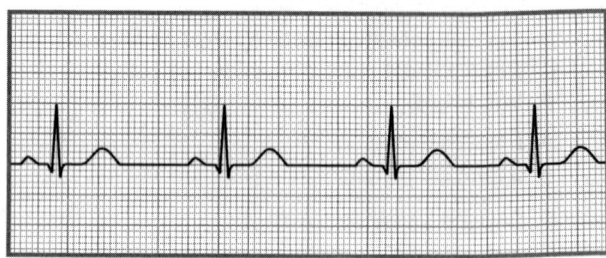

    A. Obtain blood pressure.

    B. Call rapid response team.

    C. Notify provider immediately.

    D. Administer atropine IV push.

10. A client is receiving oxygen at 60% via a simple face mask. Arterial blood gas results are: pH 7.31, PaO_2 99 mm Hg, $PaCO_2$ 51 mm Hg, and HCO_3- 28 mEq/L. Which of the following actions should the nurse implement?

    A. Request lab to repeat the test.

    B. Administer sodium bicarbonate.

    C. Decrease supplemental oxygen.

    D. Place on partial rebreather mask.

11. A nurse reviews the client's arterial blood gas results: pH 7.48, $PaCO_2$ 44 mm Hg, HCO_3- 35 mEq/L. Which of the following acid-base imbalances is present?

    A. Uncompensated metabolic alkalosis

    B. Uncompensated respiratory acidosis

    C. Fully compensated respiratory alkalosis

    D. Partially compensated metabolic acidosis

12. A client in the emergency department develops the following cardiac rhythm. The nurse performs an immediate assessment and finds the client unresponsive and pulseless. Which of the following actions is considered the priority of care?

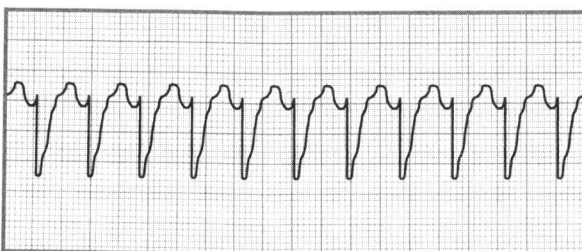

   A. Defibrillation
   B. Chest compressions
   C. Assess breath sounds
   D. Administration of amiodarone

13. A nurse assesses a client who has acute pyelonephritis. Which of the following findings would be expected? (Select all that apply.)

   A. Fever
   B. Flank pain
   C. Tachycardia
   D. Cough and dyspnea
   E. Nausea and vomiting

14. A nurse provides care to a client who has a fractured femur after falling from a ladder. Which of the following actions may reduce the incidence of fat emboli?

   A. Immobilize the extremity.
   B. Provide supplemental oxygen.
   C. Maintain a semi-Fowler's position.
   D. Administer subcutaneous heparin.

15. A client who is newly diagnosed with type 2 diabetes mellitus states, "I feel really dizzy and shaky." Which of the following actions should the nurse perform?

   A. Administer glucagon.
   B. Give 10 units of lispro.
   C. Check urine for ketones.
   D. Provide 8 oz of milk.

16. A nurse explains what to expect during a thoracentesis. Which client statement validates teaching was effective?

   A. "I need to be still during the procedure."
   B. "It will be difficult to swallow for a few hours."
   C. "A cough may develop during aspiration of fluid."
   D. "My breathing may be labored for several minutes."

17. A client's wound eviscerates following bariatric surgery. Which of the following actions should the nurse implement? (Select all that apply.)

   A. Call for help.
   B. Obtain vital signs.
   C. Reinsert protruding organs.
   D. Place in high-Fowler's position.
   E. Cover wound with moist sterile dressing.

18. A client had a modified radical mastectomy yesterday. Which of the following actions should the nurse implement to prevent transient edema of the affected arm? (Select all that apply.)

   A. Elevate arm on pillow.
   B. Administer furosemide.
   C. Apply heating pad to site.
   D. Milk drainage device tubing.
   E. Encourage gentle arm exercises.

19. A nurse provides teaching to a client who has gastroesophageal reflux disease (GERD). Which of the following instructions should be included? (Select all that apply.)

   A. Avoid tobacco products.
   B. Eat small frequent meals.
   C. Prepare a snack before bedtime.
   D. Sleep with head of the bed elevated.
   E. Refrain from caffeinated beverages.

20. A nurse assesses a client who has Guillain-Barre syndrome. Which of the following findings would be expected for this client? (Select all that apply.)

   A. Diplopia
   B. Paresthesias
   C. Thrombocytopenia
   D. Rebound tenderness
   E. Hyperactive reflexes

21. Which of the following actions should the nurse perform prior to removing a client's nasogastric tube?

   A. Inspect the tip of the tube.
   B. Auscultate for bowel sounds.
   C. Apply low intermittent suction.
   D. Measure pH of gastric contents.

22. A client who has liver failure is scheduled for a paracentesis. Which of the following actions should the nurse implement prior to the procedure? (Select all that apply.)

   A. Instruct client to void.
   B. Insert nasogastric tube.
   C. Elevate head of the bed.
   D. Measure abdominal girth.
   E. Obtain informed consent.

23. Which of the following actions should the nurse perform prior to obtaining a specimen from an indwelling urinary catheter for a client who has sepsis?

   A. Don sterile gloves.
   B. Provide catheter care.
   C. Elevate drainage bag above bladder.
   D. Clean tubing port with an antiseptic solution.

24. A nurse cares for a client who is receiving mechanical ventilation, and the high-pressure alarm sounds. Which of the following conditions can cause this to occur? (Select all that apply.)

   A. Coughing

   B. Kinked tubing

   C. Bronchospasm

   D. Tube is disconnected

   E. Occluded endotracheal tube

25. A nurse prepares for the admission of a client who has a temperature of 34° C (93° F). Which of the following rewarming methods should be implemented?

   A. Infuse warm IV fluids.

   B. Apply a heating blanket.

   C. Offer sips of warm coffee.

   D. Administer heated oxygen.

Mental Health Nursing

1. A client is newly diagnosed with a terminal illness. Which of the following should the nurse assess first?

    A. Coping skills of the client

    B. Client's perception of the diagnosis

    C. Level of support from family and friends

    D. Spiritual and cultural beliefs of the nurse

2. A home health nurse provides care to an older adult client who appears malnourished and is wearing clothes that are soiled. Which of the following interventions should the nurse implement? (Select all that apply.)

    A. Document client-caretaker interactions.

    B. Evaluate client access to basic necessities.

    C. Ask the caretaker if the client is being abused.

    D. Encourage admission to a hospital for monitoring.

    E. Report suspected client neglect to proper authorities.

3. A client who has an alcohol use disorder begins to exhibit symptoms of withdrawal. Which of the following medications should the nurse administer?

    A. Disulfiram

    B. Methadone

    C. Varenicline

    D. Phenobarbital

4. A client who is of Hispanic origin is admitted to a medical surgical unit. Which of the following factors should the nurse consider when providing culturally competent care? (Select all that apply.)

    A. Home remedies are commonly used.

    B. Maintaining eye contact is a sign of respect.

    C. Concept of time is more focused on the future.

    D. Females in the family make health care decisions.

    E. Specific foods may be requested to treat the illness.

5. A nurse provides care for a client who has anorexia nervosa. Which of the following are appropriate nursing interventions? (Select all that apply.)

    A. Rotate caregivers assigned to client.

    B. Promote cognitive-behavioral therapies.

    C. Provide a high fiber and low sodium diet.

    D. Assess for bradycardia and hypotension.

    E. Avoid client involvement in decision-making.

6. A client is talking to himself and watching a vacant area of the room. Which of the following interventions should the nurse recognize as most important?

    A. Ask the client if he is hearing voices.

    B. Monitor the client for signs of anxiety.

    C. Encourage the client to listen to music.

    D. Address the client's underlying feelings.

7. A client reports, "I have been working in a hostile environment for the past year." The nurse should recognize which of the following findings is a response to prolonged stress? (Select all that apply.)

    A. Amenorrhea

    B. Increased energy

    C. Poor attention span

    D. Decreased respirations

    E. Increased sinus infections

8. A client is newly prescribed lurasidone. Which of the following actions should the nurse implement?

    A. Obtain baseline fasting blood glucose.

    B. Instruct client to avoid wine and aged cheese.

    C. Administer test dose and observe for anaphylaxis.

    D. Inform client that temporary numbing of mouth may occur.

9. A client is prescribed sertraline for depression. Which of the following instructions should the nurse include with teaching? (Select all that apply.)

    A. "It may take 3 weeks before you feel better."

    B. "Discontinue the medication if nausea occurs."

    C. "Call your provider if you become more depressed."

    D. "You may experience symptoms of sexual dysfunction."

    E. "Sit up straight for 30 min after taking the medication."

10. An adolescent arrives to the emergency department and reports being sexually assaulted within the past hour. Which action should the nurse perform first?

    A. Perform a self-assessment.

    B. Evaluate risk for pregnancy.

    C. Place in a private room for an examination.

    D. Obtain an informed consent for photographs.

Maternal and Newborn Nursing

1. An expectant mother who plans to breastfeed is eager to learn about newborn care. Which of the following information should the nurse provide? (Select all that apply.)

   A. Schedule feedings every 4 hr.

   B. Place bumper pads in the crib.

   C. Position on back when sleeping.

   D. Expect stools to be yellow in color.

   E. Anticipate three wet diapers in 24 hr.

   F. Delay tub bath until cord has fallen off.

2. A nurse provides care for a newborn who is receiving phototherapy. Which of the following is an appropriate nursing intervention? (Select all that apply.)

   A. Weigh weekly.

   B. Apply lotion to skin.

   C. Cover male genitalia.

   D. Place mask over eyes.

   E. Monitor frequency of stools.

3. A client who is Rh-negative should receive Rho(D) immune globulin at which of the following times? (Select all that apply.)

   A. Following an amniocentesis

   B. After a spontaneous abortion

   C. Within 72 hr following delivery

   D. During a nonstress test (NST)

   E. Routinely at 28 weeks of gestation

4. A client who is at 16 weeks of gestation is scheduled for an amniocentesis. Which of the following instructions should the nurse provide?

   A. Do not drink any liquids after midnight.

   B. Empty your bladder prior to the procedure.

   C. This test will determine how well your baby is breathing.

   D. You will need to hold your breath while the needle is inserted.

5. A newborn is delivered by vaginal birth at 40 weeks of gestation. Which of the following findings should the nurse report to the provider?

   A. Heart rate 160/min and respirations 40/min

   B. Acrocyanosis and caput succedaneum

   C. Positive Babinski reflex and negative Ortolani's sign

   D. Head circumference 40 cm and chest circumference 32 cm

6. A client receives terbutaline for the management of preterm labor. Which of the following findings should the nurse report immediately?

   A. Heart rate 110/min

   B. Dyspnea and crackles

   C. Tremors and headache

   D. Blood pressure 100/60 mm Hg

7. A nurse provides education to a client who is 1 day postpartum about receiving a rubella vaccine. Which of the following instructions should be included?

   A. Breastfeeding is not recommended.

   B. An allergy to peanuts is a contraindication.

   C. A method of contraception is required for the next 30 days.

   D. Contact provider if injection site is sore within the first 24 hours.

8. A nurse should recognize which of the following signs as a manifestation of sepsis in the neonate? (Select all that apply.)

   A. Lethargy

   B. Tachypnea

   C. Hypothermia

   D. Sunken fontanel

   E. Low serum glucose

9. A client who is at 29 weeks of gestation calls the clinic to report persistent low back pain. Which of the following instructions should the nurse provide?

   A. Relax and take deep breaths.

   B. Take acetaminophen as needed.

   C. Perform gentle stretching exercises.

   D. Lie down and check for contractions.

10. A nurse provides education to a client who is 2 days postpartum about contraceptive methods. Which of the following statements indicates correct understanding?

    A. "A vaginal ring must be replaced every three months."

    B. "Injectable progestins cannot be taken when breastfeeding."

    C. "Diaphragms must be refitted with a weight gain of five pounds."

    D. "The Basal body temperature method can be influenced by stress."

Nursing Care of Children

1. A toddler has a two-day history of vomiting and diarrhea. Which of the following findings should the nurse immediately report to the health care provider?

   A. BP 68/40 mm Hg

   B. Dry mucous membranes

   C. Decreased urinary output

   D. Temperature 38.9° C (102° F)

2. A nurse discusses an Asthma Action Plan with a school-age child. Which action should the client take when symptoms are in the Yellow Zone?

   A. Drink cold fluids.

   B. Take the rescue medication.

   C. Continue with normal activities.

   D. Go to the emergency department.

3. A nurse teaches a parent how to successfully feed an infant who has an unrepaired cleft lip and palate. Which of the following instructions should the nurse provide? (Select all that apply.)

   A. Observe forehead for a wrinkled brow.

   B. Use a low-calorie formula for feedings.

   C. Burp frequently after every ounce of fluid.

   D. Hold in an upright position during feedings.

   E. Use a special feeder with a slit-cut tip nipple.

4. During a routine wellness visit, a parent expresses concern regarding the toddler's decreased appetite. Which of the following instructions should the nurse provide?

   A. Offer larger portions of food.

   B. Serve meals in the same dish.

   C. Introduce a new food each day.

   D. Promise a cookie after the meal.

5. A director of a daycare center telephones the nurse regarding concerns about a toddler who has erythema infectiosum and a red facial rash. Which of the following actions is needed?

   A. Verify immunizations are up-to-date.

   B. Prevent the child from playing in the sand box.

   C. Explain that the toddler is not likely to be contagious.

   D. Verify antibiotics are finished prior to returning to school.

6. A nurse teaches a 10-year-old child who has diabetes mellitus how to check blood glucose. Which of the following strategies would be the most effective method for learning?

   A. Watch a video about the procedure.

   B. Read a pamphlet about diabetes mellitus.

   C. Create a poster with healthy food choices.

   D. Perform a procedure after watching the nurse.

7. A nurse completes vision screening for a 5-year-old child. Which of the following findings requires further evaluation?

   A. Visual acuity of 20/15 is demonstrated in both eyes.

   B. Pupils are 4 mm and react briskly to light.

   C. One eye deviates when the child fixates on an object.

   D. The uncovered eye does not move during the cover test.

8. A nurse teaches a 5-year-old child to use an incentive spirometer. Which of the following are effective strategies to facilitate learning? (Select all that apply.)

   A. Encourage parental involvement.

   B. Allow the child to hold the spirometer.

   C. Use a doll to demonstrate the technique.

   D. Withhold television privileges if unable to perform correctly.

   E. Discuss in detail with the child how the spirometer expands the lungs.

9. A mother of a 4-year-old child requests information about the expected growth and development of a preschooler. Which of the following characteristics should the nurse discuss? Select all that apply.

   A. Resists going to bed.

   B. Prefers a variety of foods.

   C. Plays with imaginary friends.

   D. Copies shapes when drawing.

   E. Uses several words in a sentence.

10. A nurse explains how to correctly wear a bicycle helmet for a group of preschoolers. Which of the following teaching methods would be most effective?

    A. Video presentation

    B. Small group discussion

    C. One-on-one demonstration

    D. Step-by-step written instructions

Comprehensive Assessment

1. A nurse prepares to apply a sequential compression device (SCD) to a client who is on bed rest. Identify the sequence the nurse should follow. (Place the steps in selected order of performance. All steps must be used.)

    A. Wrap SCD sleeve around leg.

    B. Arrange SCD sleeve under leg.

    C. Obtain baseline circulatory assessment.

    D. Attach connector of SCD sleeve to device.

    E. Place two fingers between leg and sleeve.

    F. Observe functioning of unit for one complete cycle.

2. A client who has a spinal cord injury asks the nurse about complications of prolonged immobility. Which of the following should the nurse discuss? (Select all that apply.)

    A. Presbyopia

    B. Atelectasis

    C. Contractures

    D. Pressure sores

    E. Thrombus formation

3. A nurse provides education to a client who has a gastric ulcer. Which of the following medications decreases the secretion of gastric acid?

    A. Ranitidine

    B. Sucralfate

    C. Bismuth subsalicylate

    D. Magnesium hydroxide

4. A nurse demonstrates how to use a metered dose inhaler with a spacer. Which of the following client statements indicates understanding?

    A. "It is important to wait 5 minutes between puffs."

    B. "A whistling sound means I am breathing in too fast."

    C. "The mouthpiece will be placed in front of my tongue."

    D. "I will hold my breath for at least 3 seconds after inhaling."

5. A client is scheduled to receive an IM injection. Which of the following actions should the nurse incorporate to safely administer the medication? (Select all that apply.)

    A. Apply clean gloves.

    B. Inject at a 90° angle.

    C. Use a ½-inch needle.

    D. Select a 22-gauge needle.

    E. Identify the dorsogluteal site.

6. A nurse provides discharge instructions to a client who is newly prescribed fluoxetine. Which of the following findings should the client immediately report to the health care provider? Select all that apply.

    A. Fever

    B. Agitation

    C. Diaphoresis

    D. Hyporeflexia

    E. Hallucinations

7. A client is 2 days postoperative following surgical closure of an abdominal wound. The nurse should recognize which of the following findings is a sign of infection?

    A. WBC of 8,500/mm³

    B. Serosanguinous drainage

    C. Approximation of the wound edges

    D. Erythema of the incision line extending 2 cm

8. A nurse prepares room assignments. Which of the following rooms would be appropriate for a client who has Alzheimer's disease and a history of wandering?

    A. Private room away from exits

    B. Private room with the door closed

    C. Semiprivate room at the end of the hall

    D. Semiprivate room near the vending machine

9. A client follows the religion of Islam. During Ramadan which of the following dietary practices should the nurse anticipate?

    A. Avoiding meat and dairy.

    B. Fasting from dawn to sunset.

    C. Eating the largest meal at midday.

    D. Abstaining from eating fish with scales.

10. A nurse provides care for a toddler who has impetigo. Which action is appropriate?

    A. Allow time in the playroom.

    B. Don a mask when providing care.

    C. Place in a room with negative pressure.

    D. Wear a gown and gloves when in the room.

11. A client who is at 13 weeks of gestation reports persistent nausea and vomiting. The nurse should recognize which of the following findings requires additional investigation?

    A. Urine with ketones

    B. Brisk capillary refill

    C. Weight gain of 0.45 kg (1 lb)

    D. Blood pressure 115/75 mm Hg

12. A nurse evaluates maternal-newborn bonding. Which of the following behaviors suggests altered parental attachment?

    A. Holds neonate in the en face position.

    B. Assists father with changing soiled diaper.

    C. Names the child after a favorite musician.

    D. Continues to watch television while infant cries.

13. A client in preterm labor is receiving magnesium sulfate. The nurse should recognize which of the following findings indicates a therapeutic effect?

    A. Cervix unchanged

    B. Deep tendon reflexes 2+

    C. Presence of contractions

    D. Blood pressure 130/60 mm Hg

14. A nurse provides care for a client who is receiving oxytocin for induction of labor. Which of the following findings requires the nurse to take action?

    A. Urine output 120 mL in 4 hr

    B. FHR 110 bpm with variability

    C. Six contractions in 10 min

    D. Contraction duration 60 seconds

15. A nurse provides care for a client who is receiving TPN. Which of the following interventions reduces potential complications associated with administration?

    A. Provides additional fluids by mouth.

    B. Monitors blood glucose every other day.

    C. Maintains client in semi-Fowler's position.

    D. Performs sterile central line dressing changes.

16. A nurse prepares to administer a unit of packed RBCs to a client who has type AB positive blood. Which of the following actions should cause the charge nurse to intervene?

    A. Inserts a 20-gauge intravenous catheter.

    B. Checks client identifiers with another nurse.

    C. Prepares to administer type B negative blood.

    D. Primes tubing with dextrose 5% in 0.9% sodium chloride.

17. During care of a client who has a chest tube, the nurse should perform which of the following actions to maintain tube patency?

    A. Strip the chest tube.

    B. Provide intermittent suction.

    C. Maintain chamber at chest level.

    D. Position drainage tubing to prevent kinks.

18. A client is scheduled for coronary angiography. Which of the following laboratory findings should the nurse report to the provider?

    A. Digoxin 0.8 ng/mL

    B. Hemoglobin 12 g/dL

    C. Creatinine 1.9 mg/dL

    D. Potassium 3.8 mEq/L

19. A client is placed in the lithotomy position during a procedure. Which of the following actions should the nurse implement to prevent neurological complications?

    A. Check radial pulses.

    B. Avoid position changes.

    C. Monitor blood pressure.

    D. Ensure proper padding.

20. During the assessment of a client who is 1 day postoperative following a small bowel resection, the nurse observes petechiae scattered across the chest and abdomen. Which of the following lab values would be most important for the nurse to monitor?

    A. Albumin

    B. Bilirubin

    C. Creatinine

    D. Hemoglobin

21. A client reports continued fever and sore throat 24 hr after starting penicillin for tonsillitis. Which of the following information should the nurse provide?

    A. "Your antibiotics will need to be changed."

    B. "Come to the clinic for a repeat throat culture."

    C. "The provider will need to see you again today."

    D. "It may take a few days before symptoms improve."

22. During a preoperative assessment, a client reports the daily use of garlic oil. The nurse should be aware of an increased risk for which of the following postoperative complications?

    A. Bleeding

    B. Infection

    C. Constipation

    D. Hypertension

23. A nurse provides care for a client who experiences an acute episode of anger and aggression. Which of the following techniques should the nurse implement to de-escalate the behavior? (Select all that apply.)

    A. Set limits for the client.

    B. Communicate in a calm voice.

    C. Inform client of consequences.

    D. Maintain a close personal space.

    E. Encourage client to express feelings.

24. A nurse provides education to a client regarding the recent death of a loved one. Which of the following information should the nurse discuss?

    A. Resolving a sense of shock takes a year.

    B. Sharing your feelings of loss can be helpful.

    C. Moving through the stages of grief is predictable.

    D. Reminiscing about memories should be avoided.

25. A nurse provides education to a client who is diagnosed with myasthenia gravis. Which of the following statements indicates understanding of disease management? (Select all that apply.)

    A. "Eating slowly is important."

    B. "Difficulty breathing may occur."

    C. "Resting helps when I feel week."

    D. "Tearing of my eyes is a sign of crisis."

    E. "Sitting in the hot tub helps my muscles."

26. A nurse assesses a client who is receiving external radiation to the head and neck. Which of the following findings may be a result of therapy? (Select all that apply.)

    A. Fatigue

    B. Dry mouth

    C. Altered taste

    D. Frequent urination

    E. Difficulty swallowing

27. A client who has a recent closed head injury reports a severe headache and is restless. Which of the following is an appropriate nursing intervention?

    A. Elevate head of bed 30°.

    B. Place cool cloth to forehead.

    C. Administer morphine 2 mg IV.

    D. Prepare for a lumbar puncture.

28. A visitor develops sudden cardiac arrest in the hospital cafeteria. Which of the following are appropriate nursing interventions? (Select all that apply.)

    A. Calls for the rapid response team.

    B. Opens airway by tilting chin down.

    C. Gives two rescue breaths per minute.

    D. Compresses chest at rate of 100/min.

    E. Uses automated external defibrillator (AED).

29. A nurse provides care for a client who has been placed on suicide precautions. Which of the following are appropriate interventions? (Select all that apply.)

    A. Keep a 10 ft distance from client.

    B. Document client behavior every 2 hr.

    C. Maintain one-to-one constant observation.

    D. Ensure client's hands are always visible.

    E. Check environment for potential hazards.

30. A nurse plans care for a client who is diagnosed with Alzheimer's disease. Which of the following information should the nurse include when counseling the family? (Select all that apply.)

    A. Provide a stimulating environment.

    B. Establish a predictable daily routine.

    C. Communicate in a clear and respectful tone.

    D. Request family members visit in large groups.

    E. Research local senior services and organizations.

31. A nurse provides education to a client who is diagnosed with AIDS. Which of the following statements demonstrates teaching was effective? (Select all that apply.)

    A. "My neighbor will clean the cat's litter box."

    B. "Salad and sushi can be included in my diet."

    C. "Hamburgers should be cooked until well done."

    D. "A combination of medications will be prescribed."

    E. "I will use a spermicide and diaphragm to protect my partner."

32. A charge nurse prepares for a mass casualty. Which of the following clients would be appropriate to recommend for discharge?

    A. A middle adult client two days following a cholecystectomy

    B. An older adult client recently admitted with a syncopal episode

    C. An adolescent client who is confused after falling today at school

    D. A young adult client admitted yesterday with suspected tuberculosis

33. A nurse performs an ocular irrigation for a client who has a suspected corneal abrasion from an irritant in the eye. Identify the sequence the nurse should follow. (Place the steps in selected order of performance. All steps must be used.)

    A. Instill eye drops.

    B. Check pH of eye.

    C. Place client supine.

    D. Obtain history of exposure.

    E. Direct flow of irrigation across affected eye.

34. A nurse who works on a medical surgical unit receives a morning report. The client with which of the following laboratory results should be assessed first?

    A. Dehydration and urine specific gravity of 1.030

    B. Nephrotic syndrome and serum albumin of 3.0 g/dL

    C. Glomerular nephritis and serum potassium of 6.1 mEq/L

    D. Chronic kidney disease and glomerular filtration rate of 82 mL/min

35. A nurse provides education regarding the proper use of a car seat to the parents of an infant. Which of the following instructions should the nurse include? (Select all that apply.)

    A. Place car seat rear facing in the rear seat.

    B. Tighten harness of the car seat so it fits snugly.

    C. Put the retainer clip of harness at the level of infant's armpits.

    D. Adjust shoulder harness slots of car seat to be level with infant's ears.

    E. Avoid placing rear facing car seats in a front seat with deployable airbags.

36. A nurse plans an activity for a 4-year-old child. Which of the following is an age appropriate choice?

    A. Riding a bicycle.

    B. Playing dress-up.

    C. Building model cars.

    D. Starting a card collection.

37. A nurse plans care for a client who has COPD. Which of the following actions should the nurse include? (Select all that apply.)

    A. Encourage oral fluid intake.

    B. Maintain bed rest in the supine position.

    C. Teach to avoid extreme heat and cold temperatures.

    D. Administer pneumococcal vaccination if not previously given.

    E. Implement postural drainage with percussion and vibration.

38. A nurse plans care for a group of clients. Which task may be delegated to the licensed practical nurse (LPN)?

    A. Administer Rh immunoglobulin to a client following amniocentesis.

    B. Complete the admission assessment on a client who has pneumonia.

    C. Provide dietary teaching for a client who has a new diagnosis of celiac disease.

    D. Insert an indwelling urinary catheter for a client scheduled for a cholecystectomy.

39. A client who has advanced liver failure states, "I told my doctor to let me die if my heart stops beating or if I quit breathing. I do not want to be revived." To best ensure the client's request is honored, which of the following actions should the nurse take?

   A. Ensure the client has a health care proxy.

   B. Assure the client that end-of-life wishes will be fulfilled.

   C. Validate the do-not-resuscitate prescription is in the medical record.

   D. Verify a signed copy of the advance directives is in the medical record.

40. A nurse provides care to a client who is 48 hr postpartum and in stable condition. Which of the following tasks can be delegated to the assistive personnel (AP)? (Select all that apply.)

   A. Assist with a sitz bath.

   B. Obtain routine vital signs.

   C. Massage fundus as needed.

   D. Administer docusate sodium.

   E. Apply hydrocortisone acetate/pramoxine hydrochloride.

41. After receiving an end of shift report, which of the following clients should the nurse plan to assess first?

   A. Client who has new onset of shortness of breath

   B. Client who reports chest pain of 8 on a 0 to 10 scale

   C. Client who threatens to leave if not discharged immediately

   D. Client who is receiving a blood transfusion initiated 3 hr ago

42. A nurse reviews prescriptions for a group of clients. Which of the following procedures requires informed consent? Select all that apply.

   A. Liver biopsy

   B. Thoracentesis

   C. Appendectomy

   D. Coronary catheterization

   E. Peripheral IV catheter insertion

43. A nurse delegates to the assistive personnel (AP) the task of turning the client to the left lateral side before 0900. How should the nurse evaluate completion of the task?

   A. Ask the client for feedback regarding care.

   B. Review the client's documentation of the action taken.

   C. Observe client positioning within a set time frame.

   D. Request another nurse to follow-up at a later time.

44. A client is prescribed 0.9% sodium chloride infusion to be administered at 75 mL/hr. The macrodrip tubing drop factor is 15 gtt/mL. The nurse should adjust the IV infusion to deliver how many gtt/min? Round the answer to the nearest whole number. _____ gtt/min

45. A client who is receiving vancomycin IV suddenly develops a rash, facial flushing, and reports itching. Which of the following actions should the nurse take?

   A. Continue to monitor.

   B. Apply oxygen 4 liters/min.

   C. Obtain vancomycin peak level.

   D. Administer diphenhydramine 50 mg IV.

Practice Answers

NURSING LEADERSHIP AND MANAGEMENT

1. **Correct Answer: A**

   The nurse should recognize a spinal cord injury may exist. In any circumstance when a spinal cord injury is suspected or a possibility, the child should be calmed, reassured, and instructed not to move. No one should be allowed to move the child until the entire spine is stabilized.

2. **Correct Answer: D**

   Posting client information on a social media website is a breach of confidentiality. Nurses must not disclose client information to unauthorized individuals.

3. **Correct Answer: D**

   The Patient Self-Determination Act requires that all patients admitted to a health care facility be asked if they have an advance directive. Clients who do not have an advance directive must be given written information.

4. **Correct Answer: C**

   The client's presentation does not match the caregiver's story. A broken arm and burn marks to the chest are suspicious signs of abuse in this client. Nurses should report any suspicion of abuse, following facility policy, to the appropriate state agency.

5. **Correct Answer: C**

   The client is reporting symptoms of meningitis and will require droplet transmission precautions until a definitive diagnosis is made. Bacterial meningitis is highly contagious and potentially life-threatening.

6. **Correct Answer: B**

   Policies and procedures are maintained by each facility to establish the standard of practice for employees. These documents should be followed according to institutional guidelines.

7. **Correct Answer: D**

   Following the rule of do not use a trailing zero for doses expressed in whole number, "60" is correct. "PO" is an abbreviation that may be used and is not included in the Joint Commission Do Not Use List. "Daily" is correct, following the rule to spell out the word daily.

8. **Correct Answer: B**

   Quality improvement process is designed to correct discrepancies between developed standards and actual performance. Once a standard is developed, approved, and made available to staff, quality issues can then be identified.

9. **Correct Answer: D**

   Obtaining capillary blood glucose is within the scope of practice for the LPN. This is the most appropriate task to assign.

10. **Correct Answer: C**

    The nurse should respect the client's decision to discontinue treatment. The client has a right to decide what course of action is most appropriate to meet their goals. This response will allow the nurse to gather additional information to serve as a better advocate for the client.

11. **Correct Answer: A**

    To prevent an error, the nurse should repeat the prescription back to the provider, including the medication name, dosage, time, and route. The nurse should review all prescriptions and identify potential contraindications requiring clarification.

12. **Correct Answer: B**

    New onset of confusion is not an expected finding. Confusion can be an indication of hypoxia and requires immediate assessment to prevent additional complications.

13. **Correct Answers: A, B, D, E**

    The CDC provides an annual list of infections for surveillance. Information is used to monitor, control, and prevent the occurrence and spread of state-reportable and nationally notifiable infectious and noninfectious diseases and conditions.

14. **Correct Answer: D**

    The nurse should gather all information relevant to the situation to determine the next course of action.

15. **Correct Answer: D**

    This nursing intervention should be revised. To maximize independence, daily activities should be scheduled to follow medication administration, not prior to administering medications. The nurse should also plan rest periods for the client to prevent increased fatigue.

PHARMACOLOGY IN NURSING

1. **Correct Answer: B**

   Anticholinergic agents can cause a worsening of narrow-angle glaucoma. Acute eye pain would be concerning and needs to be reported immediately.

2. **Correct Answer: C**

   A diuretic may be prescribed when a client exhibits signs and symptoms of circulatory overload, which may occur with the transfusion of blood products. Older adults are especially at risk. Symptoms of circulatory overload include dyspnea, hypertension, bounding pulse, distended jugular veins, restlessness, and confusion.

3. **Correct Answers: A, C, D, E**

   The client should limit foods high in potassium due to spironolactone having potassium-sparing qualities. Bananas, tomatoes, avocados, and potatoes (both white and sweet) are rich sources of potassium and should be limited while taking spironolactone.

4. **Correct Answer: B**

   Acetaminophen should be used cautiously in clients who consume three or more alcoholic drinks per day because of increased risk of hepatotoxicity. The nurse should contact the health provider with this information.

5. **Correct Answer: D**

   Methylphenidate is a CNS stimulant used to treat ADHD. Effectiveness is evidenced by improvement in manifestations of ADHD, such as increased ability to focus, completing tasks, interacting with peers, and managing impulsivity.

6. **Correct Answer: A**

   The client is exhibiting signs of possible opioid overdose. Naloxone would be indicated for opioid reversal.

7. **Correct Answers: B, C, D, E**

   ACE inhibitors can cause angioedema, dry cough, hyperkalemia, and orthostatic hypotension. Swelling of the tongue and oropharynx can be life-threatening and requires emergency treatment. The provider should be notified if a cough develops. Potassium levels should be monitored. Orthostatic hypotension can especially occur with the first dose of ACE inhibitors. Clients should be instructed to change positions slowly and lie down if dizzy.

8. Correct Answer: A

Personnel preparing and administering chemotherapy should follow safe handling procedures. Special training/certification is required for administration of certain agents. If a small chemotherapy spill occurs, follow institutional procedure and use supplies contained in a chemotherapy spill kit. For large spills, Occupational Safety and Health Administration (OSHA) should be contacted.

9. Correct Answer: A

A sulfonamide allergy is a contraindication to taking sulfonylurea-type oral hypoglycemic agents (e.g., glyburide and glipizide), thiazide diuretics (such as hydrochlorothiazide), and loop diuretics (such as furosemide).

10. Correct Answer: C

The dose prescribed is morphine 2 mg, and dose on hand is 4 mg/2 mL. The nurse should administer 1 mL of morphine and discard 1 mL with another nurse as witness.

11. Correct Answer: A

When performing medication reconciliation, the nurse should notify the provider of any discrepancies between the most current medication lists compared to currently filled prescriptions to reduce error.

12. Correct Answer: B

TPN is a hyperosmolar solution that poses a risk for fluid shifts and puts the client at risk for fluid volume overload. Older adults are more vulnerable to fluid and electrolyte imbalances.

13. Correct Answer: B

Non-opioid analgesics such as acetaminophen and nonsteroidal anti-inflammatory drugs (NSAIDS) are appropriate for treating mild to moderate pain. The client is self-reporting a pain level of two (mild). Opioid analgesics such as fentanyl, morphine, and codeine are appropriate for treating moderate to severe pain.

14. Correct Answers: B, D, E, F

Constipation is a potential side effect and clients should be instructed to drink at least 2000 mL/day (unless contraindicated), and increase dietary fiber and physical exercise. Sucralfate becomes a pastelike substance that coats the ulcer and mucosal lining. Increased dietary fiber intake may reduce the likelihood of constipation caused by sucralfate administration. Sucralfate is usually taken four times a day, 1 hr before meals and at bedtime.

15. Correct Answer: B

A normal range for an activated partial thromboplastin time (aPTT) is 30 to 40 seconds. Therapeutic levels of aPTT are usually 1.5 to 2 times normal control levels. In the above scenario, the aPTT is subtherapeutic.

16. Correct Answer: 0.9 mL

Formula: dose ordered ÷ dose on hand × volume on hand = volume to administer

Calculations: 40 lb ÷ 2.2 kg = 18 kg

(2.5 mg × 18 kg) ÷ 50 mg × 1 mL = 0.9 mL

17. Correct Answer: D

The most common adverse effects are drowsiness and weakness. Adverse effects are usually mild to moderate.

18. Correct Answer: A

Clozapine and other second-generation antipsychotics can cause a group of closely linked metabolic effects: dyslipidemia, weight gain, and diabetes mellitus.

19. Correct Answer: B

Esophagitis and ulceration are the most serious adverse effects and can be prevented by remaining upright (sitting or standing) for a minimum of 30 min after administration.

20. Correct Answer: C

Clients taking this medication should avoid foods high in tyramine to prevent the life-threatening adverse effect of hypertensive crisis. Foods high in tyramine include aged cheese, smoked meats, dried fish, and overripe avocados.

21. Correct Answer: C

The infusion pump should be paused for at least 30 min before and after administering levothyroxine. Temporarily stopping a feeding when certain types of medications are administered is necessary to allow for adequate absorption. Levothyroxine is best absorbed on an empty stomach.

22. Correct Answer: B

These needles have a deflected tip that is specifically designed to penetrate the dense septum of the port without coring out small pieces. The edges of the port should be carefully palpated to identify the septum prior to placement.

23. Correct Answer: D

The nurse should hold the medication and notify the provider if the platelet count falls below 100,000/mm³. The nurse should also monitor for bleeding.

24. Correct Answer: E, D, F, C, A, B

Cleaning the port prevents the transfer of microorganisms during medication administration. The needleless tip of the syringe should be connected to the IV line to infuse the medication. The IV line should be occluded by pinching the tubing just above the injection port to aspirate for blood return. Aspirate for blood return. Release the tubing and inject medication. After injecting medication, withdraw syringe.

25. Correct Answer: A

Furosemide should be administered undiluted over 1 to 2 min. Higher doses require a continuous infusion at a rate of 4 mg/min.

FUNDAMENTALS FOR NURSING

1. Correct Answers: A, B, C, D, E

The Joint Commission requires two client identifiers, which may include the client's name, an assigned facility identification number, telephone number, birth date, or person-specific identification, including photo identification. Identifiers should be compared to the client's facility armband or MAR. Barcode scanners may be used to identify clients. Do not use the client's room number as an identifier.

2. Correct Answer: D, A, C, B, E

Assist the client to the sitting position, and allow the client to sit before standing to minimize dizziness or orthostatic changes. The chair is placed on the client's unaffected side next to the bed at a 45° angle.

Next, apply the transfer belt after sitting up. A transfer belt reduces the risk of the client falling.

Grasp the transfer belt at the client's sides to use center of gravity for movement of client.

Rock client to a standing position. The rocking motion provides momentum and minimizes muscular effort to lift client.

Request client to pivot on foot farther from chair. This action maintains support while providing adequate space for client movement.

3. Correct Answers: B, C, E

A lead apron minimizes radiation exposure of the nurse.

Visitors must stay at least 6 ft from the source and visit for no more than 30 min per day.

The sign notifies individuals of a hazard present in the room.

4. Correct Answers: A, B, C, E, F

Activity and exercise are important to maintain (or lose) weight and increase muscle strength.

Puberty occurs most frequently between the ages of 9 and 12. Students may become sexually active with the onset of puberty.

Preadolescents are entering middle school where they may be exposed to peers participating in alcohol and drug use. A "need" to fit-in increases susceptibility to peer pressure.

Peer pressure and violence increases in middle school and high school.

Eating disorders such as anorexia and bulimia most often occur in female clients during adolescence. Understanding eating disorders and healthy nutrition are important topics for this age group.

5. **Correct Answers: A, B**

   An occurrence report is created for unexpected or unusual events not consistent with the operations of the health care unit or routine care of a client. It can include events affecting a client, employee, visitor, or volunteer. Examples include: loss of property, equipment-related injuries/errors, visitor injuries, procedure/treatment errors, needlestick injuries, medication errors, accidental omission of therapies, and circumstances that lead to injury or risk for client injury.

   A visitor fall would require an occurrence report.

6. **Correct Answers: A, D, E**

   The client should avoid using hairspray or perfume while wearing a hearing aid. The residue can cause the aid to become oily and greasy.

   Batteries should be removed or disconnected when not in use.

   Follow-up with an audiologist is recommended to evaluate the effectiveness of the aid.

7. **Correct Answer: B**

   The specific ritual for bathing the body is completed by the eldest son or daughter under the direction from an older relative or temple priest.

8. **Correct Answer: C**

   A warm bath helps to relax the client prior to sleep.

9. **Correct Answers: B, C, D, E, F**

   Avoid close contact with others, including contact sports, until the infection is cleared. Do not share athletic equipment, towels, linens, clothing, or washcloths with others.

   Place soiled dressings and bandages in a sealed plastic bag before discarding in the trash.

   Keep the area covered with a dry dressing or bandage to prevent spread of the infection.

   Shower daily with an antibacterial soap; avoid taking a bath to prevent spread of the infection.

   Wash clean areas first before infected areas to avoid spreading the infection.

10. **Correct Answers: A, D, E**

    Mumps, pertussis, and various types of pneumonia require droplet precautions.

11. **Correct Answer: B**

    The client should be instructed to hold the cane on the stronger side of the body, at the level of the greater trochanter, and place 15 to 25 cm (6 to 10 in) in front of the foot.

12. **Correct Answer: D**

    Docusate sodium increases the amount of water absorbed by the stool. This helps soften the stool, making passage more comfortable.

13. **Correct Answer: C**

    The initial treatment is to relieve pressure from the heel. Pressure to an area restricts blood flow and may cause ischemia to underlying tissue, resulting in a pressure ulcer. A stage I pressure ulcer has intact skin, redness, and does not blanch with external pressure.

14. **Correct Answers: B, C, D, E**

    Report numbness or tingling. Impairment in circulation may cause decreased perfusion and peripheral nerve damage. Assess the circulation, including movement distal to the extremity, color, temperature, and increased pain.

    Keep arm elevated above the heart during the first 24 to 48 hr to prevent edema.

    The client may blow cool air from a hair dryer to help relieve itching.

    Wrap the cast with a plastic covering (such as plastic bags) prior to showering or bathing to keep the cast dry.

15. **Correct Answer: B**

    Clients who are cognitively impaired may not be able to report pain or report it accurately. Nonverbal indicators of pain include facial expressions (e.g., grimacing, wrinkled forehead), body movements (e.g., pacing, restlessness, guarding), moaning, crying, and decreased attention span.

16. **Correct Answer: C**

    The nurse should verify the accuracy of the electronic blood pressure device by comparing the initial reading with auscultation results. Some client conditions (e.g., shivering, tremors, irregular heart rate, hypotension) may affect the accuracy of electronic measurements.

17. **Correct Answers: A, B, F**

    Hard candy is considered a part of a clear liquid diet. It provides carbohydrates in the form of sugar and can relieve a dry mouth.

    Broth is a part of a clear liquid diet and provides fluid to the client along with essential minerals (such as sodium).

    Gelatin is also an element of a clear liquid diet and provides carbohydrates in the form of sugar. It can relieve thirst and prevent dehydration in the client. The nurse should remember that clear does not mean colorless.

18. **Correct Answer: C**

    Placement is verified by aspirating gastric contents and testing pH (4 or less is expected). The nurse should also assess odor, color, and consistency. Prior to first feeding, placement must be confirmed with an x-ray.

19. **Correct Answers: B, C, D, E**

    Reducing the external noise in the room can help reduce agitation in the client.

    Soothing music is a complementary therapy that can help promote relaxation and reduce agitation.

    The nurse should assess for urinary retention, constipation, and pain. These are reversible causes of agitation.

    The use of a benzodiazepine may be initiated if agitation does not decrease by reversing physical causes (e.g., constipation, urinary retention, pain).

20. **Correct Answer: B**

    In order to maintain safety of the client and others, the nurse should not leave the client alone. Strategies to handle aggressive behavior include responding quickly, remaining calm and in control, describing options clearly, and reassuring the client that staff members are present to help.

ADULT MEDICAL SURGICAL NURSING

1. **Correct Answer: D**

   Follow the Infusion Nurses Society (INS) practice recommendations. Flush with 20 mL of 0.9% sodium chloride after drawing blood. Use a 10 mL syringe for flushing a PICC line. Do not apply force if resistance is met. Flush with 10 mL of 0.9% sodium chloride before, between, and after medications.

2. **Correct Answer: B**

   Adenosine 6 mg rapid IVP (over 1 to 2 seconds) is given to convert paroxysmal supraventricular tachycardia to a normal sinus rhythm.

3. **Correct Answer: C**

   An electrocardiogram (ECG) is one of the first diagnostic tests performed for the client experiencing chest pain because it is a fast, noninvasive test to provide immediate information. The ECG graphically shows cardiac electrical activity and cardiac ischemia.

4. **Correct Answers: A, D**

   Clients who have SIADH retain fluid, which results in dilutional hyponatremia and increased urine specific gravity.

5. Correct Answer: C

A JP drain is an evacuator unit that exerts constant low pressure as long as the bulb of the device is fully compressed.

6. Correct Answer: A, E, B, D, C, F

The client should sit up in semi-Fowler's or high-Fowler's position to maximize lung expansion. The mouthpiece of the IS device is placed in the mouth and the lips; make a tight seal. Inhale slowly and maintain a constant flow during inhalation. Hold breath for 3 to 5 seconds. Exhale slowly and breathe normally for a short period between each IS breath to prevent hyperventilation and fatigue. Perform 10 IS breaths per hour while awake. At the end of these 10 breaths, instruct the client to attempt to cough twice. This assists with mobilization of secretions in the lungs.

7. Correct Answers: A, C, E

The provider should be notified of any cloudy or opaque effluent or drainage as this can be an indication of infection. Peritonitis is the major cause for discontinuance of peritoneal dialysis. Surgical asepsis (sterile technique) is employed during connection and disconnection. Infection is the most common complication of peritoneal dialysis. The dialysate should be warmed to reduce discomfort during inflow. The solution may be warmed by wrapping a heating pad around the solution bag or by using the warming chamber of the automated cycling machine.

8. Correct Answers: A, B, C, D, E

Cardiac monitoring is critical for clients with hyperkalemia. Potassium maintains resting membrane potential of cardiac muscle. Hyperkalemia can cause life-threatening cardiac dysrhythmias and cardiac arrest. Serum creatinine levels should be evaluated in clients with hyperkalemia. Elevated serum creatinine can be an indication of impaired renal function, a major cause of hyperkalemia. Glucose is required to prevent hypoglycemia caused by the insulin therapy. Intravenous regular insulin is typically infused with severe hyperkalemia. This causes a temporary shift of potassium from the serum into the cells. Sodium polystyrene sulfonate may be given for hyperkalemia. Sodium polystyrene sulfonate binds with the potassium for excretion.

9. Correct Answer: A

The rhythm on the ECG is sinus bradycardia. However, the physiological data (HR, pulse, BP, LOC, SaO$_2$) demonstrate whether or not the client is symptomatic (i.e., unstable). After any rhythm analysis, the client should always be assessed for perfusion.

10. Correct Answer: C

The supplemental oxygen should be decreased due to the PaO$_2$ level. Prolonged administration of high levels of oxygen can cause toxicity resulting in permanent damage to lung tissue. Administer oxygen at the lowest level possible to maintain oxygenation and avoid toxicity.

11. Correct Answer: A

In an uncompensated acid-base imbalance, the pH and one other value will be abnormal. In this analysis, the increased pH determines this client is alkalotic, and the increased HCO$_3$- and normal PaCO$_2$ show this is a metabolic issue.

12. Correct Answer: A

A client experiencing ventricular tachycardia who does not have a pulse should receive immediate defibrillation. Clients who are defibrillated within one minute of onset of VT have a 90% chance of being converted to a more stable rhythm.

13. Correct Answers: A, B, C, E

Fever and chills are manifestations of pyelonephritis related to inflammatory responses. Flank and back pain are manifestations related to inflammation and infection. Tachycardia and tachypnea are manifestations related to fever and/or pain. Nausea and vomiting are manifestations related to the infectious process.

14. Correct Answer: A

Immediate immobilization of the fracture in addition to early surgical fixation may reduce the incidence of fat embolism.

15. Correct Answer: D

The nurse should recognize signs and symptoms of hypoglycemia and administer 15 g of carbohydrate (e.g., 8 oz of milk; 4 oz of orange juice).

16. Correct Answer: A

The nurse should instruct the client to remain still and refrain from talking unless instructed by the provider.

17. Correct Answers: A, B, E

The nurse should call for help and the person who responds should notify the rapid response team and surgeon. One nurse should provide care to the client while another nurse notifies needed personnel. Abdominal wound evisceration is considered a surgical emergency. The nurse should stay with the client, obtaining vital signs every 5 to 10 min and closely monitoring for signs of shock. The wound should be covered with a sterile dressing moistened with warm saline. The dressing must be kept sterile and moist at all times.

18. Correct Answers: A, E

The arm on the affected side should be elevated above the level of the heart. A modified radical mastectomy involves removal of a portion of the axillary lymph nodes, which can cause transient edema. This usually resolves when collateral circulation is established, which generally occurs within a month. Gentle muscle pumping exercises (such as making a fist and releasing) can help decrease postoperative edema by causing muscle contraction, which improves circulation. This is usually started on the first postoperative day and exercises gradually increase to improve circulation and range of motion.

19. Correct Answers: A, B, D, E

All tobacco products should be avoided. Tobacco increases esophageal reflux by promoting the relaxation of the lower esophageal sphincter (LES). Excessive relaxation of the LES is the most common cause of GERD. Eating small frequent meals should be encouraged. Large meals delay gastric emptying and promote reflux by increasing the pressure and volume within the stomach. Sleeping with the head of the bed elevated should also be encouraged. This allows gravity to assist in keeping the stomach contents from entering the esophagus. Peristalsis also decreases in the supine position, thus promoting the reflux of stomach contents. Drinking caffeinated beverages should be avoided. Caffeine, along with certain other foods and beverages (e.g., chocolate, citrus fruits, alcohol), increases esophageal reflux by promoting the relaxation of the LES.

20. Correct Answers: A, B

Diplopia, as well as other cranial nerve manifestations (e.g., facial weakness, dysphagia, difficulty swallowing), and paresthesias may occur. The client may also experience other sensory manifestations such as cramping of the legs.

21. Correct Answer: B

The nurse should verify the presence of bowel sounds prior to removing the nasogastric tube to evaluate the success of abdominal decompression and the return of peristalsis.

22. Correct Answers: A, C, D, E

A distended bladder would increase the risk of an unintended puncture of the bladder. Excessive ascetic fluid may cause ineffective lung expansion and dyspnea. The head of the bed should be elevated to at least 30°. During the procedure, the client sits on the edge of the bed or in a chair. Abdominal girth is a good indicator of the degree of ascites. The girth should decrease significantly after the procedure. To measure the girth, the client lies flat and is measured around the umbilicus area at the end of exhalation. A paracentesis is an invasive procedure requiring an informed consent.

23. Correct Answer: D

Prior to obtaining a urine specimen from an indwelling urinary catheter, the port should be cleaned with an antiseptic such as povidone-iodine solution or alcohol. A sterile 5 mL syringe is then used to aspirate the urine specimen from the port.

24. Correct Answers: A, B, C, E

The high pressure alarm will sound when there is increased resistance to the delivery of a breath. This increased resistance can occur if the client coughs or "fights" the ventilator. Additional causes include kinks in the tubing (from biting), client experiencing a bronchospasm, and if the ETT becomes plugged with mucus.

25. Correct Answer: B

This client has symptoms of mild hypothermia. The treatment includes external rewarming devices such as heating blankets, warm blankets, warm packs, and convective air warmers. Treatment may also include warm, high-carbohydrate fluids that do not contain alcohol or caffeine.

MENTAL HEALTH NURSING

1. Correct Answer: B

The more clearly the problem and impact of the diagnosis can be defined, the more likely effective solutions and coping strategies will be identified. This should be the initial assessment of the nurse.

2. Correct Answers: A, B, E

The nurse should monitor and document verbal and nonverbal communication. Avoidance of eye contact, aggressive behavior, and blaming may reflect increased likelihood of neglect and/or abuse. It is important to determine if the client can access food and water or if they are dependent on the caretaker for nutrition and hydration. Dependency of older adults increases risk of neglect/abuse. Older adult clients may become vulnerable because of poor physical or mental health. Nurses are legally mandated to report suspected or actual abuse and/or neglect.

3. Correct Answer: D

Phenobarbital can be used to treat alcohol withdrawal. Other medications used to treat alcohol withdrawal include benzodiazepines (e.g., chlordiazepoxide, diazepam, lorazepam, oxazepam).

4. Correct Answers: A, E

Traditional treatment by cultural healers is often combined with Western medicine. Traditional practices may include home remedies such as the consumption of herbs. There are numerous hot/cold beliefs related to healing. These beliefs are not based on the nurse's definition of temperature but on hot and cold properties of foods and medications assigned by the culture. One example: Some Hispanic women believe that consuming "cold" foods after delivery will stop bleeding.

5. Correct Answers: B, C, D

Cognitive-behavioral therapy is recommended for a client who has anorexia nervosa. Cognitive reframing, journal writing, relaxation activities, and desensitization exercises are encouraged. A diet that is high in fiber and low in sodium is recommended to prevent constipation and fluid retention. Consider the client's preferences and ability to consume food when developing the initial eating plan. A structured eating schedule should be instituted at the start of therapy to promote new eating habits. A liquid supplement may be prescribed. Caffeine should be avoided. The client will be monitored during and after meals. The client who has anorexia nervosa should be monitored for bradycardia, hypotension, and hypothermia.

6. Correct Answer: A

If the client is hearing voices, it will be important to assess if the voices are commanding the client to harm self or others. This will require immediate safety measures.

7. Correct Answers: A, C, E

Physiologic response to chronic stress impacts the reproductive system, which may lead to infertility, amenorrhea, decreased libido, impotence, and anovulation. During times of stress, the brain's catecholamine serotonin synthesis becomes more active, impacting the way the brain utilizes serotonin. A stressful life event affects the neurotransmitter stress response and changes mood (such as causing depression), sleep, sexuality, metabolism, appetite, attention span, and memory. Corticosteroids are released during a stressful event and suppress the immune system, which increases the risk of viral and bacterial infections.

8. Correct Answer: A

The nurse should obtain a baseline fasting blood glucose and monitor periodically throughout treatment. The client should report increased thirst, urination, or appetite. Lurasidone is a second-generation (atypical) antipsychotic and metabolic syndrome may occur. New onset of diabetes mellitus or loss of glucose control in clients who have diabetes mellitus may develop.

9. Correct Answers: A, C, D

The nurse should inform the client that it may take 1 to 3 weeks for an initial therapeutic response and up to 2 months for a maximal response to medication. Sertraline is a selective serotonin reuptake inhibitor (SSRI) and has a long half-life. The nurse should instruct the client to immediately report increased depression or thoughts/intent of suicide. The nurse should inform the client that sexual dysfunction may occur and to inform the provider if the effects are intolerable. Medication dosage may be adjusted or the client's medication may be changed.

10. Correct Answer: A

The nurse should perform a self-assessment first. It is important for the nurse who works with this client to be empathetic, nonjudgmental, and objective. If the nurse has an emotional connection due to a past event or person in his life, it would be better for another nurse to care for the client.

MATERNAL AND NEWBORN NURSING

1. Correct Answers: C, D, F

The newborn should be placed supine to decrease the risk of sudden infant death syndrome (SIDS). Stools of a newborn who breastfeeds are yellow and seedy. The stools are lighter and looser than the stools of a newborn that is bottle fed. Tub baths (i.e, submersion in water) should not be given until the cord falls off. Most cords fall off within 10 to 14 days.

2. Correct Answers: C, D, E

Keep the newborn undressed during phototherapy. For a male newborn, a surgical mask (like a bikini) should be placed over the genitalia to prevent possible testicular damage from heat and light waves. The metal strip from the mask should be removed to prevent possible burning. The newborn's eyes must be protected by an opaque mask to prevent retinal damage. The newborn's eyes should be closed prior to applying the mask to prevent excoriation of the corneas. The mask should be removed periodically to assess and cleanse the eyes. Monitor elimination and daily weights for evidence of dehydration. The stools will contain some bile and be loose and green.

3. Correct Answers: A, B, C, E

   Rho(D) immune globulin is given to a mother who has an Rh-negative blood type to prevent/suppress antibody formation to an Rh-positive fetus. It is given at 28 weeks of gestation and within 72 hr following delivery. Rho(D) is given following an amniocentesis, ectopic pregnancy, chorionic villus sampling, trauma, placental abruption, placenta previa, and percutaneous umbilical cord sampling.

4. Correct Answer: B

   The nurse should instruct the client to empty the bladder prior to the procedure to reduce its size and reduce the risk of accidental puncture.

5. Correct Answer: D

   These findings should be reported to the provider because they are abnormal. The average newborn's head circumference is 33 to 35 cm. The average chest circumference is 30 to 33 cm and should also be 2 to 3 cm less than the head circumference. In this scenario, the head is larger than the expected findings and is significantly larger than the chest. The newborn should be evaluated for hydrocephalus.

6. Correct Answer: B

   Dyspnea and crackles should be reported immediately. Terbutaline stimulates cardiopulmonary effects including bronchodilation. Any signs of pulmonary edema such as dyspnea, crackles, or decreased oxygen saturation require immediate action.

7. Correct Answer: C

   Contraception must be used to avoid pregnancy for 1 month after being vaccinated because of the risk of teratogenic effects.

8. Correct Answers: A, B, C, E

   Lethargy is a manifestation of neonatal sepsis. Lethargy is determined by observing the neonate and finding limited spontaneous movements or drowsiness. A decrease in level of consciousness is the earliest indicator of a declining neurological status. For example, the neonate may have a weak cry or a weak suck. Tachypnea is a manifestation of neonatal sepsis. Sepsis causes impaired oxygenation and tissue perfusion, and the respiratory rate increases to provide more oxygen to the tissues. Hypothermia is a manifestation of neonatal sepsis. During sepsis, the neonate develops an inability to maintain a stable body temperature, which often results in hypothermia. A low serum glucose level is a manifestation of neonatal sepsis. Sepsis increases the metabolic demands and increases glucose utilization, which results in hypoglycemia.

9. Correct Answer: D

   The client should be instructed to lie down and check for contractions over 1 hr. The onset of preterm labor is often mistaken for common discomforts of pregnancy. Signs and symptoms of preterm labor include dull, intermittent back pain, uterine contractions, lower abdominal cramping, menstrual-like cramps, suprapubic or pelvic pain or pressure, and change in vaginal discharge (e.g., bloody show, rupture of amniotic membranes).

10. Correct Answer: D

    The basal body temperature method can be influenced by many variables, including stress, alcohol, fatigue, illness, and sleep patterns.

NURSING CARE OF CHILDREN

1. Correct Answer: A

   The toddler has a history of fluid loss and the nurse should place priority on the possibility of impending shock. In infants and young children, hypotension is usually a late sign of dehydration and can be a warning of cardiovascular collapse.

2. Correct Answer: B

   The Yellow Zone means caution. The child should use a quick-relief medication to prevent an asthma attack from getting worse. Indications of Yellow Zone: Peak flow numbers 50% to 80% of best peak flow, cough, wheeze, tight chest, and wakes during the night.

3. Correct Answers: A, C, D, E

   Observe for a facial signal (e.g., elevated eyebrows, wrinkled forehead, watery eyes), which is an indication the infant should stop feeding for a brief period. Burp after every ounce of liquid or two to three times during a feeding. Infants who have a cleft lip and/or palate swallow a lot of air. Hold in an upright position and support the infant's head. This position facilitates gravity to allow fluid to be swallowed rather than enter the nasal cavity. Use a special feeder that does not require suction. Many bottles use a one-way flow valve. Nipples may be long and thin or wide and round. Slits may also vary (e.g., slit-cut, X-cut, Y-cut).

4. Correct Answer: B

   During the toddler years, ritualism is important. Food may be rejected because of certain practices, such as serving food in a different dish. Serve food using the same dish, cup, or spoon every time they eat.

5. Correct Answer: C

   Erythema infectiosum (fifth disease) is caused by the human parvovirus B19 and is transmitted via contact with blood, blood products, and respiratory secretions. It is usually transmitted when hands come in contact with a contaminated surface. After the rash appears, the child is not likely to be contagious. It is usually safe for the child to go back to school.

6. Correct Answer: D

   The most effective method for learning is through participation.

7. Correct Answer: C

   Strabismus is when one eye deviates from a point of fixation. The weak eye becomes "lazy" and amblyopia may develop. If not treated, blindness from disuse may result.

8. Correct Answers: A, B, C

   Parents are the main source of support for the child and should be encouraged to participate in care. Allowing the child to hold and manipulate equipment increases familiarity and decreases anxiety. Young children think concretely. Demonstrating the procedure on a doll helps clarify misconceptions.

9. Correct Answers: A, C, D, E

   It is expected for a preschooler to resist going to bed. Other sleep disturbances include trouble going to sleep, nightmares, and waking during the night. It is also expected for a preschooler to engage in pretend play. Imaginary friends can help the child accomplish tasks, experience different situations, or provide comfort during times of loneliness. Preschoolers should be able to copy simple shapes such as circles and squares. They should also be able to use scissors to cut along a line. Preschoolers should be able to use four to five words in a sentence. This age group enjoys talking. The child may also ask a lot of questions and tell exaggerated stories.

10. Correct Answer: C

    A one-on-one demonstration would be the most effective approach for teaching preschoolers. Learning and problem solving are accomplished most effectively when they are based on what the preschooler can see and hear directly. Understanding may be enhanced through demonstrations using dolls, puppets, or role-playing.

COMPREHENSIVE ASSESSMENT

1. Correct Answer: C, B, A, E, D, F

   Obtain baseline circulatory assessment, including pulse and skin integrity of lower extremities, before applying the SCD. Arrange the SCD under the leg and align the leg position as indicated on the inner lining of the sleeve of the SCD. Wrap the SCD sleeve around the leg. The sleeve applies pressure and facilitates venous return. Place two fingers between the leg and sleeve to check fit. The sleeve should fit snugly around the leg, but not too tight. The client should not feel any numbness or tingling. Attach the connector of the SCD sleeve to the mechanical unit/device. Electrical supply is required as the sleeve does not operate independently. Observe functions for one complete cycle for proper functioning. Continue to monitor the client's skin integrity and circulation of lower extremities.

2. Correct Answers: B, C, D, E

   Stasis of respiratory secretions and weakened respiratory muscles can lead to atelectasis and hypostatic pneumonia. Decreased muscle strength, atrophy of muscles, altered joint mobility and contractures can develop. Increased pressure on the skin along with decreased circulation can lead to the formation of pressure sores. Stasis of blood in the legs occurs. The client is at an increased risk for thrombus formation.

3. Correct Answer: A

   Histamine2 (H2) receptor antagonists such as ranitidine suppress secretion of gastric acid by blocking H2 receptors of the parietal cells in the stomach.

4. Correct Answer: B

   The spacer should not make a whistling sound when the correct technique is used. The spacer makes a whistling sound when the client is breathing in too rapidly.

5. Correct Answers: A, B, D

   Application of clean gloves reduces the transfer of microorganisms and provides protection for the nurse from body fluids. The angle of insertion for an IM injection is 90°. A needle 18- to 27-gauge (usually 22- to 25-gauge) and 1 to 1.5 inches long is used for an adult. Clients who are obese or very thin may require an alteration in needle length.

6. Correct Answers: A, B, C, E

   Fluoxetine is a selective serotonin reuptake inhibitor (SSRI). Fever is a sign of serotonin syndrome. Serotonin syndrome is a potentially lethal condition that can occur 2 to 72 hours after initiation of treatment with an SSRI. Other risk factors include concurrent use of SSRIs with tricyclic antidepressants, monoamine oxidase inhibitors, and St. John's wort. Agitation, diaphoresis, and hallucinations are signs of serotonin syndrome.

7. Correct Answer: D

   Erythema of the incision line greater than 1 cm on each side of the wound may indicate infection.

8. Correct Answer: A

   When a client is admitted to a new setting, a private room (away from exits, stairs, and elevators) may be needed for a client who wanders or is agitated. Provide appropriate supervision in an area that provides maximum observation.

9. Correct Answer: B

   Clients who follow the religion of Islam may fast from dawn to sunset during Ramadan.

10. Correct Answer: D

    Impetigo is a bacterial infection of the skin caused by Staphylococcus. Contact precautions are required for caregivers and visitors and include wearing a gown and gloves. Assign the client to a private room if possible or a room with other clients who have the same infection.

11. Correct Answer: A

    Persistent nausea and vomiting past 12 weeks of gestation may indicate hyperemesis gravidarum. The most important laboratory test with hyperemesis gravidarum is urinalysis to determine if there are ketones and acetone in the urine. Clients who have excessive vomiting may have ketonuria and electrolyte imbalances.

12. Correct Answer: D

    Maternal inhibiting behaviors to bonding and attachment include ignoring the newborn or not making an effort to respond to the infant's needs.

13. Correct Answer: A

    The goal of care for preterm labor is to stop contractions and prevent cervical change.

14. Correct Answer: C

    An adverse effect of oxytocin is uterine hyperstimulation. Discontinue oxytocin if uterine hyperstimulation occurs. Clinical findings of uterine hyperstimulation include: a contraction frequency more often than every 2 min, a contraction duration longer than 90 seconds, a contraction intensity resulting in pressure greater than 90 mm Hg as shown by the intrauterine pressure catheter (IUPC), a uterine resting tone greater than 20 mm Hg between contractions, or no relaxation of the uterus.

15. Correct Answer: D

    TPN increases the risk of infection. The concentrated glucose is a medium for bacterial growth. Dressing changes for central lines should be performed using sterile technique to reduce the risk of sepsis.

16. Correct Answer: D

    The intravenous solution of dextrose 5% in 0.9% sodium chloride is not appropriate to use because it will cause clotting or hemolysis of blood cells to occur. The only solution the nurse should use during the administration of blood is 0.9% sodium chloride.

17. Correct Answer: D

    The tubing should be maintained in a position that will avoid kinks and large loops, both of which can block drainage.

18. Correct Answer: C

    The nurse should report a creatinine of 1.9 mg/dL because it is above the expected reference range of 0.6 to 1.2 mg/dL. The client is at risk for contrast-induced renal failure due to renal insufficiency.

19. Correct Answer: D

    The lithotomy position increases the risk of peroneal nerve compression, which can cause neurological complications such as foot drop. The nurse should implement measures to prevent this complication such as ensuring proper padding and position changes at regular intervals.

20. Correct Answer: D

    Petechiae can be an indication of thrombocytopenia which would be especially concerning in a post-surgical client as it will increase the risk of bleeding.

21. Correct Answer: D

    The client has been diagnosed and started on antibiotics. Fever and sore throat are expected manifestations of tonsillitis. It may take a few days for symptoms to improve. If the client had reported symptoms of airway obstruction (e.g., drooling and stridor), emergency treatment would be indicated. Antibiotics (usually penicillin or azithromycin) are prescribed for 7 to 10 days in addition to supportive care.

22. Correct Answer: A

A client who is taking garlic supplements will have an increased risk of bleeding. Garlic suppresses platelet aggregation and can also stimulate fibrinolysis.

23. Correct Answers: A, B, C, E

Setting limits can de-escalate the situation. For example, tell the client in a calm voice: "I need you to stop yelling." This de-escalation technique allows the client to respond to the nurse's calm, clear voice. The nurse approaches the client using this technique to soothe the client and promotes feelings of security and safety. One of the most important roles the nurse plays in the client's use of appropriate behaviors is that of role model and educator. Inform the client of consequences of the behavior such as loss of privileges. Describe options clearly and offer choices. Encourage the client to express feelings verbally using therapeutic communication techniques (e.g., reflective techniques, silence, active listening).

24. Correct Answer: B

Telling the story of loss and grief is therapeutic for the bereaved. Talking about feelings with trusted loved ones, friends, support/bereavement groups, and counselors who actively listen is part of the grieving process. Anger, anxiety, guilt, and loneliness are expected grief reactions that need to be expressed to someone willing to listen in a caring fashion.

25. Correct Answers: A, B, C, D

The client should eat slowly and carefully to avoid aspiration. The client may have difficulty chewing and swallowing because the muscles have become weakened. Assess the client's gag and ability to chew and swallow. Food should be cut into small pieces. The diaphragm and intercostal muscles can be affected. The client is at increased risk for muscle weakness, especially during a crisis. Planning for frequent periods of rest is necessary. The client experiences fatigue and muscle weakness. The client may experience a myasthenic crisis, cholinergic crisis, or a combination of the two (mixed). Increased lacrimation (tearing) is one of the characteristics of a mixed crisis.

26. Correct Answers: A, B, C, E

Fatigue can occur with external radiation therapy. Dry mouth (i.e., xerostomia) can occur if the salivary glands have become irradiated. This can be a long-term effect. Altered taste (i.e., dysgeusia) can occur from radiation, some clients develop an aversion to the taste of red meat. Difficulty swallowing (i.e., dysphagia) can occur with radiation therapy to the head and neck.

27. Correct Answer: A

The client is exhibiting early signs and symptoms of a change in LOC. The head of the bed should be elevated at 30° to 45°. Maintain the head in a midline position. This position facilitates the drainage of venous blood or CSF. Adjust head elevation to sustain cerebral perfusion pressure (CPP) greater than 70 mm Hg.

28. Correct Answers: A, D, E

Assess client rapidly and then call the rapid response team (EMS or rapid response team). A compression rate of 100/min and compression to ventilation ratio of 30 to 2 without a pause for ventilations should be used. Place AED pads. Follow audio instructions and deliver shock if prompted. Every minute of a sudden cardiac arrest without defibrillation decreases the survival rate by 7% to 10% (AHA). AEDs are in public places.

29. Correct Answers: C, D, E

Initiate and maintain a one-to-one observation around the clock, always having client in sight and in close proximity. There is an increased risk for suicide during staff rotation time. The client's hands should always be visible even when sleeping. Check environment for potential hazards, which could include open windows, overhead pipes that are easily accessible, glass, metal silverware, electrical cords, belts, shoelaces, tweezers, razors, shampoo, and plastic bags.

30. Correct Answers: B, C, E

The client who has memory problems will benefit most from a structured and consistent environment. Establishing a predictable routine is helpful for the client who has Alzheimer's disease. Using a low, clear, and respectful tone provides a calming effect and reduces anxiety, stress, and fear. The client who has dementia should be addressed distinctly by name when initiating interaction, and the nurse should speak slowly. Family members need to know where to get help when caring for a loved one who has Alzheimer's disease. This can include counseling, education regarding the progression of the dementia, and community-based organizations (e.g., senior day care centers, respite care, family support groups, Alzheimer's Association Safe Return).

31. Correct Answers: A, C, D

The client should implement strategies to prevent infection. Meats, fish, and eggs should be cooked to the proper temperature. The client will be prescribed highly active antiretroviral therapy, which includes a combination of medications.

32. Correct Answer: A

This client is soon to be discharged and can most likely be cared for at home with support.

33. Correct Answer: D, B, A, C, E

Obtain a history including type of irritant, treatment received, and if client has any allergies, especially to the "caine" family of medications. Evaluate visual acuity. Don gloves and check pH of affected eye (to test the agent splashed into eye). This will help to evaluate when it has been washed out. Instill proparacaine hydrochloride eye drops as prescribed to numb the eye. Place client supine and move client's head toward the affected eye. Use an eyelid speculum or have client hold eye open and direct flow of normal saline across affected eye from the nasal corner of the eye toward the outer corner of the eye. A 1000 mL bag of 0.9% sodium chloride with macrodrip IV tubing should be used.

34. Correct Answer: C

A client who has chronic kidney disease is at risk for hyperkalemia. A serum potassium level of 6.1 mEq/L puts the client at increased risk of dysrhythmias. This is the priority client.

35. Correct Answers: A, B, C, E

An infant car seat should be placed in the rear seat and be rear facing. Infants and toddlers should remain in a rear-facing car seat until the age of 2 years or the height recommended by the manufacturer. The harness of the car seat should be adjusted to fit the infant snugly. The retainer clip of the harness (of the car seat) should be positioned at the level of the infant's armpits. An infant car seat should not be placed in the front seat of a vehicle with deployable airbags.

36. Correct Answer: B

Playing pretend and dress-up is important for the imagination of preschoolers. The other activities are too advanced and may cause frustration.

37. Correct Answers: A, C, D, E

Adequate hydration keeps airways moist and thins secretions, making them easier to expectorate. Extreme heat increases the body temperature and oxygen consumption. Extreme cold can cause bronchospasms; shivering causes increased oxygen consumption. Clients with COPD are at high risk for respiratory infections because damaged airways do not effectively filter viruses and bacteria. Preventive measures are needed. Postural drainage with percussion and vibration will help loosen secretions, making them easier to expectorate.

38. Correct Answer: D

It is within the scope of practice for the LPN to perform procedures requiring aseptic and sterile techniques.

39. Correct Answer: C

This action will verify the client's end-of-life wishes have been communicated to and documented by the provider. This honors the client's wishes by preventing resuscitation. A signed advance directive provides information about the client's wishes. However, the DNR order must be documented.

40. Correct Answers: A, B

Cold and warm applications (sitz baths) are appropriate tasks to delegate to an AP. Neither the teaching related to the correct use of a sitz bath, nor the assessment of the perineal area can be delegated. Vital signs for stable clients are appropriate tasks to delegate to an AP. The nurse must identify the AP's knowledge and skills prior to delegating a task.

The RN may delegate elements of care but not the nursing process.

41. Correct Answer: A

The nurse should assess the client experiencing a new onset of shortness of breath first. The Airway, Breathing, Circulation (ABC) framework is used to determine the highest priority.

42. Correct Answers: A, B, C, D

An informed consent is required for surgical and nonsurgical procedures that carry more than a slight risk to the client. Informed consent must be freely given by a person of legal age who is mentally capable. A liver biopsy, thoracentesis, and coronary catheterization are procedures that carry a slight risk to the client. All surgical procedures require informed consent.

43. Correct Answer: C

The nurse is responsible for evaluating the outcome of the delegated task. Observing the client's position will ensure the task was completed.

44. Correct Answer: 19 gtt/min

Formula:

$$\frac{\text{Volume (mL)}}{\text{Time (min.)}} \times \frac{\text{Drop Factor}}{\text{(gtt/mL)}} = \frac{\text{Y (Flow Rate}}{\text{in gtt/min)}}$$

Calculation:

$$\frac{75\ \text{mL}}{60\ \text{min}} \times 15\ \text{gtt/mL} = 18.75 = 19\ \text{gtt/min}$$

45. Correct Answer: D

If red man syndrome occurs, discontinue the vancomycin infusion and administer diphenhydramine. To prevent red man syndrome, infuse vancomycin at a slow rate.